ANDREAS J. KESEL

THE POTENTIAL HEALING OF CANCER WITH P53 (RE)ACTIVATORS

TWO NEW DRUGS EXPLOITING CANCER'S *WARBURG* EFFECT

© 2023 Andreas Johannes Kesel

ISBN Softcover: 978-3-384-00311-9
ISBN Hardcover: 978-3-384-00312-6

Druck und Distribution im Auftrag des Autors:
tredition GmbH, Heinz-Beusen-Stieg 5, 22926 Ahrensburg,
Germany

TABLE OF CONTENTS

CHAPTER ONE

BIOGRAPHY OF THE AUTHOR

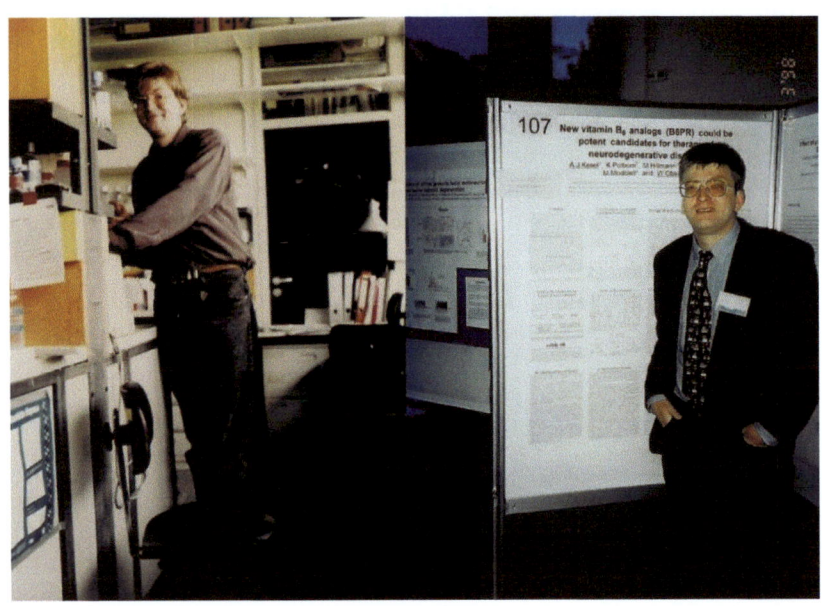

1990 ABITUR. 1991–1993 CHEMISTRY SCHOOL DR. ERWIN ELHARDT, STUDY OF CHEMICAL-TECHNICAL ASSISTANT (CTA). 1993 PRACTICAL TRAINING, MAX-PLANCK-INSTITUTE FOR BIOCHEMISTRY, MARTINSRIED, GERMANY, DEPARTMENT OF PROTEIN CHEMISTRY OF DR. FRIEDRICH LOTTSPEICH, IN THE FORMER LABORATORY OF DR. PEHR VICTOR EDMAN (ADVISOR: KERSTIN ANDERSSON, GENERAL TRAINING IN PROTEIN CHEMISTRY, ELECTROPHORESIS, AND PROTEIN SEQUENCING BY THE *EDMAN* METHOD). 1993 PRACTICAL TRAINING, MAX-PLANCK-INSTITUTE FOR NEUROBIOLOGY, MARTINSRIED, GERMANY, DEPARTMENT OF NEUROIMMUNOLOGY OF PROF. DR. DR. H.C. HARTMUT WEKERLE (ADVISOR: DR. ANTONIO IGLESIAS, TRAINING IN MOLECULAR BIOLOGY AND DNA SEQUENCING). 1993–1995 WORK AS CHEMICAL-TECHNICAL ASSISTANT AT MAX-PLANCK-INSTITUTE FOR BIOCHEMISTRY IN THE DEPARTMENT

OF VIRUS RESEARCH OF PROF. DR. DR. DR. H.C. PETER HANS HOFSCHNEIDER, WITH SPECIAL TRAINING IN THE MOLECULAR BIOLOGY OF HUMAN HEPATITIS B VIRUS. 1995–2000 STUDY OF PHARMACY AT LUDWIG-MAXIMILIANS-UNIVERSITY, MUNICH, GERMANY. 2004–2005 STUDY OF PHARMACY AT JULIUS-MAXIMILIANS UNIVERSITY OF WÜRZBURG, GERMANY. 2006–2011 DOCTORAL STUDY AT JULIUS-MAXIMILIANS UNIVERSITY OF WÜRZBURG, GERMANY, IN THE DEPARTMENT OF PHARMACEUTICAL CHEMISTRY OF PROF. DR. ULRIKE HOLZGRABE. 2011–2015 PUBLICATION WORK AS PRIVATE RESEARCHER IN MUNICH, GERMANY. 2015–2017 WORK AS CHIEF MEDICINAL CHEMIST FOR POP TEST ONCOLOGY LLC OF RANDICE LISA ALTSCHUL, CLIFFSIDE PARK, NJ, USA. 1998 ELECTION AS AN EXTERNAL MEMBER OF THE NEW YORK ACADEMY OF SCIENCES, NEW YORK, USA. 2005 MEMBER OF THE AMERICAN CHEMICAL SOCIETY, DIVISION OF MEDICINAL CHEMISTRY. 18 PUBLICATIONS AND/OR CONGRESS ABSTRACTS IN PEER-REVIEWED JOURNALS. 29 CO-AUTHORED PATENTS.

PUBLICATIONS OF THE AUTHOR

[1] Eberhard Hildt, Stephan Urban, Andreas Kesel, Peter Hans Hofschneider. *Functional characterization of baculovirus-derived MHBs^t*, Molecular Biology of Hepatitis B Viruses, October 3–6 **1994**, Institut Pasteur, Paris, France (Chair: Marie Annick Buendia, Alan McLachlan).

[2] Stephan Urban, Eberhard Hildt, Christoph Eckerskorn, Andreas Kesel, Peter Hans Hofschneider. *Mass Spectrometric Analysis of Baculovirus-Derived HBX*, Molecular Biology of Hepatitis B Viruses, October 3–6 **1994**, Institut Pasteur, Paris, France (Chair: Marie Annick Buendia, Alan McLachlan).

[3] Andreas J. Kesel, Stephan Urban, Walter Oberthür. *Interconvertible (Z/E)-Stereoisomers of a Vitamin B₆ Coenzyme Analog Derived from Pyridoxal 5'-Phosphate and Rhodanine*, Tetrahedron **1996**, *52*, 14787–14800.

[4] Andreas J. Kesel, Isolde Sonnenbichler, Kurt Polborn, Lutz Gürtler, Wolfgang E. F. Klinkert, Manuel Modolell, Andreas K. Nüssler, Walter Oberthür. *A New Antioxidative Vitamin B₆ Analogue Modulates Pathophysiological Cell Proliferation and Damage*, Bioorg. Med. Chem. **1999**, *7*, 359–367.

[5]   Andreas J. Kesel. *A System of Protein Target Sequences for Anti-RNA-viral Chemotherapy by a Vitamin B_6-Derived Zinc-Chelating Trioxa-adamantane-triol*, Bioorg. Med. Chem. **2003**, *11*, 4599–4613.

[6]   Andreas J. Kesel. *Synthesis of retinoid vitamin A–vitamin B_6 conjugate analogues for antiviral chemotherapy*, Biochem. Biophys. Res. Commun. **2003**, *300*, 793–799.

[7]   Julian A. Tanner, Bo-Jian Zheng, Jie Zhou, Rory M. Watt, Jie-Qing Jiang, Kin-Ling Wong, Yong-Ping Lin, Lin-Yu Lu, Ming-Liang He, Hsiang-Fu Kung, Andreas J. Kesel, Jian-Dong Huang. *The Adamantane-Derived Bananins Are Potent Inhibitors of the Helicase Activities and Replication of SARS Coronavirus*, Chem. Biol. (Cell Chem. Biol.) **2005**, *12*, 303–311.

[8]   Andreas J. Kesel. *Synthesis of Novel Test Compounds for Antiviral Chemotherapy of Severe Acute Respiratory Syndrome (SARS)*, Curr. Med. Chem. **2005**, *12*, 2095–2162.

[9]   Andreas J. Kesel. *The Bananins: New Anticorona-RNA-Viral Agents with Unique Structural Signature*, Anti-Infective Agents Med. Chem. **2006**, *5*, 161–174.

[10] Andreas J. Kesel. *Broad-spectrum antiviral activity including human immunodeficiency and hepatitis C viruses mediated by a novel retinoid thiosemicarbazone derivative*, Eur. J. Med. Chem. **2011**, *46*, 1656–1664.

[11] Andreas J. Kesel. *An Update on the Bananins: Anti-RNA-Viral Agents with Unique Structural Signature*, Anti-Infective Agents **2013**, *11*, 1–21.

[12] Andreas J. Kesel, Hans-Christoph Weiss, Andreas Schönleber, Craig W. Day, Dale L. Barnard, Mervi A. Detorio, Raymond F. Schinazi. *Antiviral agents derived from novel 1-adamantyl singlet nitrenes*, Antivir. Chem. Chemother. **2013**, *23*, 113–128.

[13] Andreas J. Kesel, Zhuhui Huang, Michael G. Murray, Mark N. Prichard, Laura Caboni, Daniel K. Nevin, Darren Fayne, David G. Lloyd, Mervi A. Detorio, Raymond F. Schinazi. *Retinazone inhibits certain blood-borne human viruses including Ebola virus Zaire*, Antivir. Chem. Chemother. **2014**, *23*, 197–215.

[14] Andreas Schönleber, Sander van Smaalen, Hans-Christoph Weiss, Andreas J. Kesel. *N—H···O and C—H···F hydrogen bonds in the incommensurately modulated crystal structure of adamantan-1-ammonium*

4-fluorobenzoate, Acta Crystallogr. B Struct. Sci. Cryst. Eng. Mater. **2014**, *70*, 652–659.

[15] Francesco Saettini, Matteo F. Olivieri, Andreas J. Kesel, Laura Bonalume, Francesca Marzari. *Dermatology in ancient Greece: The myth of Melampus and the use of Helleborus*, V[th] Congresso Nazionale SiDerP (Società Italiana di Dermatologia Pediatrica – Italian Society of Pediatric Dermatology), April 16–18 **2015**, Florio Park Hotel, Palermo, Italy.

[16] Andreas J. Kesel, Craig W. Day, Catherine M. Montero, Raymond F. Schinazi. *A new oxygen modification cyclooctaoxygen binds to nucleic acids as sodium crown complex*, Biochim. Biophys. Acta **2016**, *1860*, 785–794.

[17] Matteo F. Olivieri, Francesca Marzari, Andreas J. Kesel, Laura Bonalume, Francesco Saettini. *Pharmacology and psychiatry at the origins of Greek medicine: The myth of Melampus and the madness of the Proetides*, J. Hist. Neurosci. **2017**, *26*, 193–215.

[18] Andreas J. Kesel. *The Spermine Phosphate-Bound Cyclooctaoxygen Sodium Epigenetic Shell of Euchromatin DNA Is Destroyed by the Epigenetic Poison Glyphosate*, Preprints **2017**, 2017010086, https://doi.org/10.20944/preprints201701.0086.v4.

[19] Andreas J. Kesel. *The Spermine Phosphate-Bound Cyclooctaoxygen Sodium Epigenetic Shell of Euchromatin DNA Is Destroyed by the Epigenetic Poison Glyphosate*, Arch. Clin. Biomed. Res. **2023**, *7*, 171–190, https://doi.org/10.26502/acbr.50170331.

[20] Andreas J. Kesel. *The Epigenetic Protection Shell of Euchromatin DNA. Selenium Content — Detoriation by Glyphosate*, 1ˢᵗ ed., tredition GmbH, Ahrensburg, Germany, 2023, ISBN 978-3347944442.

PATENTS OF THE AUTHOR

[1] Andreas J. Kesel, Walter Oberthür. (Z)-5-[[3-Hydroxy-2-methyl-5-[(phosphonooxy)methyl]-4-pyridinyl]methylen]-2-thioxo-4-thiazolidinon, Verfahren zu dessen Herstellung und Verwendung. **Ger. Pat.** DE 196 45 974 C1 (1998). Filed 1996/11/07.

[2] Andreas J. Kesel, Walter Oberthür. Mono-, oligo-, and polymeric Knoevenagel condensation products useful e.g. in pharmaceuticals, cosmetics and assay procedures. **Ger. Pat.** DE 198 19 820 A1 (2000). Filed 1998/05/04.

[3] Andreas J. Kesel, Walter Oberthür. NEW KNOEVENAGEL CONDENSATION PRODUCTS, METHOD FOR THEIR PRODUCTION AND THEIR

USE. **PCT/WIPO Pat. Appl.** WO/1998/020013 A1 (1998). Filed 1997/11/07.

[4] Andreas J. Kesel, Walter Oberthür. NEW KNOEVENAGEL CONDENSATION PRODUCTS, METHOD FOR THEIR PRODUCTION AND THEIR USE. **Eur. Pat. Appl.** EP 0 937 089 A1 (1999). Filed 1997/11/07.

[5] Andreas J. Kesel, Walter Oberthür. MONOMERIC, OLIGOMERIC AND POLYMERIC KNOEVENAGEL CONDENSATION PRODUCTS. **PCT/WIPO Pat. Appl.** WO/1999/057124 A1 (1999). Filed 1999/04/30.

[6] Walter Oberthür, Andreas J. Kesel. ANTIOXIDATIVE VITAMIN B_6 ANALOGS. **PCT/WIPO Pat. Appl.** WO/2000/066599 A1 (2000). Filed 2000/04/28.

[7] Andreas J. Kesel, Walter Oberthür. MONOMERIC, OLIGOMERIC AND POLYMERIC KNOEVENAGEL CONDENSATION PRODUCTS. **Eur. Pat. Appl.** EP 1 075 481 A1 (2001). Filed 1999/04/30.

[8] Walter Oberthür, Andreas J. Kesel. NEW ANTIOXIDATIVE VITAMIN B_6 ANALOGS. **Eur. Pat. Appl.** EP 1 173 451 A1 (2002). Filed 2000/04/28.

[9] Walter Oberthür, Andreas J. Kesel. Antioxidative vitamin B$_6$ analogs. **U.S. Pat. Appl.** 6,369,042 B1 (2002). Filed 1999/11/10.

[10] Randice L. Altschul, Neil D. Theise, Andreas J. Kesel, Myron Rapkin, Rebecca O'Brien, Anthony R. Arment. PHARMACEUTICAL COMPOSITIONS AND METHODS. **PCT/WIPO Pat. Appl.** WO/2017/023694 A1 (2017). Filed 2016/07/28.

[11] Randice L. Altschul, Neil D. Theise, Andreas J. Kesel, Myron Rapkin, Rebecca O'Brien, Anthony R. Arment. PHARMACEUTICAL COMPOSITIONS AND METHODS. **U.S. Pat. Appl.** US 2017/0051007 A1 (2017). Filed 2016/07/28.

[12] Randice L. Altschul, Neil D. Theise, Andreas J. Kesel, Myron Rapkin, Rebecca O'Brien, Anthony R. Arment. PHARMACEUTICAL COMPOSITIONS AND METHODS. **U.S. Pat. Appl.** US 9,598,459 B2 (2017). Filed 2016/07/28.

[13] Randice L. Altschul, Neil D. Theise, Andreas J. Kesel, Myron Rapkin, Rebecca O'Brien, Anthony R. Arment. PHARMACEUTICAL COMPOSITIONS AND METHODS. **U.S. Pat. Appl.** US 2017/0128465 A1 (2017). Filed 2016/12/06.

[14] Randice L. Altschul, Neil D. Theise, Andreas J. Kesel, Myron Rapkin, Rebecca O'Brien, Anthony R. Arment. PHARMACEUTICAL COMPOSITIONS AND METHODS. **U.S. Pat. Appl.** US 9,855,284 B2 (2018). Filed 2016/12/06.

[15] Randice L. Altschul, Neil D. Theise, Andreas J. Kesel, Myron Rapkin, Rebecca O'Brien, Anthony R. Arment. THERAPEUTIC AGENTS AND METHODS:. **PCT/WIPO Pat. Appl.** WO/2018/067520 A2 (2018). Filed 2017/10/03.

[16] Randice L. Altschul, Neil D. Theise, Andreas J. Kesel, Myron Rapkin, Rebecca O'Brien, Anthony R. Arment. Pharmaceutical Compositions and Methods. **U.S. Pat. Appl.** US 2018/0185392 A1 (2018). Filed 2017/11/29.

[17] Randice L. Altschul, Neil D. Theise, Andreas J. Kesel, Myron Rapkin, Rebecca O'Brien, Anthony R. Arment. Pharmaceutical Compositions and Methods. **Eur. Pat. Appl.** EP 3 400 233 A1 (2018). Filed 2016/07/28.

[18] Randice L. Altschul, Neil D. Theise, Andreas J. Kesel, Myron Rapkin, Rebecca O'Brien, Anthony R. Arment. PHARMACEUTICAL

COMPOSITIONS AND METHODS. **U.S. Pat. Appl.** US 10,238,666 B2 (2019). Filed 2017/11/29.

[19] Randice L. Altschul, Neil D. Theise, Andreas J. Kesel, Myron Rapkin, Rebecca O'Brien, Anthony Arment. PHARMACEUTICAL COMPOSITIONS AND METHODS. **U.S. Pat. Appl.** 2019/0134062 A1 (2019). Filed 2019/01/08.

[20] Randice L. Altschul, Neil D. Theise, Andreas J. Kesel, Myron Rapkin, Rebecca O'Brien, Anthony R. Arment. THERAPEUTIC AGENTS AND METHODS. **Eur. Pat. Appl.** EP 3 534 910 A2 (2019). Filed 2017/10/03.

[21] Randice L. Altschul, Neil D. Theise, Andreas J. Kesel, Myron Rapkin, Rebecca O'Brien, Anthony R. Arment. THERAPEUTIC AGENTS AND METHODS:. **U.S. Pat. Appl.** 2019/0381038 A1 (2019). Filed 2017/10/03.

[22] Randice L. Altschul, Neil D. Theise, Andreas J. Kesel, Myron Rapkin, Rebecca O'Brien, Anthony Arment. PHARMACEUTICAL COMPOSITIONS AND METHODS. **U.S. Pat. Appl.** US 10,517,881 B2 (2019). Filed 2019/01/08.

[23] Randice L. Altschul, Neil D. Theise, Andreas J. Kesel, Myron Rapkin, Rebecca O'Brien, Anthony Arment. PHARMACEUTICAL COMPOSITIONS AND METHODS. **U.S. Pat. Appl.** 2020/0101087 A1 (2020). Filed 2019/11/21.

[24] Randice L. Altschul, Neil D. Theise, Andreas J. Kesel, Myron Rapkin, Rebecca O'Brien, Anthony R. Arment. THERAPEUTIC AGENTS AND METHODS. **U.S. Pat. Appl.** US 11,040,037 B2 (2021). Filed 2017/10/03.

[25] Randice L. Altschul, Neil D. Theise, Andreas J. Kesel, Myron Rapkin, Rebecca O'Brien, Anthony R. Arment. THERAPEUTIC AGENTS AND METHODS. **U.S. Pat. Appl.** 2021/0353623 A1 (2021). Filed 2021/04/28.

[26] Randice L. Altschul, Neil D. Theise, Andreas J. Kesel, Myron Rapkin, Rebecca O'Brien, Anthony R. Arment. THERAPEUTIC AGENTS AND METHODS. **U.S. Pat. Appl.** US 11,224,599 B2 (2022). Filed 2021/04/28.

[27] Randice L. Altschul, Neil D. Theise, Andreas J. Kesel, Myron Rapkin, Rebecca O'Brien, Anthony R. Arment. THERAPEUTIC AGENTS AND

METHODS. **U.S. Pat. Appl.** 2022/0298203 A1 (2022). Filed 2021/11/22.

[28] Randice L. Altschul, Neil D. Theise, Andreas J. Kesel, Myron Rapkin, Rebecca O'Brien, Anthony Arment. PHARMACEUTICAL COMPOSITIONS AND METHODS. **U.S. Pat. Appl.** US 11,576,921 B2 (2023). Filed 2019/11/21.

[29] Randice L. Altschul, Neil D. Theise, Andreas J. Kesel, Myron Rapkin, Rebecca O'Brien, Anthony Arment. PHARMACEUTICAL COMPOSITIONS AND METHODS. **U.S. Pat. Appl.** 2023/0142627 A1 (2023). Filed 2022/10/31.

ACKNOWLEDGEMENTS

The author wants to heartily thank K. Gurova (Roswell Park Comprehensive Cancer Center, Buffalo, NY, USA) for the cytochrome c assays of **PT162**, **PT166** and **PT167**. I heartily thank R.F. Schinazi [Center for AIDS Research (now: Center for ViroScience and Cure), Laboratory of Biochemical Pharmacology, Department of Pediatrics, Emory University School of Medicine, Atlanta, GA, USA, and (up to 2016) the Veterans Affairs Medical Center, Decatur, GA, USA, and Children's Healthcare of Atlanta, Atlanta, GA, USA] for the HIV-1$_{LAI}$ testings of **PT162**. In addition, the author wishes to heartily thank H. Braunschweig and his associated Senior Researchers T. Kupfer and K. Radacki (Institute for Anorganic Chemistry, Julius-Maximilians-University of Würzburg, Germany) for the X-ray crystallographic solving of the crystal and molecular structure of **PT166**. I am grateful to E. Billings, M. Tobea, and, especially, B. Webb (The Scripps Research Institute, Center for Metabolomics and Mass Spectrometry, San Diego, CA, USA) for the LC/MS investigation service of the **PT167** specimen after more than six years storage in the refrigerator. I cordially thank C. Schnieders, G. Schnieders, R. Schnieders and T. Konrath (DEUTERO GmbH, Kastellaun, Germany) for measuring the

500 MHz spectrum of **PT167** after more than six years storage in the refrigerator. The author is deeply indepted to T. Westfeld, E.-M. May, D. Wiegel, W. Wübbolt, O. Meier, R. Sachs, A. Karbach, W. Bergmeier, J. Moldenhauer and H.-J. Hühn (Currenta GmbH & Co. OHG, Leverkusen, Germany) for analytical services. I am obliged to K. Hecker, K. Meuser and K. Hecker (HEKAtech GmbH, Wegberg, Germany) for expert elemental analyses.

DEDICATION

THE AUTHOR DEDICATES THIS BOOK TO HIS LATE FATHER DR. RER. NAT. GÜNTHER KESEL AND TO HIS LOVELY MOTHER HILDEGARD FRIEDA FRANZISKA KESEL, WITHOUT THEIR SUPPORT THE AUTHOR'S WORK WOULD NOT HAVE BEEN POSSIBLE. THIS BOOK IS ALSO DEDICATED TO THE AUTHOR'S SOULMATE FARKAS GYÖNGYI, THE PEARL OF THE WOLF.

PREFACE AND ABSTRACT

This book is based on the patents listed in the Patents of the Author Section (pp. XVI–XXII): [15,20,21,24–27].

In 1930 *Otto Heinrich Warburg* (1883–1970) published [1] his theory on the origin of cancer cells based on a series of preceding investigations [2–4]. He summarized his theory on the origin of cancer cells in 1956 [5]. This theory was coined the *Warburg* hypothesis [6]. The essence of this hypothesis on the origin of cancer is that, under aerobic conditions, malignant tissues metabolize approximately tenfold more glucose to lactate in a constant time window than primary tissues, a phenomenon known as the *Warburg* 'malignant' effect. *Warburg* claimed that cancer cells heavily rely on aerobic glycolysis as an energy source for malignant growth, rather than on the aerobic respiration, thereby claiming a defect in cancer cell respiration. The *Warburg* hypothesis was heavily debated for many years since its introduction [6], especially regarding the respiratory defect misinterpreted by *Warburg* himself [6], and only in recent years many details of the *Warburg* hypothesis were confirmed as correct [7–10]. Importantly, the *Warburg* effect itself, which was proved to constitute a fact *in vivo* [11], has to be differentiated from the complete *Warburg* hypothesis which was the cause of ongoing scientific debate [see 12–14].

In 2002 it was shown that human cancer cells indeed suffer from defects in cellular respiration, either a marked depletion in cellular mitochondrial content or a selective repression in expression of the catalytic β-subunit of mitochondrial Complex V F-type ATPase (β-F_1-ATPase) concurrent with an increase in the expression of the glycolytic enzyme glyceraldehyde 3-phosphate dehydrogenase [7]. Both mechanisms impair mitochondrial respiration and give support for the *Warburg* hypothesis [7]. In rat rhabdomyosarcoma R1H cells mitochondrial function was found to be deficient by a dysregulation of the mitochondrial protein–to–cardiolipin ratio [10]. Mitochondrial respiration of R1H cells was significantly impaired, joined by the incapacity of the rhabdomyosarcoma cells to differentiate into mature striated skeletal muscle cells [10]. The intriguing abnormalities in cardiolipin content were confirmed *in vivo* utilizing brain tumors grown in mice [9]. The compositional cardiolipin abnormalities involved an abundance of immature molecular species and deficiencies of mature molecular species, suggesting major defects in cardiolipin synthesis and remodeling in rodent brain tumor tissue [9]. The tumor cardiolipin abnormalities were also associated with significant reductions in both individual and linked electron transport chain activities [9]. The acidic phospholipid cardiolipin [1,3-bis(*sn*-3'-phosphatidyl)-*sn*-glycerol, 1,3-diphosphatidyl-*sn*-glycerol] is known to anchor cytochrome *c* together with cytochrome *c* oxidase at the inner mitochondrial membrane [15–18]. Abnormalities in cardiolipin content and composition thus strongly impair cellular mitochondrial respiration by impairment of cytochrome *c*/cytochrome *c* oxidase function(s) of Complexes III (coenzyme Q – cytochrome *c* reductase) and IV (cytochrome *c* oxidase) of the electron transport chain [9].

The intrinsic pathway of programmed cell death (apoptosis) triggers cytochrome *c* release from the inner mitochondrial membrane into the cytosol [19] where cytochrome *c* associates with apoptotic protease activating factor 1 (Apaf-1, apoptotic peptidase activating factor 1) and procaspase 9 to form the apoptosome [19]. The apoptosome in turn activates the effector caspases 3, 6 and 7 to execute programmed cell death [19]. In cancer cells this mechanism is defective or inefficient [20]. Therefore, in cancer therapy one possibility to selectively and completely kill cancer cells is to induce their apoptosis over the intrinsic pathway by pharmacological intervention [20]. Targeting mitochondria by antineoplastic drugs was suggested as a novel strategy for cancer therapy [20]. Recently, I isolated a lipophilic polyammonium cation, compound **1**, as a by-product of the reaction of 1-aminoadamantane (amantadine) with 1,3-bis(chloromethyl)benzene (α,α'-dichloro-*m*-xylene) in refluxing absolute ethanol. Amantadine is known as an antiparkinsonian (*N*-methyl-D-aspartate ionotropic glutamate receptor antagonist) drug [21] and chemotherapeutic antiviral drug inhibiting influenza A virus M2 protein transmembrane proton channel [22]. This synthesis was inspired by potential binding of a polyammonium cationic drug to DNA and/or p53 tumor suppressor protein tetramerization domain [23]. It was found that compound **1** (**PT162, NSC 796018**), a new compound never synthesized before [according to Chemical Abstracts Service (CAS®) SciFinder® search], induced apoptosis in all cell lines of the National Cancer Institute (NCI) Developmental Therapeutics Program (DTP) 60-cancer cell 5-dose testing, excluding leukemia cell lines, in the micromolar range of growth inhibition 50% (**GI50**). I decided to merge compound **1** (**PT162, NSC 796018**) with the colchic(in)oid compound **2** (**PT166, NSC 750423**) which showed submicromolar **GI50** in the NCI DTP 60-cancer cell 5-dose testing, but did not induce cancer cell apoptosis. Compound **2** (**PT166, NSC 750423**) was synthesized from colchicine and thiosemicarbazide in an one-step procedure and represents a new compound never synthesized before [according to Chemical Abstracts Service (CAS®) SciFinder® search] just as compound **1** (**PT162, NSC 796018**). Compound **1** (**PT162, NSC 796018**) reacted with compound **2** (**PT166, NSC 750423**) under impact of sodium hydroxide (NaOH) to give compound **3**. Compound **3** (**PT167, NSC 799315**), a new compound never synthesized before [according to Chemical Abstracts Service (CAS®) SciFinder® search], showed submicromolar **GI50** in the NCI DTP 60-cancer cell 5-dose testing constantly in most cell lines including leukemia cells. Importantly, compound **3** (**PT167, NSC 799315**) was able to induce apoptosis in all investigated cancer cells, including leukemia cell lines, with a Mean of Inhibition Data (**MID**) for total growth inhibition (**TGI**, growth inhibition 100%) of 4.57 µM, and a **MID** for lethal concentration 50% (**LC50**) of 15.85 µM. I report here the chemistry and NCI DTP 60-cancer cell 5-dose testing data for compound **1** (**PT162, NSC 796018**), compound **2** (**PT166, NSC 750423**) and compound **3** (**PT167, NSC 799315**), and demonstrate the apoptotic release of cytochrome c into the cytosol and activation of effector caspases induced by compounds **1** and **3**. I propose that compound **1** and compound **3** induce apoptosis according to the *Warburg* hypothesis of pre-damaged respiration as a hallmark of cancer by exploiting the defect in mitochondrial cardiolipin–cytochrome c association in cancer cells.

The purpose of this book is to propose a new strategy to heal human cancer completely with two entirely new drug compounds exploiting cancer's *Warburg* effect characterized by a defective mitochondrial aerobic respiration, substituted for by cytosolic aerobic fermentation/glycolysis of glucose into L-(+)-lactic acid. The two essentially new drugs **P(op)T(est)162** and **PT167** were discovered and developed by *Andreas J. Kesel* and internationally patented by PopTest Oncology LLC/Palisades Therapeutics. The *in vitro* antineoplastic highly efficacious drug **PT167** represents a covalent combination of **PT162** and **PT166**. The intermediate drug **PT166** is an entirely new colchic(in)oid derivative synthesized from colchicine. **PT166**'s structure was determined by X-ray crystallography. **PT162** and **PT167** were active *in vitro* versus 60 cancer cell lines of the National Cancer Institute (NCI) Developmental Therapeutics Program (DTP) 60-cancer cell testing. **PT162** and **PT167** both not only stop the growth of cancer cells to ±0% (cancerostatic effect), but completely kill all 60 cancer cells to a level of −100% (tumoricidal effect). **PT162** and **PT167** induce mitochondrial apoptosis (under cytochrome *c* release) in all cancer cells tested by (re)activating (in most cancers impaired) p53 function which results in a decrease of cancer's dysregulated cyclin D1 and an induction of the cell cycle-halting cyclin-dependent kinase inhibitor $p21^{Waf1}/p21^{Cip1}$.

Keywords: cancer growth, tumor metastasis, cancer's *Warburg* effect, p53, p53 (re)activators, mitochondrial apoptosis, cytochrome *c* release, tumoricidal drug effect.

INTRODUCTION

Adenosine 5′-triphosphate (ATP) is required for normal cell proliferation and survival and comes primarily from two sources. The first is glycolysis, which comprises a series of reactions that metabolizes D-(+)-glucose to pyruvate in the cytoplasm to produce a net of 2 molecules ATP from each D-(+)-glucose. The other is the citric acid cycle (CAC), also known as the *Krebs* cycle, *Szent Györgyi–Krebs* cycle or the tricarboxylic acid cycle (TCA cycle), which uses pyruvate formed from glycolysis in a series of reactions that donate electrons *via* nicotinamide adenine dinucleotide (NADH/H$^+$) and flavin adenine dinucleotide (FADH$_2$) to the respiratory chain complexes in the mitochondria. With oxygen (O$_2$) serving as the final electron acceptor, electron transfer across the mitochondrial inner membrane creates a proton gradient which forms 36 molecules ATP *per* one D-(+)-glucose molecule by catalysis of F_1F_O–ATP synthase. In conditions of oxygen limitation, such as within muscles under prolonged exercise, pyruvate is not utilized in the citric acid cycle (CAC), but is converted into L-(+)-lactic acid ('Fleischmilchsäure') by lactate dehydrogenase (LDH) in a process termed anaerobic glycolysis.

Many cancer cells consume D-(+)-glucose heavily and produce L-(+)-lactic acid rather than catabolizing D-(+)-glucose *via* the citric acid cycle (CAC) which is normal for generating ATP in non-hypoxic healthy cells. The avid uptake of D-(+)-glucose by tumors is the prerequisite for the detection and monitoring of human cancers by 2-deoxy-2-[^{18}F]fluoroglucose positron emission tomography (PET). More than 90 years ago, *Otto Heinrich Warburg* (1883−1970) observed that thin slices of human and animal tumors *ex vivo* displayed high levels of D-(+)-glucose uptake and L-(+)-lactate production. The shift toward L-(+)-lactate production in cancers, even in the presence of adequate oxygen, is termed the *Warburg* effect or aerobic glycolysis [1−8]. These observations have been confirmed, although the nuances of aerobic glycolysis and its molecular characteristics are still under investigation. Tumors display aerobic glycolysis partly through activation of (proto-)oncogenes or loss of tumor suppressors, which is then further intensified by stabilization of the evolutionary conserved hypoxia-inducible factor (HIF) *via* adaptive response to hypoxic microenvironment or through pathways that stabilize HIF under non-hypoxic conditions. Recent advances in genomics and proteomics have provided insights into molecular mechanisms that contribute to the *Warburg* effect and tumorigenesis [6−10]. Molecular mechanisms provide significant molecular insights into many aspects of the *Warburg* effect such as the role of (proto-)oncogenes [*AKT* (protein product: protein kinase B), *MYC* proto-oncogene, and *HRAS* (protein product: H-Ras GTPase protein)], tumor suppressors [succinate dehydrogenase (SDH) and fumarate hydratase (FH)], and of the novel HIF pathway including pyruvate dehydrogenase kinase (E.C. 2.7.11.2) isozyme 1 (PDK1). In addition to oncogenic activation of aerobic glycolysis, the activation of HIF, a transcription factor that is stabilized in response to hypoxia, also significantly contributes to the conversion of D-(+)-glucose to L-(+)-lactate. HIF-1 consists of an oxygen sensitive HIF-1α subunit that heterodimerizes with HIF-1β to bind DNA. In conditions of high oxygen partial pressure, HIF-1α is hydroxylated by a specific prolyl hydroxylase [hypoxia-inducible factor prolyl hydroxylase 2 (HIF-PH2) or prolyl hydroxylase domain-containing protein 2 (PHD2), an enzyme encoded by the *EGLN1* gene; also known as hypoxia-inducible factor-proline dioxygenase, HIF prolyl-hydroxylase (E.C. 1.14.11.29)] using α-ketoglutarate derived from the citric acid cycle (CAC) [(HIF-1α protein-incorporated) (2S)-L-proline + α-ketoglutaric acid + O_2 → (2S,4R)-*trans*-4-hydroxyproline + succinate + $CO_2\uparrow$]. The hydroxylated HIF-1α subunit is recognized by the *von Hippel−Lindau* (VHL) protein and prone to degradation in the 26S proteasome, such that HIF-1α is continuously synthesized and degraded in equilibrium under non-hypoxic conditions. Hypoxia is a pathophysiologic stimulus of anaerobic glycolysis promoting stabilization of HIF-1 and its direct *trans*-activation of glycolytic enzyme genes. Hence, adaptation to the hypoxic tumor microenvironment results in increased D-(+)-glucose uptake and L-(+)-lactate production. In addition to hypoxia, oncogenic events have been linked to stabilization of HIF in the presence of adequate oxygen. Activation of the (c-)*Src* proto-oncogene [protein product: proto-oncogene tyrosine-protein kinase Src] increased *in vivo* tumorigenicity as well as HIF-1 levels under non-hypoxic conditions [24]. The oncogenic *HRAS* oncogene product (H-Ras GTPase protein) has been reported to increase the level of HIF-1 [25], and phosphatidylinositol 3-kinase [phosphoinositide 3-kinase (PI3K), phosphatidylinositol-4,5-bisphosphate 3-kinase (E.C. 2.7.1.153)] signaling may stabilize HIF-1 [24]. In renal cell carcinoma VHL tumor suppressor gene mutations disrupt its function which is necessary for the oxygen-dependent prolyl hydroxylation and proteasomal degradation of HIF-1 [26]. Moreover, mutations of the citric acid cycle (CAC) tumor suppressors, SDH and FH, have also been linked to the stabilization of HIF. In particular, prolyl hydroxylation of HIF-1α requires α-ketoglutarate as a substrate which is converted to succinate, such that deficiency of SDH or FH decreases α-ketoglutarate supply and increases succinate level, thereby inhibiting the degradation of HIF-1 [27]. Taken together, activation of certain oncogenic pathways stabilizes HIF-1 protein under non-hypoxic conditions, resulting in activation of glycolytic metabolism. However, activation of glycolytic flux alone would not account for the *Warburg* effect, which is also associated with diminished mitochondrial function that has been thought to decrease passively due to the lack of oxygen. Two recent studies provide insight into the *Warburg* effect through a novel HIF-1-mediated mechanism that actively inhibits mitochondrial function [28,29]. PDK1, which is one of four iso(en)zymes, was identified as a direct HIF-1 target gene in hypoxic cells. PDK1 phosphorylates and inactivates the mitochondrial pyruvate dehydrogenase (PDH) complex. Suppression of PDH by PDK1 inhibits the conversion of pyruvate to acetyl-coenzyme A (acetyl-CoA), thereby compromising mitochondrial function and respiration. Because non-hypoxic stabilization of HIF through oncogenic events has been observed in many types of tumors, PDK1 levels may be upregulated in non-hypoxic tumor cells by HIF which would dissociate pyruvate from PDH and result in the increased L-(+)-lactate production. A recent immunohistochemical study further provided evidence that PDK1 expression is elevated in non-small-cell lung cancers [30]. PDH expression seems to be reduced in high PDK1-expressing cancer cells. These studies suggest that PDK1 activation may be a key regulatory trait contributing to the *Warburg* effect. The activation of (proto-)oncogenes, such as *AKT, MYC*, and *HRAS*, along with the stabilization of HIF, could enhance aerobic glycolysis or the *Warburg* effect in tumor cells by inducing glycolytic flux and compromising mitochondrial function [8,31].

The protein p53, also known as tumo(u)r protein TP53, cellular tumo(u)r antigen p53, or transformation-related protein 53 (TRP53) is a regulatory protein that is often mutated in human cancers [32−35]. The p53 proteins (originally thought to be a single protein) are essential in vertebrates for preventing cancer formation [32−35]. As such, p53 has been described as 'the guardian of the genome' because of its role in conserving genome stability by preventing genome mutation [34,36]. Hence *TP53* is classified as a tumo(u)r suppressor gene [32−37]. The *TP53* gene is the most frequently mutated gene in human cancer (mutated in > 50% of investigated human cancers) [38−41], indicating that the *TP53* gene plays a crucial role in preventing cancer formation in human individuals. The *TP53* gene encodes a protein that binds to DNA consensus sequences [33], regulates gene expression, and induces apoptosis in consequence to mutational DNA damage, thus preventing transmission/inheritance of genomic mutations to the next generation of cells by cell division/mitosis [32−37]. In addition to the full-length protein, the human *TP53* gene encodes at least 12 protein isoforms (including splice variants) [42−45]. The *TP53* gene is expressed in every human cell type, except in red blood cells (erythrocytes) which lack a nucleus [45].

In humans, the *TP53* gene is located on the short arm of chromosome 17 (17p13.1) [46,47]. The gene (20 kb) spans eleven exons, with a non-coding exon 1 and a very long first intron of 10 kb overlapping the *Hp53int1* gene [human protein 53 intron 1; 1,125 base pairs (bp)] [35]. The coding sequence contains five regions showing a high degree of conservation in vertebrates, predominantly in exons 2, 5, 6, 7, and 8, but the sequences found in invertebrates show only distant resemblance to mammalian *TP53* [35].

p53 was identified in 1979 by *Sir David P. Lane & Lionel V. Crawford* [48], *Arnold J. Levine & Daniel I.H. Linzer* [49], and *Lloyd J. Old, Albert B. DeLeo & Colleagues* [50]. p53 had been assumed before to exist as the target of the SV40 virus (*Polyomaviridae*, *Betapolyomavirus*; simian vacuolating virus 40, simian virus 40) which is tumorigenic. SV40 virus' oncogenic potential involves suppression of the transcriptional properties of p53 [48,49] and retinoblastoma [p(105-)Rb] [51] tumor suppressor proteins by the SV40 large T antigen [48,49,51]. The name p53 was coined in 1979 [50], describing the apparent molecular mass of the protein on sodium dodecyl sulfate–polyacrylamide gel electrophoresis (SDS–PAGE).

The murine *TP53* gene was first cloned by *Peter V. Chumakov & Colleagues* (Academy of Sciences of the U.S.S.R., Moscow, Russia) in 1982 [52], and, independently, in 1983 by *Arnold J. Levine, Moshe Oren & David Givol* [53,54]. The human *TP53* gene was cloned in 1984 [42], and the full-length clone was identified in 1985 [55].

The 393 amino acid (aa) protein p53 has seven domains:
1. The acidic N-terminal transcription-activation domain 1 (TAD1), also known as activation domain 1 (AD1), which activates transcription factors; the N-terminus contains two complementary transcriptional activation domains, with the major one at residues 1–42 and a

minor one at residues 55–75, specifically involved in the regulation of several pro-apoptotic genes [35].

2. Transcription-activation domain 2 (TAD2), also known as activation domain 2 (AD2), important for apoptotic activity: residues 43–63.

3. PXXP proline-rich domain important for the apoptotic activity of p53 by nuclear exportation *via* mitogen-activated protein kinase (MAP kinase or MAPK) factors: residues 64–92 [56].

4. Central DNA-binding (core) domain (DBD), contains one zinc dication (Zn^{2+}) and several arginine amino acids: residues 102–306; this region is responsible for binding the p53 co-repressor LMO3 (LIM domain only protein 3); LMO3 acts as a co-repressor of p53, suppressing p53-dependent transcriptional regulation without inhibition of its DNA-binding activity [57].

5. Nuclear localization signal (NLS) domain, residues 316–325.

6. (Homo)oligomerization domain (OD): residues 307–355; homotetramerization is essential for the activity of p53 *in vivo*.

7. C-terminal negative regulation domain (Neg) involved in downregulation of DNA binding of the DBD central domain: residues 364–393 [58].

Mutations that deactivate p53 in cancer usually occur in the DBD. Most of these mutations destroy the ability of the protein to bind to its target DNA sequences, and thus prevent transcriptional activation of these genes. As such, mutations in the DBD are recessive loss–of–function mutations. Molecules of p53 with mutations in the OD dimerize with wild-type p53 (p53α), and prevent p53α from activating transcription. Therefore, OD mutations have a dominant negative effect on the function of p53.

Wild-type p53 (p53α) protein is a labile polypeptide, joining structured/folded and unstructured regions that act in a synergistic manner [59]. SDS−PAGE analysis of p53 indicates it to be a 53 kDa protein. However, the actual mass of the full-length p53 protein (p53α) based on the sum of molecular masses of its amino acid residues is only 43.65 kDa. This difference is due to the high number of proline residues in the protein, which slow its migration on SDS−PAGE, thus making it to appear heavier than it actually is. Wild-type p53 (p53α) represents a phosphoprotein, which is multiply phosphorylated when p53 activation occurs by multiple stressors [60,61], especially at L-serine (S) aa 20 (Ser20, S20) by casein kinase 1 (CK1) [60]. CK1 was identified as the human herpesvirus 6B (HHV-6B)-induced protein kinase that targets the Ser20 site on p53 [60]. The wild-type p53 DBD core binds one zinc dication (Zn^{2+}) very tightly [62,63]. p53 DBD exhibits two unusual properties — one of the highest zinc affinities of any eukaryotic protein and extreme instability in the absence of zinc — which are predicted to balance p53 at the top of folding/unfolding in the cell, with a major determinant being available zinc concentration [62]. Protein p53 binds zinc extremely tightly when folded, but is intrinsically unstable in the absence of zinc at 37 °C. Whether the wild-type p53 protein folds in the cell is largely determined by the concentration of available zinc. Consequently, zinc dysregulation in the cell as well as a large percentage of tumorigenic p53 mutations can cause p53 to lose zinc and its tumor-suppressing activity, and misfold [63].

As with 95% of human genes, *TP53* encodes more than one protein [44,45]. All these p53 proteins are called the p53 isoforms. These proteins range in apparent size from 26 to 53 kDa. Several isoforms were discovered in 2005 [44], and so far 12 human p53 isoforms have been identified (p53α, p53β, p53γ, Δ40p53α, Δ40p53β, Δ40p53γ, Δ133p53α, Δ133p53β, Δ133p53γ, Δ160p53α, Δ160p53β, Δ160p53γ) [44,45]. p53 isoforms are expressed in a tissue-dependent manner, and p53α is never expressed alone [44,45].

The full length p53α isoform protein can be subdivided into different protein domains. Starting from the N-terminus, there are first the N-terminal *trans*-activation domains (TAD 1 and TAD 2) which are needed to induce a subset of p53 target genes. These domains are followed by the proline-rich domain (PXXP), whereby the aa motif PXXP is repeated (P is L-proline, and X can be any amino acid). It is required among other for p53-mediated apoptosis [64]. Some isoforms lack the proline-rich domain, such as Δ133p53β/γ, and Δ160p53α/β/γ; hence, some isoforms of p53 are not able to mediate apoptosis, emphasizing the multiple roles of the *TP53* gene [65]. Central is the DBD which enables the sequence-specific DNA-binding. The C-terminal domains complete the p53α protein. They include the NLS, the nuclear export signal (NES), and the OD. The NLS and NES are responsible for the subcellular compartmentalization of p53. Through the OD, p53 can form a homotetramer and then bind to DNA targets. Among the p53 isoforms some domains can be missing, but all of them share most of the highly conserved DBD.

The isoforms are formed by several mechanisms. The β and the γ isoforms are generated by multiple splicing of intron 9, which leads to a different C-terminus. Furthermore, the usage of an internal promoter in intron 4 produces the Δ133p53 and Δ160p53 isoforms which lack the TAD domains (Δ133p53α/β/γ, Δ160p53α/β/γ) and a part of the DBD (Δ160p53α/β/γ). Moreover, alternative initiation of translation at ATG triplet codon aa 40 or ATG triplet codon aa 160 produce the Δ40p53 and Δ160p53 isoforms, respectively. Due to the isoformic nature of p53 proteins, there have been several sources of evidence showing that mutations within the

TP53 gene giving rise to mutated isoforms are causative agents of various cancer phenotypes, from mild to severe, due to single mutation in the *TP53* gene. Recents studies show that p53 isoforms are differentially expressed in different human tissues, and the loss−of−function or gain−of−function mutations within the isoforms can provoke tissue-specific cancer, or provide cancer stem cell malignancy in different cell types [44,45,64−66].

p53 plays an important role in regulation of, or progression through, the cell cycle, in apoptosis and maintenance of genomic stability, by several mechanisms:

- p53 can activate DNA repair proteins when DNA has suffered sustained damage. Thus, it may be an important factor in aging.
- p53 can arrest growth by holding the cell cycle at the G_1/S boundary on DNA damage recognition — if it stops the cell cycle here for long enough time, the DNA repair machinery will have time to fix the damage and the cells will be allowed to continue the cell cycle.
- p53 can initiate apoptosis (programmed cell death) if DNA damage proves to be irreparable.
- p53 is essential for the senescence response to shortened telomeres [67,68].
- p53 acts as an inhibitor of angiogenesis generally mediated by vascular endothelial growth factor A (VEGF-A) [69−71].
- p53 plays an important role in the differentiation and maintenance of human stem cells throughout embryonal development and adult human life [72−79].

In human embryonic stem cells (hESCs) p53 is maintained at low inactive levels [72]. This is because activation of p53 leads to rapid differentiation of hESCs [73]. Studies have shown that p53 knock-out delays differentiation and that introducing p53 causes spontaneous differentiation [72,73].

p53 promotes differentiation of hESCs and plays a key role in cell cycle as a differentiation regulator. When p53 becomes stabilized and activated in hESCs, it induces the cyclin-dependent kinase inhibitor $p21^{Waf1}/p21^{Cip1}$ to establish an elongation of G_1 cell cycle phase. This typically leads to abolition of S phase entry, which stops the cell cycle in G_1 cell cycle phase and leads to differentiation. An investigation in mouse embryonic stem cells has recently shown, however, that the expression of p53 does not necessarily lead to differentiation [74]. Protein p53 also activates microRNA 34a (miR-34a) and microRNA 145 (miR-145) which then repress the hESCs pluripotency factors, further promoting differentiation [72]. In adult stem cells, p53 regulation is important for maintenance of stemness in adult stem cell niches. Stress signals such as hypoxia affect levels of p53 in these niche cells through the hypoxia inducible factors HIF-1α and HIF-2α. While HIF-1α stabilizes p53, HIF-2α suppresses it [75]. Suppression of p53 plays important roles in cancer stem cell phenotype, induced pluripotent stem cells (iPS cells, iPSCs), and other stem cell functions such as *blastema* formation [*blastema* (ancient Greek: βλάστημα, 'offspring') = mass of cells capable of growth and regeneration into organs or body parts]. Cells with decreased levels of p53 have been shown to reprogram into stem cells with a much greater efficiency than normal cells [76,77]. Published investigations suggest that the lack of cell cycle arrest and apoptosis gives more cells the chance to be reprogrammed [76,77]. Decreased levels of p53 were also shown to be a crucial aspect of *blastema* formation in the legs of salamanders [78]. p53 regulation is very important in acting as a barrier between stem cells and the differentiated stem cell state, as well as a barrier between stem cells being functional or malignant, respectively [79].

Protein p53 acts as a cellular stress sensor. In unstressed cells, p53 levels are kept low through a continuous degradation of p53. A protein called Mdm2 (Mouse double minute 2 homolog, E3 ubiquitin-protein ligase Mdm2, also called HDM2 in humans) binds to p53 [80,81], preventing its action and transporting it from the nucleus to the cytosol. Mdm2 also acts as an ubiquitin ligase and covalently attaches ubiquitin to p53 and thus marking p53 for degradation in the 26S proteasome [82]. However, ubiquit(in)ylation of p53 is reversible. A ubiquitin-specific protease, the ubiquitin-specific-processing protease 7 (USP7), also known as ubiquitin carboxyl-terminal hydrolase 7 or herpesvirus-associated ubiquitin-specific protease (HAUSP), can cleave ubiquitin from p53 [83], thereby saving it from proteasome-dependent degradation *via* the ubiquitin ligase pathway. Ubiquitin carboxyl-terminal hydrolase 42 (USP42) has also been shown to deubiquitinate p53 and may be required for the ability of p53 to respond to stress [84]. Mdm2 protein recognizes and binds to the N-terminal *trans*-activation domain (TAD) of the p53 tumor suppressor protein and acts as an inhibitor of p53 transcriptional activation [85]. On activation of p53, Mdm2 is also activated and dissociates from p53, setting up a feedback loop [86]. p53 levels can show oscillations (or repeated pulses) in response to certain stresses, and these pulses can be important in determining whether the cells survive the stress, or die [86]. p53 is normally kept at low levels by being constantly marked for degradation by Mdm2 [80–88]. Once p53 is activated in response to a myriad of stressors — including DNA damage and other stress factors [oxidative stress, ultraviolet (UV) radiation damage of DNA, DNA double-strand breaks, heat shock, osmotic shock, kidney failure (duty for hemodialysis) [89], starvation, (2′-deoxy)ribonucleotide depletion, deregulated oncogene expression] — various pathways will lead to the dissociation of the p53 and Mdm2 complex [80−88]. Once activated, p53 protein will induce cell cycle arrest, to allow either repair/survival of the cell or apoptosis to eliminate the damaged cell, respectively [80−88].

Certain viral pathogens (SV40 virus, human papillomavirus, *Epstein−Barr* herpesvirus, human adenovirus) can also affect the human p53 protein that is is expressed from the human *TP53* gene. One such example, human papillomavirus (*Papillomaviridae*; HPV), encodes a protein, E6, which binds to the p53 protein and inactivates it [90]. This mechanism, in synergy with the inactivation of the cell cycle regulator p105-Rb by the HPV protein E7 [91], allows for repeated cell division manifested clinically as warts. HPV is believed to cause cancer by integrating its genome into nuclear DNA. Some of the early genes expressed by HPV, such as E6 and E7, act as oncogenes that promote malignant transformation and tumor growth [90,91]. HPV genome integration into human chromosomal DNA can also cause carcinogenesis by promoting genomic instability associated with alterations in DNA copy number. The E6 papillomaviral gene produces a protein (also called E6) that simultaneously binds to two host cell proteins, p53 and E6-associated protein [ubiquitin-protein ligase E3A (UBE3A), also known as E6AP ubiquitin-protein ligase (E6AP)] [92−94]. E6AP is an E3 ubiquitin ligase, an enzyme whose purpose is to tag proteins with a post-translational modification, a polypeptide called ubiquitin. By binding both proteins, E6 induces E6AP to attach a chain of ubiquitin molecules to p53, thereby marking p53 for proteasomal degradation [92−94]. Protein p53 also induces the cyclin-dependent kinase inhibitor $p21^{Waf1}/p21^{Cip1}$ protein which blocks the formation of the cyclin D1−D3/Cdk4(6) and cyclin E/Cdk2 complexes, thereby preventing the phosphorylation of p105-Rb tumor suppressor protein [95,96], and, in consequence, halting cell cycle progression by preventing the activation of E2F transcription factors (*E2F* is a group of genes that encode a family of transcription factors in higher eukaryotes; three of them are activators: E2F1, E2F2, and E2F3a; six others act as suppressors: E2F3b, E2F4−8; all of them are involved in the cell cycle regulation and synthesis of DNA in mammalian cells; for activators, E2F1 binding to p105-Rb has been shown to mask its *trans*-activation domain responsible for transcription activation [95,96]). The cyclin D1−D3/Cdk4(6) and cyclin E/Cdk2 complexes phosphorylate p105-Rb and related pocket proteins allowing them to disassociate from E2F1 [95,96]. Thus, the degradation of p53 induced by E6 promotes deregulated cell division, cell growth and cell survival, all characteristics of malignant transformation. It is important to note, that while the interaction between E6, E6AP and p53 was the first to be characterized, there are multiple other proteins in the host cell which interact with E6 [94] and contribute to the induction of cancer [94]. Certain HPV types, in particular types 16, 18, 31, and 45, can also lead to progression from a benign wart to low- or high-grade cervical dysplasia, which are reversible forms of pre-malignant lesions. Persistent infection of the cervix over the years can cause irreversible changes leading to carcinoma *in situ* and, eventually, invasive cervical cancer. This results from the action(s) of HPV genes, especially those encoding the oncoproteins E6 and E7 which are the two viral products that are preferentially retained and expressed in cervical cancers by integration of viral DNA into the host chromosomal DNA.

Another example is the tumorigenic *Epstein−Barr* herpesvirus [*Herpesviridae*, *Gammaherpesvirinae*, *Lymphocryptovirus*; human herpesvirus 4 (HHV-4), EBV]. *Epstein−Barr* virus nuclear antigen 5 (EBNA-5, EBNA-LP) binds to p53 and inhibits its *trans*-activating function [97,98], and EBNA-5 (EBNA-LP) binds to p105-Rb tumor suppressor protein [97]. Moreover, *Epstein−Barr* virus nuclear antigen 2 (EBNA-2) and *Epstein−Barr virus* latent membrane protein 1 (LMP-1) induce p53 expression *via* nuclear factor κB (NFκB) *trans*-activation [99]. Oncogenic human adenoviral (*Adenoviridae, Mastadenovirus*; human adenoviruses) protein adenovirus early region 1A (E1A) also targets p53 [100−103] and p105-Rb tumor suppressor proteins [100,104]. Adenoviral E1A raises p53 protein expression [100−103]. Conversely, oncogenic human adenoviral protein adenovirus early region 1B (E1B) targets p53 and inhibits the apoptosis induction mediated by p53 [100,103]. During human adenovirus infection, the E1A region expresses two major proteins, 243R and 289R, that differ by 46 aa that are present in 289R. Comparison of the aa sequences of 243R and 289R between serotypes suggests the presence of three conserved domains 1, 2, and 3 (CD1, CD2, and CD3) [102]. Expression of E1A has been shown to cause an increase in the level of p53 protein and induce p53-dependent apoptosis [101]. Stabilization of p53 requires the N-terminus or CD1 of E1A and occurs through modification of a ubiquitin-protease pathway [102,105].

Protein p53 (re)activators target either (i) mutant p53 proteins by restoring misfolded mutant p53 protein activity, or (ii) E3 ubiquitin-protein ligase Mdm2−p53 protein−protein interaction(s) acting as Mdm2 antagonists, or (iii) Mdmx−p53 protein−protein interaction(s) acting as Mdmx antagonists [106−109]. Mdmx (MDMX, Mdm4, Hdmx), a structural homologue of Mdm2, has no ubiquit(in)ylation activity but is able to bind to the N-terminus of p53 and inactivate it directly, or to aid Mdm2 in ubiquit(in)ylating p53 by heterodimerization with Mdm2 [87,107].

Protein p53α seems to have evolved to be thermodynamically and kinetically unstable at body temperature in humans, which may allow for tighter control of p53 protein levels [107]. Many oncogenic mutations inactivate p53 function by disrupting the direct binding to specific DNA (known as contact mutants) or by preventing the proper folding of the central DBD of p53 (known as structural mutants) [107]. Many of these mutant p53 proteins are temperature-sensitive, which has encouraged attempts to discover molecules that can restore mutant p53 activity by acting as p53 chaperones. This concept has recently proved to be successful in *Gaucher*'s disease, a lysosomal storage disorder [110], in which small-molecules were found to restore the activity of the mutant glucocerebrosidase enzyme by causing its stabilization [110]. These observations have led to generic methods of identifying protein targets of small-molecule drugs *via* their chaperoning function, where the binding of a small-molecule chaperone to its target protein selectively increases its resistance to denaturation induced by high temperatures [107].

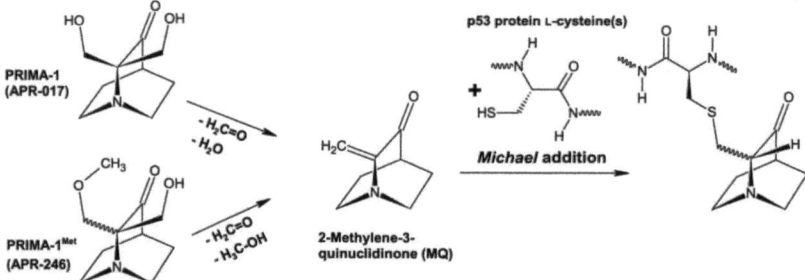

Fig. I. The mechanism by which **PRIMA-1** [**APR-017**, 2,2-bis(hydroxymethyl)-3-quinuclidinone] and **PRIMA-1**^Met (**APR-246**) are activated *in vivo* to 2-methylene-3-quinuclidinone (MQ). MQ binds to mutant p53 misfolded DBD core L-cysteine (Cys, C) residues aa Cys124/Cys277 by *Michael* addition to the α,β-unsaturated ketone, and restores wild-type p53 function upon binding to mutant p53 [111−113].

PRIMA-1 [APR-017, 2,2-bis(hydroxymethyl)-3-quinuclidinone, 2,2-bis(hydroxymethyl)-1-azabicyclo[2.2.2]octan-3-one; developed at the Karolinska Institute, Stockholm, Sweden] [111,112] (Fig. I) and its structural analogue **PRIMA-1**[Met] [APR-246, (2RS)-2-(hydroxymethyl)-2-(methoxymethyl)-3-quinuclidinone, (2RS)-2-(hydroxy-methyl)-2-(methoxymethyl)-1-azabicyclo[2.2.2]octan-3-one; developed by Aprea Therapeutics, Doylestown, PA, USA] [113] (Fig. I) have been shown to restore mutant p53 (R273H and R175H) activity *in vitro* and *in vivo*. In 2002, small-molecule screening identified [111] **PRIMA-1** (acronym for: p53 reactivation with induction of massive apoptosis-1), a drug that restored wild-type p53 function upon binding to mutant p53. **PRIMA-1** triggered *in vitro* apoptosis in Saos-2 osteosarcoma cells transduced to express the aa R273H mutant protein p53[R273H], and suppressed *in vivo* tumor formation by these cells. **PRIMA-1** inhibited prion-like amyloid aggregation of mutant p53 in cancer cells [112]. Pharmacologically, **PRIMA-1** and **PRIMA-1**[Met] are actually prodrugs; their mutual active metabolite, 2-methylene-3-quinuclidinone (MQ) [111,112] (Fig. I), reacts covalently with thiol (R−SH, mercaptan) groups of L-cysteine (Cys, C) residues Cys124 and Cys277 [113] (Fig. I) in the misfolded core DBD of mutant p53, restoring wild-type p53 conformation. Only a minority of the reported mutant p53-reactivating small-molecules succeeded into clinical trials. The first to reach a clinical trial was **PRIMA-1**[Met], an *O*-methylated derivative of **PRIMA-1**, also known as **APR-246**. **APR-246** demonstrated better activity than **PRIMA-1** *in vitro*

Fig. II (next page). The organic chemical structure formulae of the mutant p53 (re)activators **P53R3** [114], **SCH529074** [115], and **Bifunctional ligand L**[I] (**NSC 788648**) [116], in comparison to **PT162** (**NSC 796018**) and **PT167** (**NSC 799315**) [this work]. **PT162** and **PT167** share chemical property resemblance to **P53R3**, **SCH529074**, and **L**[I].

XLVII

Bifunctional ligand L' (NSC 788648)

PT167 (NSC 799315)

SCH529074

P53R3

PT162 (NSC 796018)

and in preclinical studies, with increased apoptotic effects in acute myeloid leukemia (AML) cell lines and patient primary cells. Additionally, **APR-246** promoted apoptosis in cell lines derived from small-cell lung carcinoma (SCLC), and delayed tumor growth in mice injected with SCLC-derived cell lines.

P53R3 [114] (Fig. II) is a 4-aminoquinazoline-type molecule which was originally identified using p53 DNA-binding assays [114]. This compound, a 2-({4-[bis(4-chlorophenyl)methyl]piperazin-1-yl}methyl)quinazolin-4-amine derivative, restores sequence-specific DNA-binding to several p53 hot spot mutants, but also improves the recruitment of wild-type p53 to target gene promoters. Analogously, **SCH529074** [115] (Fig. II) represents another 4-aminoquinazoline-type molecule, also a 2-({4-[bis(4-chlorophenyl)methyl]piperazin-1-yl}methyl)quinazolin-4-amine derivative like **P53R3**. **SCH529074** reactivates mutant p53 and also binds to p53 DBD, interrupting Mdm2-mediated ubiquitination of wild-type p53 [115]. A striking p53 reactivator is the compound 2-({bis[(pyridin-2-yl)methyl]amino}methyl)-6-iodo-4-(1,3-benzothiazol-2-yl)phenol = **Bifunctional ligand L^I (NSC 788648)** [116] (Fig. II). The drug bears zinc-metallochaperone features and strongly interacts with mutant p53 [116]. The insertion of an iodine atom into the compound structure (Fig. II) promotes inhibition of mutant p53 aggregation, restores Zn^{2+}-binding to mutant p53, and reactivates wild-type p53 transcriptional function [116]. The effects were observed both *in vitro* and *in vivo*. The **Bifunctional ligand L^I** evoked only minimal toxicity to non-cancerous tissues, showing a selective cytotoxicity to mutant p53 tumors [116]. **PT162** and **PT167** share chemical property resemblance to **P53R3**, **SCH529074**, and **L^I** (Fig. II). They are all cationic charged at physiological pH 7.40 and bear strongly hydrophobic contact regions (Fig. II).

PT162 (**NSC 796018**) and **PT167** (**NSC 799315**) may have three antineoplastic mechanisms−of−action: (i) their binding to mutant p53 core DBD like **P53R3**, **SCH529074**, and **Bifunctional ligand L^I**, thereby restoring sequence-specific DNA-binding of p53 mutants, inhibiting mutant p53 prion-like amyloid aggregation, restoring Zn^{2+}-binding to mutant p53 DBD, and reactivating wild-type p53 transcriptional activity, (ii) their binding to the tetramerization OD of mutant p53 by ionic and hydrophobic interaction(s), thereby restoring the tetramerization of OD mutant p53, reinstalling the target promoter DNA-binding and transcriptional activation properties of OD mutant p53, and (iii) their binding to mitochondrial cardiolipin, thereby interrupting the anchoring of cytochrome c (and cytochrome c oxidase, Complex IV) at the inner mitochondrial membrane, inducing cytochrome c release into the cytosol with triggering of mitochondrial apoptosis (intrinsic pathway).

The first antineoplastic mechanism−of−action of **PT162** (**NSC 796018**) and **PT167** (**NSC 799315**) is analogous to the antineoplastic mechanism−of−action of **P53R3**, **SCH529074**, and **Bifunctional ligand L^I**, by binding to and restoring of proper folding at the core DBD of mutant p53 proteins [114−116]. The second mechanism−of−action of **PT162** (**NSC 796018**) and **PT167** (**NSC 799315**) involves the restoration of tetramerization and, consequently, DNA-binding ability of p53 tetramerization OD mutants. Protein p53 <u>must</u> tetramerize to be able to bind to promoter DNA cognate sequences in the genes of p53 transcriptional *trans*-activation targets [23,117].

About half of human tumors carry inactivating mutations in the *TP53* gene [38−41]. Unlike other tumor suppressor genes, such as *RB1*, *APC*, *BRCA1*, and *CDKN2A*, which are inactivated primarily by deletion or nonsense mutations, 74% of *TP53* tumor-derived mutations are point mutations that change a single aa. More than 95% of these missense mutations occur in the DBD; they fall into two main categories, commonly termed DNA contact and structural/conformational mutations. In contrast, ~17% of germ line p53 mutations in people with *Li–Fraumeni* syndrome [118,119] and *Li–Fraumeni*-like syndromes [119] affect aa in the p53 tetramerization OD, even though it consists only of a short aa segment (~30 aa), whereas ~80% of germ line mutations affect DBD aa residues (*Li–Fraumeni* syndrome [118,119] is a rare, autosomal dominant, hereditary disorder that predisposes carriers to multiple cancer development; the syndrome is linked to germline mutations of the *TP53* tumor suppressor gene; it was named after two American physicians, *Frederick P. Li* and *Joseph F. Fraumeni Jr.*, who first recognized the syndrome after reviewing the medical records and death certificates of 648 childhood rhabdomyosarcoma patients [118]). The p53 DBD is six times as long as the p53 tetramerization OD. This finding implies that germ line mutations exist at similar frequencies in the p53 tetramerization OD and the p53 DBD, and both domains are essential for p53-mediated activity [23].

The p53 tetramerization OD consists of a β-strand (Glu326–Arg333), a tight turn (Gly334), and an α-helix (Arg335–Gly356) [23]. The structure of the p53 tetramerization OD was determined by nuclear magnetic resonance (NMR) spectroscopy [120] (Fig. III, Fig. IV) and X-ray crystallography [121]. Two monomers form a dimer through their antiparallel β-sheets and α-helices, and two dimers become a tetramer through the formation of an unusual four-helix bundle. Ala-scanning of the p53 tetramerization OD revealed that 9 hydrophobic residues constitute critical determinants of its stability and oligomerization status [23]. An earlier study of tumor-derived mutants R337H, R337C, or L344P from patients with *Li–Fraumeni*-like syndrome

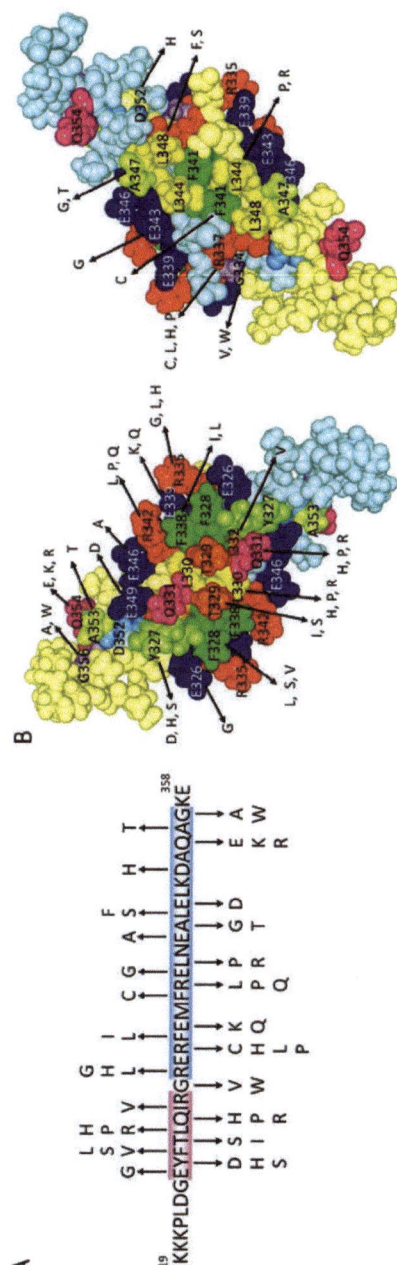

Fig. III. The wild-type protein p53 tetramerization OD and frequent cancer cell mutations occurring in the protein p53 tetramerization OD, adapted from [23]. **A**, aa sequences and the positions of the missense mutations in the tetramerization domain of p53, β-strand aa are highlighted in <u>red</u>, α-helical aa are highlighted in <u>blue</u>. **B**, space-filling model of p53 tetramerization OD (RCSB Protein Data Bank code: 3SAK; https://doi.org/10.2210/pdb3SAK/pdb [122]). The aa residues of the mutation site in the p53 tetramerization OD and the location of these residues in the tetrameric structure are shown. Anionic L-glutamic acid (Glu, E) aa residues are shown in <u>blue</u>, hydrophobic L-phenylalanine (Phe, F) aa residues are in <u>green</u>, L-tyrosine (Tyr, Y) aa residues are in <u>lighter green</u>, hydrophobic L-leucine (Leu, L) aa residues are in <u>yellow</u>, L-alanine (Ala, A) aa residues are in <u>light green</u>, L-glutamine (Gln, Q) aa residues are in <u>purple</u>, cationic L-arginine (Arg, R) aa residues are in <u>red</u>. The primary dimer is depicted, and the other dimer is removed from it, to give a direct view of the interior of the protein. The right dimer was obtained by rotating the structure in the left picture by 180° around the horizontal axis [23].

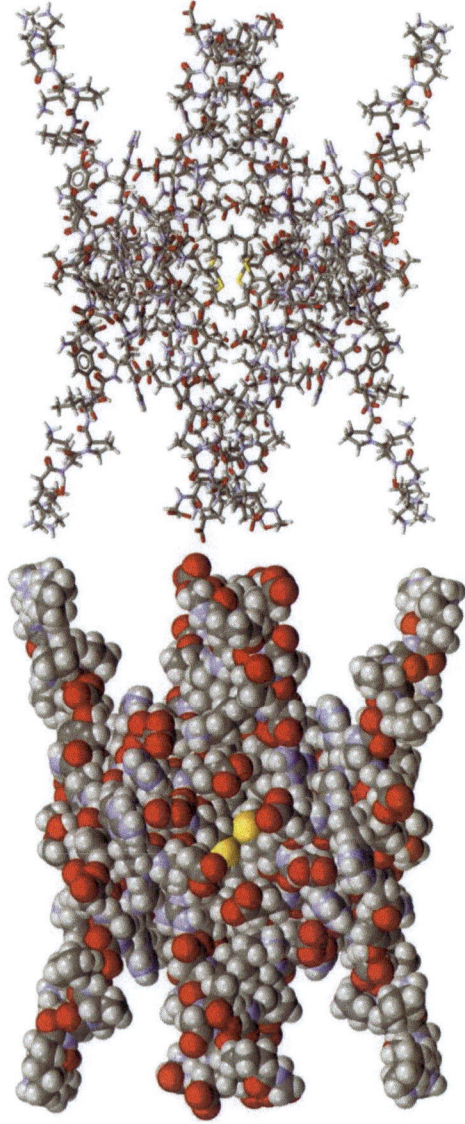

Fig. IV. The wild-type protein p53 tetramerization OD solved as high-resolution multi-dimensional nuclear magnetic resonance (NMR) structure (RCSB Protein Data Bank code: 3SAK; https://doi.org/10.2210/pdb3 SAK/pdb [120,122]). **Top,** capped-stick model of the p53 tetramerization OD. **Bottom,** space-fill model of the p53 tetramerization OD. The 42 aa sequence of the p53 OD fragment is: 319-KKKPLDGEYFTLQIRGRE RFEMFRELNEALELKD AQAGKEPG-360, in this sequence anionic Glu (E) and Asp (D) aa residues are shown in blue, hydrophobic Phe (F) and Tyr (Y) aa residues are in green, hydrophobic Leu (L) aa residues are in orange, Ala (A) aa residues are in light green, Gln (Q) and Asn (N) aa residues are in purple, cationic Arg (R) and Lys (K) aa residues are in red, Met (M) aa residues are in yellow; β-strand aa stretches are underlined, α-helical aa stretches are set *italic*.

revealed a propensity for dramatic destabilization; the presence of the R337H mutation entailed pH-dependent instability of the mutant p53 tetramer [23]. Leu344 occurs in the α-helix, and after introducing a helix-breaking proline (L344P) p53 could not form tetramers. R337C forms dimers and tetramers at low temperature; however, even though its tetrameric structure is destabilized significantly at physiological temperatures, it is only partially inactivated in several functional assays [23]. The p53 proteins with these mutations, as with other p53 tetramerization OD mutations (*e.g.* L330H, R337L, R342P, E349D, and G334V), exhibit an overall decrease in DNA binding and *trans*-activation activity [23]. Wild-type p53 binds DNA as a tetramer, each subunit recognizing five nucleotides of the 20 nucleotide-long promoter cognate DNA target site [117]. The wild-type p53 tetramerization OD high-resolution NMR structure (Fig. III, Fig. IV) reveals a surface of many anionic (Glu, Asp) and hydrophobic (Phe, Tyr, Leu, Ile, Ala, Met) aa residues. This feature predisposes the p53 OD sequence 319-**KKKPLDG EYFTLQIRG*RERFEMFRELNEALELKDA QAG*K**EPG-360 (β-strand stretches underlined, α-helical stretches set *italic*) as ideal binding partner of the cationic and hydrophobic molecules **PT162** (**NSC 796018**) and **PT167** (**NSC 799315**) (Fig. II), based on ionic plus−minus charge attraction and hydrophobic interaction(s). **PT162** (**NSC 796018**) presents as a pentacation and **PT167** (**NSC 799315**) represents a trication at physiological pH 7.40, and the 31 aa p53 tetramerization OD peptide (aa 326−356) is overally negative charged and strongly hydrophobic [Net: 7 negative charges (E, D), 5 positive charges (R, K), 13 hydrophobic residues (F, Y, L, I, A, M)].

The third mechanism−of−action of **PT162** (**NSC 796018**) and **PT167** (**NSC 799315**) is based on the chemical structure of cardiolipin [1,3-bis(*sn*-3′-phosphatidyl)-*sn*-

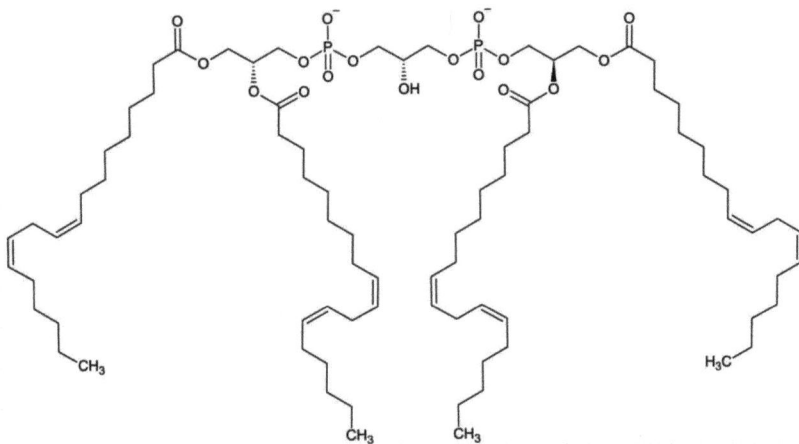

Fig. V. The organic chemical structural formula of cardiolipin [1,3-bis(*sn*-3′-phosphatidyl)-*sn*-glycerol, 1,3-diphosphatidyl-*sn*-glycerol]. The molecule is optically active, representing the L,L-form. Pictured is the predominant dianionic species in the inner mitochondrial membrane with $C_{18:2}$ [linoleic acid, (9Z,12Z)-9,12-octadecadienoic acid] at each of the four acyl positions, as isolated from bovine heart, bovine heart cardiocyte mitochondria, and rat liver [123−125].

glycerol, 1,3-diphosphatidyl-*sn*-glycerol] [123−125] (Fig. V). Cardiolipin is dianionic and strongly hydrophobic, making it a perfect binding partner of the cationic and hydrophobic molecules **PT162 (NSC 796018)** and **PT167 (NSC 799315)** (Fig. II), based on ionic plus−minus charge attraction and hydrophobic interaction(s). By binding to cardiolipin and disrupting the tight association between cytochrome *c* and cardiolipin at the inner mitochondrial membrane in mitochondria, **PT162 (NSC 796018)** and **PT167 (NSC 799315)** trigger mitochondrial apoptosis (programmed cell death, intrinsic pathway), characterized by cytochrome *c* release from mitochondria into the cytosol and caspase 3 activation [19,20]. This is accompanied by **PT162 (NSC 796018)**- and **PT167 (NSC 799315)**-mediated p53 activation, therefrom resulting cyclin-dependent kinase inhibitor

Waf1/Cip1/CDKN1A ($p21^{Waf1}$/$p21^{Cip1}$) induction leading to cell cycle arrest, and disruption of the malignant cell *Warburg* effect by **PT162** (**NSC 796018**)- and **PT167** (**NSC 799315**)-rescued/restored p53 influence on mitochondrial respiration enzyme Complex IV [induction of <u>s</u>ynthesis of <u>c</u>ytochrome *c* <u>o</u>xidase 2 (*SCO2*) gene] [126,127].

The cyclin-dependent kinase inhibitor Waf1/Cip1/Sdi1/CAP20/MDA-6/CDKN1A ($p21^{Waf1}$/$p21^{Cip1}$), also known as cyclin-dependent kinase inhibitor 1A or Cdk-interacting protein 1, is a cyclin-dependent kinase inhibitor (CKI) that is capable of inhibiting all cyclin/cyclin-dependent kinase (Cdk) complexes (CDKCs), though is primarily associated with inhibition of cyclin E/Cdk2 [128−130]. The gene of $p21^{Waf1}$/$p21^{Cip1}$ represents a major target of p53 *trans*-activation activity [131] and thus is associated with linking DNA damage to cell cycle arrest. The $p21^{Waf1}$/$p21^{Cip1}$ gene promoter contains several p53 response elements that govern direct binding of p53 protein tetramers, resulting in transcriptional activation of the gene *CDKN1* coding for $p21^{Waf1}$/$p21^{Cip1}$, located on chromosome 6 (6p21.2) in humans [132]. Protein $p21^{Waf1}$/$p21^{Cip1}$ is a predominant inhibitor of p53-dependent and p53-independent apoptosis [133]. DNA damage and oxidative stress (*e.g.* H_2O_2) activate two pathways, one involving p53-dependent apoptosis, and the other one involving p53-dependent activation of $p21^{Waf1}$/$p21^{Cip1}$ that protects cells from apoptosis.

$p21^{Waf1}$/$p21^{Cip1}$ is a potent CKI [128−130]. The $p21^{Waf1}$/$p21^{Cip1}$ protein binds to, and inhibits the activity of, cyclin E/Cdk2, cyclin A/Cdk1 (Cdk1 is also known as CDC2), cyclin B/Cdk1, cyclin A/Cdk2, cyclin D1−D3/Cdk2 and cyclin D1−D3/Cdk4(6) complexes [128−130], and thus functions as a regulator of cell cycle progression at the G_1/S (cyclin E/Cdk2) and G_2/M (cyclin A/Cdk1, cyclin B/Cdk1) phase boundaries. The binding of p21 to Cdk complexes occurs through the p21 N-terminal domain, which is homologous to other Cip/Kip Cdk inhibitors like cyclin-dependent kinase inhibitor 1B (p27^{Kip1}, encoded by the *CDKN1B* gene) and cyclin-dependent kinase inhibitor 1C (p57^{Kip2}, encoded by the *CDKN1C* gene). Specifically it contains a Cy1 motif in the N-terminal half, and weaker Cy2 motif in the C-terminal domain, that allow it to bind Cdk in a region that blocks its ability to complex with cyclins and thus prevent Cdk activation. During late G$_1$ phase, cyclin-dependent kinase complexes (CDKCs) bind and phosphorylate members of the retinoblastoma (p105-Rb) protein family [134]. Members of the p105-Rb protein family are tumor suppressors, which prevent uncontrolled cell proliferation that would occur during tumor formation. However, p105-Rbs are also thought to repress the genes required for the transition from G$_1$ phase to S phase. When the cell is ready to transition into the next phase the CDKCs cyclin D1/Cdk4 and cyclin D1/Cdk6 monophosphorylate p105-Rb, followed by hyperphosphorylation (14 *O*-phosphate) catalysed by the cyclin E/Cdk2 CDKC. Once phosphorylation occurs, transcription factors are then released to irreversibly inactivate p105-Rb and progression into the S phase of the cell cycle progresses. p21 as a tumor suppressor governs p105-Rb phosphorylation [134]. Formation of the RB−E2F complexes depends on the phosphorylation status of p105-Rb. The activity of the cyclin-dependent kinase inhibitor Waf1/Cip1/CDKN1A (p21^{Waf1}/p21^{Cip1}) leads to hypophosphorylated p105-Rb. Hypophosphorylated p105-Rb binds to E2F transcription factor dimers. RB−E2F complexes repress transcription of numerous cell cycle genes, many of which are required for G$_1$/S transition [134].

The cyclin E/Cdk2 CDKC formed in the G$_1$ phase aids in the initiation of DNA replication during S phase. At the end of S phase, cyclin A is associated with Cdk1 and Cdk2.

During G_2 phase, cyclin A is degraded, while cyclin B is synthesized and cyclin B/Cdk1 complexes form. Not only are cyclin B/Cdk1 complexes important for the transition into M phase, but these CDKCs play a role in regulatory and structural processes: chromosomal condensation, fragmentation of *Golgi* network, and breakdown of nuclear lamina. Inactivation of the cyclin B/Cdk1 complex through the degradation of cyclin B is necessary for exit out of the M phase (mitosis) of the cell cycle.

p105-Rb is a central regulator of the cell cycle [134]. Functionally, the RB family of transcription factors/tumor suppressors represents transcriptional co-repressors. It forms complexes with the E2F family of transcription factors. Importantly, the resulting RB−E2F complexes switch E2F promoter sites from activator to repressor sites [134]. RB binds preferentially E2F1, E2F2, and E2F3, but can also attach to E2F4 and E2F5. These factors form complexes with the DP dimerization partners DP1 or DP2 to form the E2F component of RB−E2F complexes [134]. The E2F component of these complexes contacts the DNA via E2F transcription factor binding sites in the gene promoters. RB−E2F complexes downregulate transcription of genes [134]. Classical RB−E2F target genes often control the cell cycle by contributing to DNA replication and the transition from the G_1 to S phase. Specifically, genes such as DNA polymerase α (*POLA1*), cyclin A (*CCNA2*), thymidine kinase (*TK1*), dihydrofolate reductase (*DHFR*), cyclin-dependent kinase 1 Cdk1/CDC2 (*CDK1*), and minichromosome maintenance complex component 3 and 5 (*MCM3* and *MCM5*; DNA replication-licensing factors) are considered *bona fide* RB−E2F targets [134].

When the cyclin-dependent kinase inhibitor $p21^{Waf1}/p21^{Cip1}$ is complexed with Cdk2, the cell cannot continue to the next phase of cell division. A mutant p53 will no longer bind DNA in an effective way, and, as a consequence, the p21^{Waf1}/p21^{Cip1} protein will not be available to act as the 'stop signal' for cell division. Studies with human embryonic stem cells (hESCs) [135] commonly describe the nonfunctional p53–p21 axis of the G$_1$/S checkpoint pathway with subsequent relevance for cell cycle regulation and the DNA damage response (DDR). Importantly, p21^{Waf1}/p21^{Cip1} mRNA is clearly present and upregulated after the DDR in hESCs, but p21^{Waf1}/p21^{Cip1} protein is not detectable [135]. In hESCs p53 activates numerous microRNAs (*e.g.* miR-302a, miR-302b, miR-302c, and miR-302d) that directly inhibit the p21^{Waf1}/p21^{Cip1} expression in hESCs [135]. As a proliferation inhibitor, p21^{Waf1}/p21^{Cip1} is thought to play an important role in preventing tumor development. This notion is supported by data indicating that p21^{Waf1}/p21^{Cip1}-null mice are more prone to spontaneous and induced tumorigenesis [133], and p21^{Waf1}/p21^{Cip1} synergizes with other tumor suppressors to protect against tumor progression in mice [133]. The p21^{Waf1}/p21^{Cip1} protein binds directly to CDKCs that drive forward the cell cycle and inhibits their kinase activity, thereby causing cell cycle arrest to allow DNA repair by DDR after DNA damage has taken place. p21^{Waf1}/p21^{Cip1} can also mediate growth arrest associated with differentiation and a more permanent growth arrest associated with cellular senescence.

p21^{Waf1}/p21^{Cip1} interacts with proliferating cell nuclear antigen (PCNA) [136], a DNA polymerase accessory factor, and plays a regulatory role in S phase DNA replication and DNA damage repair [136]. In addition to its ability to bind cyclin/Cdk complexes, p21^{Waf1}/p21^{Cip1} contains a C-terminal binding site for PCNA, and is found in quaternary complexes containing p21^{Waf1}/p21^{Cip1}, PCNA, and cyclin/Cdk in normal cells [133]. PCNA plays an essential role in DNA replication and different types of DNA repair, including nucleotide excision repair (NER), mismatch repair, and base excision repair (BER). Through its direct interaction with PCNA, p21^{Waf1}/p21^{Cip1} can block DNA synthesis catalysed by DNA polymerase δ [133]. Specifically, p21^{Waf1}/p21^{Cip1} has a high affinity for the PIP-box binding region on PCNA, binding of p21^{Waf1}/p21^{Cip1} to this region is proposed to block the binding of processivity factors necessary for PCNA-dependent S phase DNA synthesis, but not PCNA-dependent NER. As such, p21^{Waf1}/p21^{Cip1} acts as an effective inhibitor of S phase DNA synthesis, though permits NER, leading to the proposal that p21^{Waf1}/p21^{Cip1} acts to preferentially select polymerase processivity factors depending on the context of DNA synthesis. p21^{Waf1}/p21^{Cip1} protein was reported to be specifically cleaved by CASP3-like caspases, which thus leads to a dramatic activation of Cdk2, and may be instrumental in the execution of apoptosis following caspase activation. However p21^{Waf1}/p21^{Cip1} may inhibit apoptosis and does not induce cell death on its own [133].

Studies on p53-dependent cell cycle arrest in response to DNA damage identified p21^{Waf1}/p21^{Cip1} as the primary mediator of downstream cell cycle arrest. Notably, *el-Deiry et al.* [131] identified a protein p21 (WAF1) which was present in cells expressing wild type p53 but not in those with mutant p53; moreover, constitutive expression of p21^{Waf1}/p21^{Cip1} led to cell cycle arrest in a number of cell types. *Dulić et al.* [137] found that γ-irradiation of fibroblasts induced a p53- and p21-dependent cell cycle arrest; here p21^{Waf1}/p21^{Cip1} was found bound to inactive cyclin E/Cdk2 complexes [137]. Working in mouse models, it was also shown that, whilst mice lacking p21^{Waf1}/p21^{Cip1} were healthy [138], spontaneous tumours developed in them [133], and G$_1$ checkpoint control was compromised in cells derived from these mice [138]. Taken together, these investigations defined <u>p21^{Waf1}/p21^{Cip1}</u> as <u>the primary mediator of p53-dependent cell cycle arrest</u> in response to DNA damage. Recent work [139] exploring p21^{Wafl}/p21^{Cip1} activation in response to DNA damage at a single cell level have demonstrated that pulsatile p53 activity leads to subsequent pulses of p21^{Wafl}/p21^{Cip1}, and that the strength of p21^{Wafl}/p21^{Cip1} activation is cell cycle phase-dependent [139]. Moreover, studying p21^{Wafl}/p21^{Cip1} levels in populations of cycling cells, not exposed to DNA damaging agents, have shown that DNA damage occurring in mother cell S phase can induce p21^{Wafl}/p21^{Cip1} accumulation over both mother G$_2$ and daughter G$_1$ phases which subsequently induces cell cycle arrest [140].

p21^{Wafl}/p21^{Cip1} is negatively regulated by ubiquitin ligases, both over the course of the cell cycle and in response to DNA damage. Specifically, over the G$_1$/S transition it has been demonstrated that the E3 ubiquitin ligase complex SCF^{Skp2} induces degradation of p21^{Wafl}/p21^{Cip1} [141,142]. SCF^{Skp2} [Skp, cullin, F-box-containing complex (or SCF complex) is a multi-protein E3 ubiquitin ligase complex that catalyses the ubiquitination of proteins destined for 26S proteasomal degradation; it consists of: a variable F-box protein (FBP) like Skp2, S-phase kinase-associated protein 1 (Skp1), cullin 1 (CUL1), and RING-box protein 1 (RBX1, Rbx1, ROC1)]. Studies have also demonstrated that the E3 ubiquitin ligase complex CRL4^{Cdt2} degrades p21^{Wafl}/p21^{Cip1} in a PCNA-dependent manner over S phase, necessary to prevent p21^{Wafl}/p21^{Cip1}-dependent re-replication [143], as well as in response to UV irradiation [144]. CRL4^{Cdt2} is the CUL4A (cullin 4A)−DDB1 (DNA damage-binding protein 1)−RBX1 complex. At the N-terminus, CUL4A binds to the β-propeller of the DDB1 adaptor protein which interacts with numerous DDB1−CUL4−Associated Factors (DCAFs). As a result, the N-terminus is crucial for the recruitment of substrates for the ubiquitin ligase complex. At the C-terminal end, CUL4A interacts with the RBX1/ROC1 protein *via* its

RING domain. Recent work [140] has now found that in human cell lines SCF^{Skp2} degrades $p21^{Waf1}/p21^{Cip1}$ towards the end of G_1 phase, allowing cells to exit a quiescent state, whilst $CRL4^{Cdt2}$ acts to degrade $p21^{Waf1}/p21^{Cip1}$ at a much higher rate than SCF^{Skp2} over the G_1/S transition and subsequently to maintain low levels of $p21^{Waf1}/p21^{Cip1}$ throughout S phase.

Cytoplasmic $p21^{Waf1}/p21^{Cip1}$ expression can be significantly correlated with lymph node metastasis, distant metastases, advanced TNM stage [TNM Classification of Malignant Tumors (TNM), a classification of cancer staging that stands for: size or direct extent of the primary tumor (T), degree of spread to regional lymph nodes (N), presence of distant metastasis (M)], depth of invasion, and OS (overall survival rate) [145]. A study [146] on immunohistochemical markers in malignant thymic epithelial tumors shows that the level of $p21^{Waf1}/p21^{Cip1}$ expression was negatively correlated with survival and significantly correlated with World Health Organization (WHO) type B2/B3 mixed type thymoma manifestation. In case of high $p21^{Waf1}/p21^{Cip1}$ levels of expression, when combined with low p27 and high p53 expression levels, the DFS (disease-free survival) in malignant thymic epithelial tumor patients decreases [146].

$p21^{Waf1}/p21^{Cip1}$ mediates the resistance of hematopoietic stem cells to an infection with human immunodeficiency virus type 1 (*Retroviridae*, *Orthoretrovirinae*, *Lentivirus*; HIV-1) by complexing with the HIV-1 integrase and thereby aborting chromosomal integration of the HIV-1 DNA provirus [147]. HIV-1-infected individuals who naturally suppress viral replication have elevated levels of $p21^{Waf1}/p21^{Cip1}$ and its associated mRNA [148]. $p21^{Waf1}/p21^{Cip1}$ expression affects at least two stages in the HIV-1 life cycle inside $CD4^+$ T cells, significantly limiting production of new viruses, in contrast to the situation in macrophages [149]. The inhibitory action of p53 on HIV-1 replication is well established [150–152].

PT162 (**NSC 796018**) clearly inhibits HIV-1$_{LAI}$ replication in CD4$^+$ T lymphocytes (Chapter Four, Section 4; see Appendix, Table S1) by inducing p53 and its associated cyclin-dependent kinase inhibitor p21^{Waf1}/p21^{Cip1} [153]. The latter factor p21^{Waf1}/p21^{Cip1} is induced by p53 activation [131] and inhibits HIV-1 replication [154]. In addition, tumor suppressor protein p53 interacts with HIV-1 *trans*-activator protein Tat [155–157], HIV-1 Nef accessory protein [158], and HIV-1 Vpr accessory protein [159,160]. HIV-1 kills CD4$^+$ T lymphocytes by inducing p53-mediated mitochondrial apoptosis [161]. The small-molecule chemical 9-aminoacridine (9AA) inhibited HIV-1 replication in peripheral blood lymphocyte (PBL) cells by inducing p21^{Waf1}/p21^{Cip1} expression *via* p53 (re)activation [162]. In HIV-1-infected CD4$^+$ T lymphocytes p53 was inactivated through binding to HIV-1 Tat protein [162,163].

Human cyclin D exists as the three homologues cyclin D1 (295 aa, encoded by the *CCND1* gene), cyclin D2 (289 aa, encoded by the *CCND2* gene), and cyclin D3 (292 aa, encoded by the *CCND3* gene) [164–166]. The *CCND1* gene encodes the cyclin D1 protein [alternative names: B-cell lymphoma 1 protein (Bcl-1), BCL-1 oncogene, PRAD1 oncogene, D11S287E]. The human *CCND1* gene is located on the long arm of chromosome 11 (11q13.3) [164–167]. *CCND1* captures 13,319 bp (with five exons) and translates into a 295 aa protein. Cyclin D1 was originally cloned as PRAD1 or D11S287E in 1991 as a breakpoint rearrangement with the parathyroid hormone (PTH, parathormone, parathyrin) locus in benign parathyroid adenoma [167], and was shown to be required for progression through the G$_1$ phase of the cell cycle to induce cell migration [168], angiogenesis [169], and to induce the *Warburg* effect [170]. Cyclin D1 is expressed in all adult human tissues with the exception of cells derived from bone marrow stem cells (both lymphoid and myeloid) [164,165]. The synthesis of cyclin D1 is initiated during G_1 cell cycle phase and drives the G_1/S phase transition [171]. Cyclin D1 is one of the major cyclins assuming its functional importance [172]. It interacts with four Cdks: Cdk2, Cdk4, Cdk5, and Cdk6 [172]. In proliferating cells, cyclin D1/Cdk4 and cyclin D1/Cdk6 CDKCs accumulation is of great importance for cell cycle progression. Cyclin D1 has no effect on G_1/S transition unless it forms a complex with Cdk4(6). The cyclin D1/Cdk4(6) CDKCs monophosphorylate p105-Rb, which releases E2F-driven expression of cell cycle genes (*e.g.* cyclin E and cyclin A) important for progression into S phase [172]. Cyclin D1 possesses a tertiary structure similar to other cyclins, called the cyclin fold. This contains a core of two compact domains with each having five α-helices [172]. The first five-helix bundle is a conserved cyclin box, a region of about 150 aa residues in all cyclins, which is needed for Cdk-binding and activation. The second five-helix bundle is composed of the same arrangement of helices, but the aa sequence of the two subdomains differs. Cyclin D1 protein shows the following domains [172]:

- LXCXE p105-Rb-binding motif.
- LLXXXL co-activator-binding motif which binds an LXXLL motif in the steroid receptor co-activators SRC1 and AIB1.
- 1st cyclin box (aa 3−151) in G_1/S-specific cyclin D1 that mediates Cdk-binding, and is necessary for interaction with the CKIs $p21^{Waf1}$/$p21^{Cip1}$, $p27^{Kip1}$, and $p57^{Kip2}$.
- 2nd cyclin box (aa 156−265) in G_1/S-specific cyclin D1.
- C-terminal PEST sequence that is rich in L-proline, L-glutamic acid, L-serine, and L-threonine, which marks the protein for rapid turn-over.

- L-threonine residue (T286) that controls nuclear export and protein stability, when phosphorylated at T286 by MAPKs cyclin D1 is degraded in the 26S proteasome.

All three D-type cyclins (D1, D2, D3) exhibit the same 1st cyclin box α-helix [172].

Independent of Cdk-binding, cyclin D1 binds to nuclear receptors [including estrogen receptor α (ERα) [173], thyroid hormone receptor (TR) [174], peroxisome proliferator-activated receptor γ (PPARγ) [175], and androgen receptor (AR) [176]] to regulate cell proliferation, growth, and differentiation. Cyclin D1 enhances ERα activity, through interactions with ERα and its co-regulators SRC1 [nuclear receptor coactivator 1 (NCOA1)] and AIB1 [nuclear receptor coactivator 3 (NCOA3)]. Cyclin D1 also binds to histone acetyltransferases (HATs) like P/CAF (p300/CBP-associated factor), and to histone deacetylases (HDACs) like HDAC1, HDAC2, HDAC3, and HDAC5, to regulate cell proliferation and cell differentiation genes in the early-G_1 to mid-G_1 phase [174−177].

Increasing cyclin D1 levels during the G_1 phase is induced by mitogenic growth factors primarily through Ras-mediated pathways, and by hormones [174,178]. These Ras-mediated pathways lead to the increase in transcription of cyclin D1, and inhibit its proteolysis and export from the nucleus [174,178]. The expression of cyclin D1 is induced by growth factors including epidermal growth factor (EGF), insulin-like growth factors 1 and 2 (IGF-1 and IGF-2), amino acids, lysophosphatidic acid (LPA) [174], and hormones including androgens (testosterone, 5α-dihydrotestosterone, androsterone), all-*trans* retinoic acid (ATRA), and the PPARγ ligand (15-deoxy-$\Delta^{12,14}$-prostaglandin J_2) [174]. Many oncogenic signals induce cyclin D1 expression through distinct DNA sequences at the *CCND1* gene promoter, including Ras [rat sarcoma virus small GTPase; three human

Ras genes: *HRAS* (from *Harvey* rat sarcoma virus, codes for GTPase HRas = transforming protein p21), *KRAS* (from *Kirsten* rat sarcoma virus, codes for GTPase KRas), *NRAS* (neuroblastoma Ras viral oncogene homolog)], (c-)Src (Src non-receptor tyrosine kinase family: Src, Yes, Fyn, Fgr, Lck, Hck, Blk, Lyn, Frk), (c-)Erb-B2 [human epidermal growth factor receptor 2, EGFR2 (HER2/neu), receptor tyrosine-protein kinase erbB2, CD340], β-catenin (catenin β-1), oncogenic signal transducer(s) and activator(s) of transcription (STATs; STAT3, STAT5A), and SV40 polyomavirus small T antigen [174].

Cyclin D1 is degraded by the 26S proteasome upon phosphorylation of T286 and subsequent ubiquit(in)ylation *via* the CRL4^{Cdt2}–AMBRA1 (activating molecule in beclin 1-regulated autophagy, autophagy and beclin 1 regulator 1) E3 ubiquitin ligase complex [179,180]. CRL4^{Cdt2} is the CUL4A (cullin 4A)–DDB1 (DNA damage-binding protein 1)–RBX1 complex. AMBRA1 was first identified as DDB1 and CUL4-associated factor 3 (DCAF3) [181].

Growth factors {*e.g.* epidermal growth factor (EGF), fibroblast growth factors (FGFs), platelet-derived growth factors (PDGFs), transforming growth factor-α (TGF-α), neurotrophins [nerve growth factor (NGF), brain-derived neurotrophic factor (BDNF), neurotrophin-3 (NT-3) and neurotrophin-4 (NT-4)]} stimulate the Ras/Raf/MEK/ERK signal transduction pathway [182–186] that controls cyclin levels: mitogen [*e.g.* epidermal growth factor (EGF)]→receptor-linked tyrosine kinase (*e.g.* epidermal growth factor receptor (EGFR, Erb-B1, HER1)→Shc/Grb2/SOS-1-activated Ras (GTP-Ras)→MAP3K [mitogen-activated protein (MAP) kinase kinase kinase (MAPKKK); (c-)Raf1]→MAP2K [MAP kinase kinase (MAPKK, MEK); MEK1, MEK2]→MAP kinase [MAPK; ERK1 (p44 extracellular signal-regulated kinase 1,

MAPK3), ERK2 (p42 extracellular signal-regulated kinase 2, MAPK1)]→(c-)Myc↑cyclines↑(p21^{Waf1}/p21^{Cip1})↓ [187,188]. Apart from EGFR, other cell surface mitogen receptors that can activate the Ras/Raf/ERK pathway include, *e.g.*, Trk A/B (tropomyosin receptor kinase A and B; nervous system neurotrophin receptor), fibroblast growth factor receptors (FGFRs) and platelet-derived growth factor receptor (PDGFR). MAPK activates the (proto-oncogenic) transcription factor (c-)Myc which controls transcription of genes important in cell cycle (activated Myc: cyclin A↑, cyclin E↑, cyclin D1↓) [187,188].

Cyclin D1 is regulated by the downstream pathway of mitogen receptors *via* the Ras/Raf/MEK/ERK signal transduction cascade [189−193] involving Ras, Rac-1 (Ras-related C3 botulinum toxin substrate 1) and protein kinase C isoforms (PKC ε, λ, ζ) [194], and the Wnt/β-catenin/Tcf/LEF-1 (lymphoid enhancing factor 1, lymphoid enhancer-binding factor 1) pathway [195] incorporating the PI3K/Akt [protein kinase B (PKB)]/IκB (inhibitor κB)/IKKα (IKK1, IκB kinase α) pathway [195,196]. The MAPK ERK1/2 activates the downstream transcription factors (c-)Myc, AP-1 [activator protein 1 = heterodimer of (c-)Jun and (c-)Fos], and (c-)Fos which in turn activate the transcription of the Cdk4, Cdk6, and cyclin D1 genes [197,198]. Rho family GTPases (Rac-1) [199], integrin-linked kinases (ILKs) [200] and focal adhesion kinase [FAK; also known as: PTK2 protein tyrosine kinase 2 (PTK2)] [201], activate cyclin D1 gene in response to integrins. The CKIs p27^{Kip1} and p21^{Waf1}/p21^{Cip1} are also promoters of the cyclin D1/Cdk4(6) CDKCs [202]. Without p27^{Kip1} and p21^{Waf1}/p21^{Cip1}, cyclin D1 levels are reduced and the corresponding CDKCs are not formed at detectable levels [202]. Cyclin D1/Cdk4 also enables the activation of cyclin E/Cdk2 complex by sequestering p21^{Waf1}/p21^{Cip1} and p27^{Kip1}, allowing entry into the S phase [203].

In eukaryotes, overexpression of translation initiation factor 4E (eIF4E) leads to an increased level of cyclin D1 protein and an increased amount of extranuclear cyclin D1 mRNA [204]. This is because eIF4E promotes the extranuclear export of cyclin D1 mRNAs [205].

Inhibition of cyclin D1 *via* inactivation or degradation leads to cell cycle exit and differentiation. Inactivation of cyclin D1 is triggered by several CKIs like $p21^{Waf1}/p21^{Cip1}$, $p27^{Kip1}$, $p57^{Kip2}$, and the INK4 family ($p16^{INK4A}$, $p15^{INK4B}$, $p18^{INK4C}$, $p19^{INK4D}$) [203,206,207]. The INK4 family (Inhibitors of Cdk4) is composed of four proteins, $p16^{INK4A}$, $p15^{INK4B}$, $p18^{INK4C}$, and $p19^{INK4D}$, that specifically bind to only Cdk4 and Cdk6 and inhibit their interaction with D-type cyclins, thus preventing their activation [203,206,207]. In contrast, the other members of the Cip/Kip CKI family, $p21^{Waf1}/p21^{Cip1}$, $p27^{Kip1}$, and $p57^{Kip2}$, bind to both Cdk and cyclin subunits and have the ability to inhibit all CDKCs [203,206,207]. INK4 family proteins are activated in response to hyperproliferative stress that inhibits cell proliferation due to overexpression of *e.g. HRAS* and *MYC*. Hence, INK4 family proteins bind to cyclin D-dependent Cdk4 and Cdk6 only and inactivate the whole CDKCs. Glycogen synthase kinase 3 β (GSK3β) causes cyclin D1 degradation by inhibitory phosphorylation at T286 of the cyclin D1 protein [208−210]. GSK3β itself is negatively regulated by the Wnt/β-catenin/Tcf/LEF-1 and PI3K/Akt/IκB/IKKα pathway(s) [195,196,208], in form of phosphorylation of GSK3β at its L-serine 9 (S9) by activated Akt (PKB) resulting in inhibition of GSK3β activity [208]. GSK3β-dependent phosphorylation of cyclin D1 at T286 promotes the nuclear−to−cytoplasmic redistribution of cyclin D1 during S phase of the cell cycle [209]. Removal of cyclin D1 from the nucleus during S phase appears essential for regulated cell division [209]. $p21^{Waf1}/p21^{Cip1}$ promotes the nuclear accumulation of cyclin D1 complexes *via* inhibition of cyclin D1 nuclear export [210]. *In vivo* $p21^{Waf1}/p21^{Cip1}$ can inhibit GSK3β-triggered cyclin D1 nuclear export and phosphorylation-dependent nuclear–to–cytoplasmic shuttling [210]. The ability of $p21^{Waf1}/p21^{Cip1}$ to inhibit cyclin D1 nuclear export correlates with its ability to bind to T286-phosphorylated cyclin D1, thereby preventing cyclin D1/ chromosomal region maintenance 1 [CRM1; also known as exportin 1 (XPO1)] export factor association [210].

Very importantly, activation of p53 protein represses cyclin D1 expression [211], directly at the *CCND1* gene promoter, through downregulation of Bcl-3 (B-cell lymphoma factor 3; atypical member of the IκB family, transcriptional co-activator of the NFκB subunit p52 [212]) and increased association of the NFκB subunit p52 with histone deacetylase 1 (HDAC1) [211,213]. The oncoprotein Bcl-3 induces cyclin D1 expression [214]. Upon induction of p53 a specific repression of cyclin D1 promoter activity, correlating with a decrease in cyclin D1 protein and mRNA levels, was observed [211]. This repression was dependent on the proximal NFκB binding site in the cyclin D1 promoter, which has been shown to bind the p52 NFκB subunit. p53 inhibited the expression of Bcl-3 oncoprotein and also reduced p52/Bcl-3 complex levels [211].

Cyclin D1 is dysregulated in cancer [172,215–217]. Evidence that cyclin D1 is required for tumorigenesis was indicated by the inactivation of cyclin D1 by cDNA antisense construct [218] or gene deletion [219]. Preventing or reducing cyclin D1 gene utilization reduced breast tumor [218,219] and gastrointestinal tumor [220] growth *in vivo*. Cyclin D1 overexpression is sufficient for the induction of mammary tumorigenesis [221], attributed to the induction of cell proliferation, increased cell survival by inhibition of apoptosis [222], induction of chromosomal instability [223,224], restraint of autophagy [225,226], and multiple non-canonical functions [227]. Overexpression is induced as a result of gene amplification, growth factor- or oncogene-induced cyclin D1 expression by Ras [197], Src [228], (c-)Erb-B2 (HER2/neu, EGFR2) [218], STAT3 [229], STAT5A [230], impaired protein degradation, or chromosomal translocation. Gene amplification is responsible for overproduction of cyclin D1 protein in head−and−neck squamous cell carcinoma, non-small-cell lung cancer, endometrial cancer, malignant melanoma, pancreatic cancer, breast cancer, colorectal cancer, pituitary adenomas, bladder cancer, and esophageal carcinoma [172]. In mantle cell lymphoma (MCL), cyclin D1 overexpression is the result of a chromosomal t(11;14)(q13;q32) IgH (immunoglobulin heavy chain) locus (14q32.3) translocation with *CCND1* (11q13.3) [172,216], and this rearrangement accounts for more than 90% of MCL patients, making this translocation a hallmark of MCL [216]. Multiple myeloma (MM) has the same t(11;14)(q13;q32) IgH locus (14q32.3) translocation with *CCND1* (11q13.3) [231], observed at a frequency of ~16%, which accounts for cyclin D1 overexpression in ~30–50% of MM cases [172,216].

Cyclin D1 overexpression has been shown to correlate with early cancer onset and tumor progression [172,232], and it can lead to oncogenesis by increasing anchorage-independent growth and angiogenesis *via* VEGF-A production [233]. Cyclin D1 overexpression can also downregulate Fas expression [233], leading to increased resistance to antineoplastic chemotherapy and protection from apoptosis. Increased levels of cyclin D1 can be caused by various types of dysregulation [172,232], including:

- Amplification of the *CCND1* gene with concomitant overexpression of cyclin D1 protein [172,232].
- Chromosomal t(11;14)(q13;q32) IgH locus (14q32.3) translocation with *CCND1* (11q13.3) [172,216,231].

- Mutations in the degradation motif recognized by the CRL4^{Cdt2}–AMBRA1 E3 ubiquitin ligase (P287S, P287T, deletion Δ289−292), or mutations in the F-box protein FBXO4 (Fbxo4) [172,216].
- Disruption of nuclear export and proteolysis of cyclin D1 by point mutation of its T286 phosphorylation site (T286R) or its complete deletion Δ266−295 [172].
- Induction of cyclin D1 gene transcription by oncogenic Ras, (c-)Src, (c-)ErbB2, and STAT3/5A signal transduction pathways (like already discussed).
- Splice variant cyclin D1b (cyclin D1 isoform) [216,234] overexpression, *e.g.* in breast, prostate, and esophageal cancer [172,234]; in contrast to cyclin D1 (= cyclin D1a), cyclin D1b is encoded by a mRNA where intron 4 is not spliced, resulting in a unique C-terminus. As a result of this alternative splicing, cyclin D1b loses its T286 phosphorylation site encoded in exon 5 that directs its ubiquit(in)ylation-dependent degradation; the consequence is cyclin D1b accumulation in the nucleus and ultimately tumorigenesis [172,216,234].

Cyclin D1 overexpression is correlated with shorter cancer patient survival and increased metastasis [235,236]. *CCND1* gene overexpression was detected in [172,232]:

- Non-small-cell lung cancer (18–76%) [172,216,237,238].
- Head−and−neck squamous cell carcinoma (20–68%) [172,236].
- Pancreatic carcinoma (42−82%) [172,239].
- Melanoma (30−65%) [172].
- Endometrial cancer (40−56%) [172].
- Bladder cancer (15%) [240].
- Colorectal cancer (55%) [172].
- Pituitary adenoma (49%) [241,242].
- Breast carcinoma (50–70%) [172,243–245].

Cyclin D1 overexpression is strongly correlated to estrogen receptor-positive (ER$^+$) breast cancer [172,243–245] and deregulation of cyclin D1 is associated with antineoplastic hormone (*e.g.* tamoxifen) therapy resistance in therapy-refractory breast cancer [246,247]. Repression of cyclin D1 and upregulation of p21^{Waf1}/p21^{Cip1} was induced by **PT162** (**NSC 796018**) and reported for other cytotoxic drugs [248].

Apoptosis [from ancient Greek: ἀπόπτωσις, 'the falling off' (or 'dropping off')] [249] is a tightly regulated programmed cell death (PCD) or genetically programmed cell 'suicide'. The term was coined by *John F.R. Kerr, Andrew D.H. Wyllie & Sir Alastair R. Currie* in 1972 [249]. Two major forms of apoptosis are discriminated, (i) the extrinsic or receptor-mediated pathway, and (ii) the intrinsic pathway or mitochondrial apoptosis [19,20,250–253].

For the extrinsic pathway the tumor necrosis factor-α (TNF-α) signal transduction cascade [254] is discriminated from the Fas pathway [activation-induced cell death (AICD)] [255]. TNF-α is a cytokine produced mainly by activated macrophages, and is the major extrinsic mediator of apoptosis. Most cells in the human body have two receptors for TNF-α: tumor necrosis factor receptor 1 (TNFR1) [also known as tumor necrosis factor receptor superfamily member 1A (TNFRSF1A) and CD120a; a ubiquitous membrane receptor that binds TNF-α], and tumor necrosis factor receptor 2 (TNFR2) [also known as tumor necrosis factor receptor superfamily member 1B (TNFRSF1B) and CD120b]. The binding of TNF-α to TNFR1 has been shown to initiate the pathway that leads to caspase activation *via* the intermediate adaptor proteins TNF receptor-associated death domain (TRADD, TNF receptor type 1-associated DEATH domain protein) which recruits additional adaptor proteins, one of the receptor-interacting protein (RIP) family (RIPK1, receptor-interacting serine/threonine-protein kinase 1), and

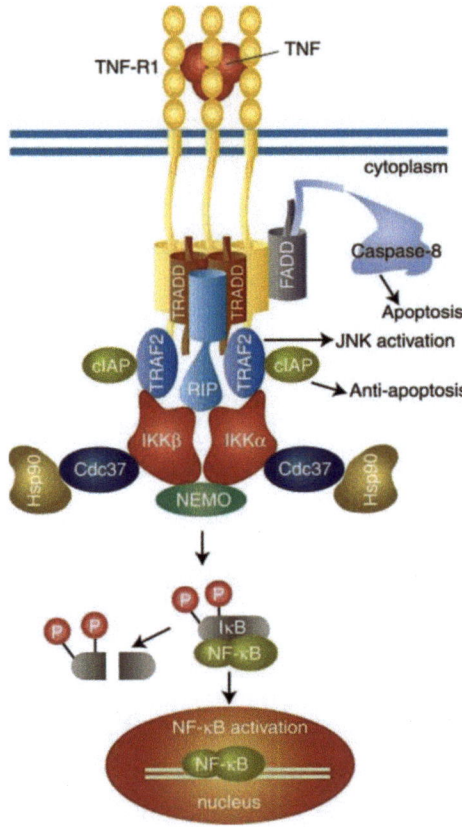

Fig. VI. The tumor necrosis factor-α (TNF-α) signal transduction cascade leading to extrinsic apoptosis (taken from [254]). Upon binding of TNF-α to its receptor TNFR1 the TNFR1-associated intracellular adaptor TRADD complex activates the FADD adaptor which in turn activates procaspase 8 and forms FasR−DISC to activate caspase 8, which activates the downstream effector caspase 3. cIAP1 and cIAP2 (IAPs) can inhibit TNF-α signaling by binding to the TRAF1/TRAF2 heterodimer. Binding of TNF-α to TNFR1 associated with TRADD and TRAF1/TRAF2 can also indirectly lead, through association with/activation of IκB kinase α/β/NEMO (IKKα/β/γ), to the anti-apoptotic activation of transcription factor NFκB.

Fas-associated death domain protein (FADD, MORT1). FADD is an adaptor protein that bridges members of the TNF receptor superfamily, such as TNFR1 and the Fas receptor, to procaspases 8 and 10 to form the death-inducing signaling complex (DISC) during apoptosis [254] (Fig. VI).

The cellular inhibitor of apoptosis proteins 1 and 2 (cIAP1 and cIAP2) can inhibit TNF-α signaling by binding to TRAF1/TRAF2 heterodimer (TNF receptor-associated factor 1 and 2). cIAP1 (human gene *BIRC2*) belongs to the IAP family of proteins (IAPs, inhibitor of apoptosis proteins) and therefore contains at least one BIR (baculoviral IAP repeat) domain. cIAP2 (BIR-containing protein 3, human gene *BIRC3*) also belongs to the IAP family. The protein factor FLIP {CASP8 and FADD-like apoptosis regulator (CFLAR), c-FLIP [FADD-like interleukin 1β-converting enzyme (FLICE)-like inhibitory protein, human gene *CFLAR*]}, representing a degenerate caspase homologue, inhibits the activation of caspase 8 (cysteinyl aspartic acid-protease 8). Binding of TNF-α to TNFR1 associated with TRADD and TRAF1/TRAF2 heterodimer can also indirectly lead, through association with/activation of IκB kinase α/β (IKKα/β), to the anti-apoptotic activation of transcription factor NFκB involved in cell survival and inflammatory responses (Fig. VI). The core of the IKK complex consists of two catalytic subunits, IKKα and IKKβ, and a regulatory subunit, NFκB essential modulator (NEMO, IKKγ, human gene *IKBKG*) (Fig. VI, Fig. VII). In addition, the IKKα/β/γ complex contains a kinase-specific chaperone consisting of heat shock protein 90 (Hsp90) and Cdc37 (Hsp90 co-chaperone Cdc37, human gene *CDC37*) that plays a role in shuttling the complex from the cytoplasm to the membrane (Fig. VI, Fig. VII). However, signaling through TNFR1 might also induce apoptosis in a caspase-independent manner. The link between TNF-α and apoptosis shows why an abnormal production of TNF-α plays a fundamental role in several human diseases, especially in autoimmune diseases.

The TNF-α receptor superfamily also includes death receptors (DRs), such as DR4 and DR5. These receptors bind to the protein TRAIL and mediate apoptosis. Death receptor 4 (DR4), also known as TRAIL receptor 1 (TRAILR1, Apo2) and tumor necrosis factor receptor superfamily member 10A (TNFRSF10A), is a cell surface receptor of the TNF receptor superfamily that binds TRAIL and mediates apoptosis. Death receptor 5 (DR5) is also known as TRAIL receptor 2 (TRAILR2) or tumor necrosis factor receptor superfamily member 10B (TNFRSF10B). TNF-related apoptosis-inducing ligand [TRAIL, Apo2 ligand (Apo2L), CD253, TNFSF10] is a cytokine that is produced and secreted by most normal tissue cells which causes apoptosis primarily in tumor cells by binding to DR4 and DR5 [254].

The Fas (first apoptosis signal) receptor [Apo1, cluster−of−differentiation 95 (CD95), Fas, FasR, apoptosis antigen 1 (APO-1, APT), TNFR superfamily member 6 (TNFRSF6)] is a transmembrane protein of the TNF family which binds the Fas ligand (FasL, CD95L, CD178). The interaction between FasR and FasL results in the formation of the FasR−DISC, which contains the FasR, FADD, procaspase 8 (and procaspase 10) [255] (Fig. VII). In some types of cells (type I), processed caspase 8 directly activates other members of the caspase family, and triggers the execution of apoptosis of the cell. In other types of cells (type II), the FasR−DISC starts a feedback loop that relies on caspase 8-mediated cleavage of the pro-apoptotic Bcl-2 family member Bid to truncated Bid (tBid) [256] and spirals into increasing release of pro-apoptotic factors (*e.g.* cytochrome *c*, SMAC/DIABLO) from mitochondria and to drive the formation of the caspase 9-activating apoptosome. Active caspase 9 activates the executioner caspase 3, which in turn activates caspase 8 outside the FasR−DISC, thereby completing a positive feedback loop. This is called AICD, a programmed cell death caused by the interaction of FasR and FasL. The binding of FasL to FasR triggers homotrimerization of FasR, whose cytoplasmic domain is then able to bind the death domain of the adaptor protein FADD. Procaspase 8 binds to FADD's death effector domain (DED) and proteolytically self-activates as caspase 8. Activated caspase 8 is released into the cytosol, where it activates the caspase cascade that initiates apoptosis [255] (Fig. VII).

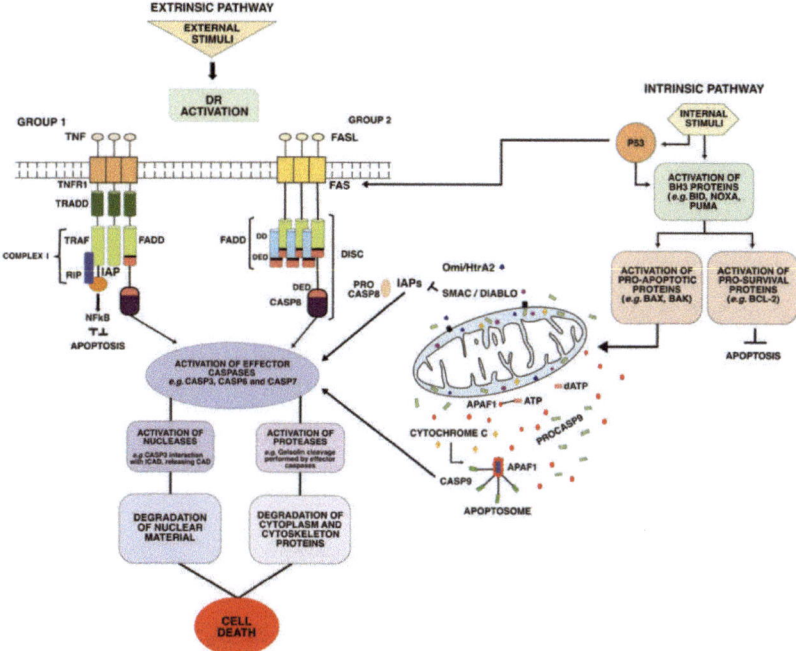

Fig. VII. The comparison of extrinsic and intrinsic pathways of apoptosis (taken from [253]). Left, the TNF-α/TNFR1-mediated induction of extrinsic apoptosis. Middle, the FasL/FasR-mediated induction of extrinsic apoptosis. Right, (p53-mediated) intrinsic mitochondrial apoptosis.

There is an additional pathway that involves CD8⁺ cytotoxic T lymphocyte-mediated cytotoxicity, the transmembrane pore-forming molecule perforin, and the serine proteases granzyme A/B-dependent killing of the cell [252]. The perforin/granzyme pathway can induce apoptosis *via* either granzyme B or granzyme A. The extrinsic, intrinsic, and granzyme A/B pathways converge on the same terminal execution pathway [252].

The intrinsic pathway or mitochondrial apoptosis [19,20,250–253] originates due to internal cellular stress. These internal stimuli, such as DNA damage or endoplasmic reticulum stress, induce the p53-dependent activation of BH3-

only (Bcl-2 homology 3, LXXXGD motif) proteins, which include **Bid** (BH3 interacting-domain death agonist), **Bim** (Bcl-2-like protein 11, Bcl-2 interacting mediator of cell death), **Bad** (Bcl-2-associated death promoter, Bcl-2-associated agonist of cell death), **Bik** (Bcl-2-interacting killer), **Bmf** (Bcl-2-modifying factor), **Noxa** (phorbol-12-myristate-13-acetate-induced protein 1), **PUMA** (p53 upregulated modulator of apoptosis, Bcl-2-binding component 3), and **HRK** (activator of apoptosis harakiri). Bcl-2 family proteins interact and activate Bcl-2 family anti-apoptotic or pro-apoptotic proteins, which may lead to the interruption of apoptotic cell death or to apoptosis. In the first case, anti-apoptotic proteins [**Bcl-2** (B-cell lymphoma protein 2), **Bcl-x$_L$** (B-cell lymphoma-extra large, Bcl-2-like protein 1), **Bcl-w** (Bcl-2-like protein 2), **Mcl-1** (induced myeloid leukemia cell differentiation protein), **A1/Bfl-1** (Bcl-2-related protein A1)] are activated, thereby interrupting cell death mechanisms. In the second case, the activation of pro-apoptotic proteins **Bax** (Bcl-2-associated X protein) or **Bak** (Bcl-2 homologous antagonist/killer) lead to mitochondrial outer membrane permeabilization (MOMP), considered a point of no return due to the release of proteins involved in the activation of caspases in the cytoplasm. This is accompanied by the collapse of the mitochondrial membrane potential $\Delta\psi_m$ and the gradual acidification of the environment around the mitochondria. Among proteins released through MOMP, there is cytochrome c, involved in the formation of apoptosomes, the pro-apoptotic protein **SMAC** (second mitochondria-derived activator of caspases) [= **DIABLO** (direct IAP binding protein with low pI)], and the **Omi/HtrA2** peptidase (high temperature requirement protein A2, Omi stress-regulated endoprotease, serine proteinase OMI), which interact with inhibitory proteins (IAPs) to activate procaspases such as procaspase 3 and procaspase 7. The release of the pro-apoptotic proteins SMAC/DIABLO and Omi/HtrA2 peptidase inhibits the negative regulation carried out by inhibitor of apoptosis proteins (IAPs) upon procaspases (Fig. VII). The release of cytochrome c in the cytoplasm activates the formation of the apoptosome, a cytosolic multiprotein complex that is composed of cytochrome c, apoptotic protease activating factor 1 (**Apaf-1**), and procaspase 9. The formation of this complex starts from the association of cytochrome c to the cytoplasmic protein structure composed of inactive Apaf-1 monomers. The assembly of the wheel-shaped heptameric apoptosome complex with sevenfold symmetry then takes place under hydrolysis of bound 2′-deoxyadenosine 5′-triphosphate (dATP) (or ATP) to dADP (or ADP) [257,258]. After binding and activation of procaspase 9, the complete apoptosome is formed. This activation occurs through binding of procaspase 9 to the caspase recognition/recruitment domain (CARD) of the Apaf-1 adapter protein which leads to activation of procaspase 9 to caspase 9 which must be bound to the apoptosome for being proteolytically active [257,258]. Next, the initiator caspase 9 (CASP9) cleaves and activates execution caspases, such as caspase 3 (CASP3) and caspase 7 (CASP7), through proteolysis that rearranges critical protein loops in the formation of active sites. When activated, execution caspases can cleave and activate other execution caspases in a feedback system during the execution phase.

A total of 25 genes in the Bcl-2 family were identified up to 2008 [259]. Named after the founding member of the family, which was isolated as a gene involved in B-cell lymphoma (hence, the human gene name *BCL2*), the Bcl-2 family is comprised of well over a dozen proteins, which have been classified into three functional groups. Members of the first group, such as Bcl-2 and Bcl-x_L, are characterized by four short, conserved Bcl-2 homology (BH) domains (BH1, BH2, BH3, BH4). They also possess a C-terminal

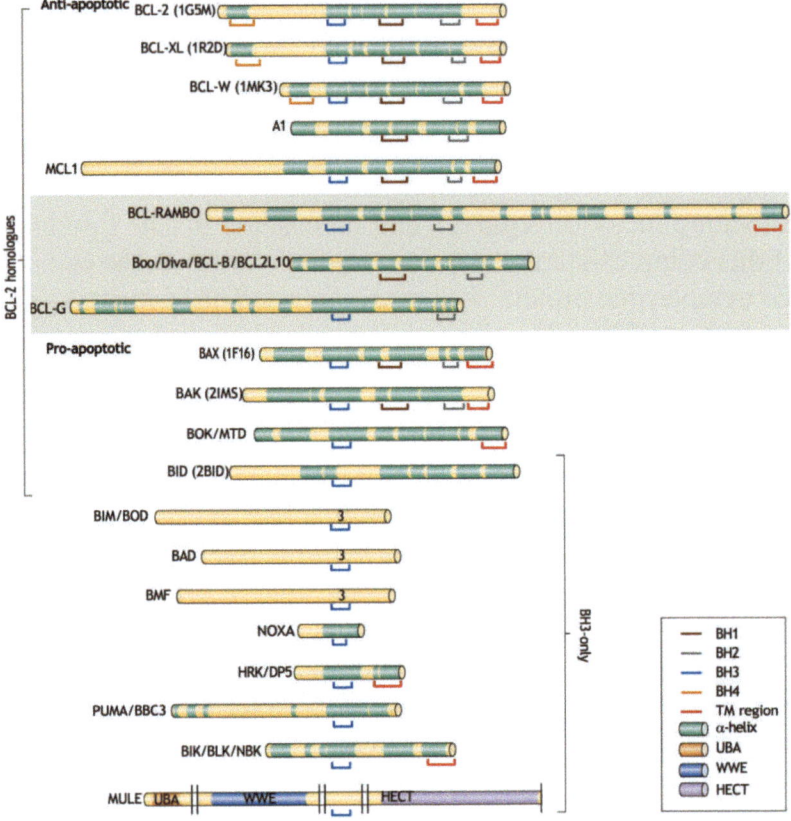

Fig. VIII. The comparison of Bcl-2 family proteins with sequence alignment of core Bcl-2 family proteins and BH3-only proteins (taken from [259]). Green bars depict α-helical segments from the determined structures or from secondary structure prediction. Red lines label regions of predicted transmembrane (TM) domains. Sequence homologies of the BH1 (brown lines), BH2 (grey lines), BH3 (blue lines) and BH4 (orange lines) regions are shown. The BH1, BH2 and BH3 domains fold to line a hydrophobic pocket that can bind BH3-only peptides. The BH3 domain, particularly among the BH3-only proteins, mediates interaction between the BH3-only proteins and core Bcl-2 family proteins and thereby promotes apoptosis. The upper five proteins [Bcl-2, Bcl-x_L, Bcl-w, A1/Bfl-1 (A1) and Mcl1] are generally anti-apoptotic. The three proteins in the shaded area are less well studied and cannot be categorized at this time. The lower 12 proteins are considered to be pro-apoptotic. MULE contains a ubiquitin-associated domain (UBA), the Trp–Trp–Glu interaction module (WWE) and a HECT ubiquitin ligase domain. Bid has a unique role as both a Bcl-2 homologue and a BH3-only protein and links the intrinsic and extrinsic apoptosis pathways. Bim (also known as Bod), Bad and Bmf are unstructured proteins.

hydrophobic tail, which localizes the proteins to the outer surface of mitochondria, and, occasionally, of the endoplasmic reticulum, with the bulk of the protein facing the cytosol. The key feature of group I members is that they all possess anti-apoptotic activity, and protect cells from death [259]. In contrast, group II consists of Bcl-2 family members with pro-apoptotic activity [259]. Members of this group, which include Bax and Bak, have a similar overall structure to group I proteins, containing the hydrophobic tail but lack the N-terminal BH4 domain. Group III consists of a large and diverse collection of proteins whose only common feature is the presence of the ~12–16 aa BH3 domain (BH3-only proteins). Although some members of group III, including Bid, are indeed divergent homologues of Bcl-2 and Bax, others share little sequence or structural similarity with group I and II, suggesting that the BH3 domain in these proteins has arisen through convergent evolution.

All proteins belonging to the Bcl-2 family contain either a BH1, BH2, BH3, or BH4 domain. All anti-apoptotic proteins contain BH1 and BH2 domains, some of them contain an additional N-terminal BH4 domain (Bcl-2, Bcl-x_L, Bcl-w), which is also seen in some pro-apoptotic proteins like Bcl-x_S, Diva, Bok-L and Bok-S [259] (Fig. VIII). On the other hand, all pro-apoptotic proteins contain a BH3 domain necessary for dimerization with other proteins of Bcl-2 family and crucial for their killing activity, some of them also contain BH1 and BH2 domains (Bax, Bak). The BH3 domain is also present in some anti-apoptotic protein, such as Bcl-2 or Bcl-

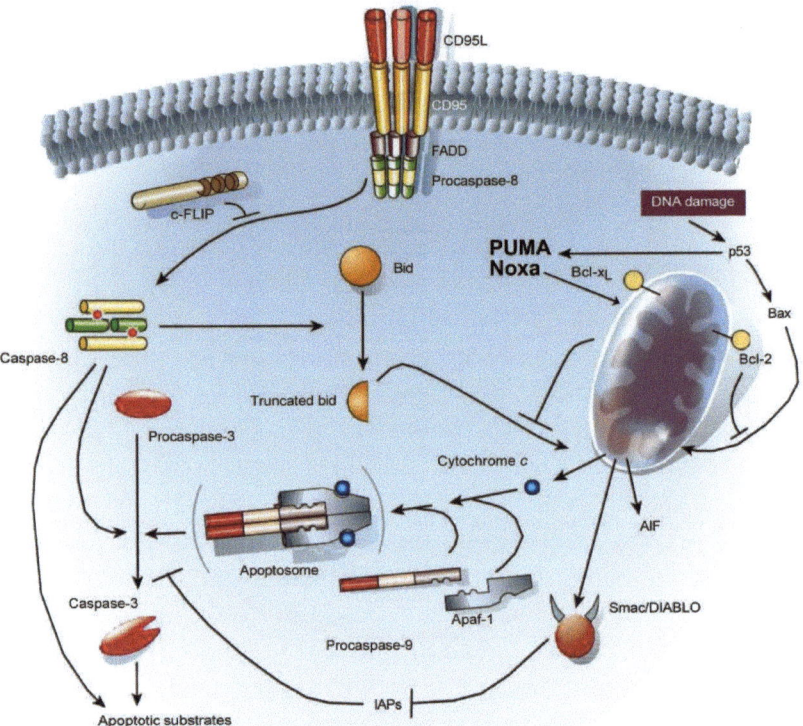

Fig. IX. The principal highlights of apoptosis (modified from [19]). Shown at the top is a typical cellular lipid bilayer membrane with FasR (CD95) and FasL (CD95L) transmembrane-coupled to FADD and procaspase 9 to trigger the <u>extrinsic pathway of apoptosis</u>. The interaction between FasR and FasL results in the formation of the FasR−DISC, which contains the FasR, FADD, procaspase 8 (and procaspase 10) [255]. In some types of cells (type I), processed caspase 8 directly activates other members of the caspase family (*e.g.* caspase 3), and triggers the execution of apoptosis of the cell. In other types of cells (type II), the FasR−DISC starts a feedback loop that relies on caspase 8-mediated cleavage of the pro-apoptotic Bcl-2 family member Bid to truncated Bid (tBid) [256] and spirals into increasing release of pro-apoptotic factors (*e.g.* cytochrome *c*, SMAC/DIABLO) from the mitochondrion (shown middle right) and to drive the formation of the caspase 9-activating <u>apoptosome</u>. The p53 upregulated modulator of apoptosis (<u>PUMA</u>) also known as Bcl-2-binding component 3 (BBC3), is a pro-apoptotic protein, member of the Bcl-2 protein family. In humans, the Bcl-2-binding component 3 protein is encoded by the *BBC3* gene. The expression of PUMA is regulated by the tumor suppressor p53. PUMA is involved in p53-dependent and p53-independent apoptosis induced by a variety of signals, and is regulated by transcription factors, not by post-translational modifications. After its activation, PUMA interacts with anti-apoptotic Bcl-2 family members, *e.g.* Bcl-2 and Bcl-x_L, thus liberating Bax and/or Bak which are then able to signal apoptosis to the mitochondrion. Phorbol-12-myristate-13-acetate-induced protein 1 is a protein that in humans is encoded by the *PMAIP1* gene, and is also known as Noxa. The expression of Noxa is induced by p53, and Noxa has been shown to be involved in p53-mediated apoptosis. The protein factor c-FLIP, representing a degenerate caspase homologue, inhibits the activation of caspase 8 (cysteinyl aspartic acid-protease 8). Bcl-2 and Bcl-x_L are anti-apoptotic Bcl-2 family factors, whereas Bax and Bak are BH3-only pro-apoptotic factors which can be activated by p53, triggering the mitochondrial pathway of apoptosis. The mitochondrion-associated apoptosis-inducing factor (AIF) is involved in initiating a caspase-independent pathway of apoptosis (positive intrinsic regulator of apoptosis) by causing DNA fragmentation and chromatin condensation.

x_L. The three functionally important Bcl-2 homology regions (BH1, BH2 and BH3) are in close spatial proximity. They form an elongated cleft that may provide the binding site for other Bcl-2 family members [259] (Fig. VIII).

The principal pathways of apoptosis are summarized as highlighted steps in **Fig. IX**. In overall conclusion, **PT162 (NSC 796018)** and **PT167 (NSC 799315)** both trigger the mitochondrial pathway of apoptosis after transcriptional (re)activation of p53 protein. **PT166 (NSC 750423)** is not able to trigger mitochondrial apoptosis, instead it represents a colchic(in)oid mitotic poison locking cells in anaphase of mitosis, probably binding to the well-known colchicine-binding site at β-tubulin [260–265]. There is no hint from my data that **PT167 (NSC 799315)** can also occupy the colchic(in)oid-binding site at β-tubulin, probably the molecule is too large for that binding site. Therefore, **PT166 (NSC 750423)** only stops tumor cell growth to ±0% growth index, but the cancer cells are all present still. In contrast, **PT162**

(NSC 796018) and **PT167** (NSC 799315) both completely destroy the tumor cells to nearly −100% of their growth index by 'genetically programmed suicide'.

Importantly, **PT162** (NSC 796018) and **PT167** (NSC 799315) are tumoricidal versus both wild-type p53 protein-expressing tumor cell lines and mutant p53 protein-expressing or none p53-expressing cancer cell lines. This pointed to p53-independent induction of mitochondrial apoptosis by **PT162** (NSC 796018) and **PT167** (NSC 799315) through their binding to mitochondrial cardiolipin based on ionic plus−minus charge attraction and hydrophobic interaction(s), thereby disrupting the membrane-anchoring of cytochrome *c* and cytochrome *c* oxidase enzymes in the inner mitochondrial membrane leading to cytochrome *c* release into the cytosol. **PT162** (NSC 796018) and **PT167** (NSC 799315) can be classified as essentially new antineoplastic drugs exploiting the cancer's *Warburg* effect [266−268]. Cancer cell mitochondria exhibit abnormalities in their cardiolipin content, composition, and metabolism [9,10,269−272]. Therefore, cancer cell mitochondria bear a weakened interaction of cardiolipin with cytochrome *c* and cytochrome *c* oxidase enzymes at the inner mitochondrial membrane. This fact is exploited by **PT162** (NSC 796018) and **PT167** (NSC 799315) through binding to cancer cell's cardiolipin, terminally interrupting its weakened interactions with respiratory chain enzymes preceding mitochondrial apoptosis.

References

[1]   O. Warburg, The metabolism of tumours, translated by F. Dickens, Constable, London, 1930.

[2]   O. Warburg, K. Posener, E. Negelein, Über den Stoffwechsel der Carcinomzelle, *Biochem. Z. (Berl.)* **152** (1924) 309–344.

[3]   O. Warburg, Über den Stoffwechsel der Carcinomzelle, *Naturwissenschaften* **12** (1924) 1131–1137.

[4]   O. Warburg, F. Wind, E. Negelein, The metabolism of tumors in the body, *J. Gen. Physiol.* **8** (1927) 519–530.

[5]   O. Warburg, On the origin of cancer cells, *Science* **123** (1956) 309–314.

[6]   W.H. Koppenol, P.L. Bounds, C.V. Dang, Otto Warburg's contributions to current concepts of cancer metabolism, *Nat. Rev. Cancer* **11** (2011) 325–337.

[7]   J.M. Cuezva, et al., The bioenergetic signature of cancer: A marker of tumor progression, *Cancer Res.* **62** (2002) 6674–6681.

[8]   J.-w. Kim, C.V. Dang, Cancer's molecular sweet tooth and the Warburg effect, *Cancer Res.* **66** (2006) 8927–8930.

[9]   M.A. Kiebish, X. Han, H. Cheng, J.H. Chuang, T.N. Seyfried, Cardiolipin and electron transport chain abnormalities in mouse brain tumor mitochondria: Lipidomic evidence supporting the Warburg theory of cancer, *J. Lipid Res.* **49** (2008) 2545–2556.

[10] V.E. Jahnke, et al., Evidence for mitochondrial respiratory deficiency in rat rhabdomyosarcoma cells, *PLoS One* **5** (2010), e8637, doi:10.1371/journal.pone.0008637.

[11] C.F. Cori, G.T. Cori, The carbohydrate metabolism of tumors. II. Changes in the sugar, lactic acid, and CO_2-combining power of blood passing through a tumor, *J. Biol. Chem.* **65** (1925) 397–405.

[12] S. Weinhouse, On respiratory impairment in cancer cells, *Science* **124** (1956) 267–269.

[13] O. Warburg, Reply to the Editor, *Science* **124** (1956) 269–270.

[14] D. Burk, A.L. Schade, Letter to the Editor, *Science* **124** (1956) 270–272.

[15] P.J. Quinn, R.M.C. Dawson, Interactions of cytochrome *c* and [^{14}C]carboxymethylated cytochrome *c* with monolayers of phosphatidylcholine, phosphatidic acid and cardiolipin, *Biochem. J.* **115** (1969) 65–75.

[16] S.B. Vik, G. Georgevich, R.A. Capaldi, Diphosphatidylglycerol is required for optimal activity of beef heart cytochrome *c* oxidase, *Proc. Natl. Acad. Sci. U. S. A.* **78** (1981) 1456–1460.

[17] S.H. Speck, C.A. Neu, M.S. Swanson, E. Margoliash, Role of phospholipid in the low affinity reactions between cytochrome *c* and cytochrome oxidase, *FEBS Lett.* **164** (1983) 379–382.

[18] M. Rytömaa, P. Mustonen, P.K.J. Kinnunen, Reversible, nonionic, and pH-dependent association of cytochrome *c* with cardiolipin-phosphatidylcholine liposomes, *J. Biol. Chem.* **267** (1992) 22243–22248.

[19] M.O. Hengartner, The biochemistry of apoptosis, *Nature* **407** (2000) 770–776.

[20] I.R. Indran, G. Tufo, S. Pervaiz, C. Brenner, Recent advances in apoptosis, mitochondria and drug resistance in cancer cells, *Biochim. Biophys. Acta* **1807** (2011) 735–745.

[21] W. Danysz, C.G. Parsons, J. Kornhuber, W.J. Schmidt, G. Quack, Aminoadamantanes as NMDA receptor antagonists and antiparkinsonian agents – Preclinical studies, *Neurosci. Biobehav. Rev.* **21** (1997) 455–468.

[22] W.L. Davies, et al., Antiviral activity of 1-adamantanamine (amantadine), *Science* **144** (1964) 862–863.

[23] R. Kamada, T. Nomura, C.W. Anderson, K. Sakaguchi, Cancer-associated p53 tetramerization domain mutants. Quantitative analysis reveals a low threshold for tumor suppressor inactivation, *J. Biol. Chem.* **286** (2011) 252–258.

[24] G.L. Semenza, Targeting HIF-1 for cancer therapy, *Nat. Rev. Cancer* **3** (2003) 721–732.

[25] C. Chen, N. Pore, A. Behrooz, F. Ismail-Beigi, A. Maity, Regulation of *glut1* mRNA by hypoxia-inducible factor-1. Interaction between H-*ras* and hypoxia, *J. Biol. Chem.* **276** (2001) 9519–9525.

[26] W.G. Kaelin Jr., Molecular basis of the VHL hereditary cancer syndrome, *Nat. Rev. Cancer* **2** (2002) 673–682.

[27] M.A. Selak, et al., Succinate links TCA cycle dysfunction to oncogenesis by inhibiting HIF-α prolyl hydroxylase, *Cancer Cell* **7** (2005) 77–85.

[28] I. Papandreou, R.A. Cairns, L. Fontana, A.L. Lim, N.C. Denko, HIF-1 mediates adaptation to hypoxia by actively down-regulating mitochondrial oxygen consumption, *Cell Metab.* **3** (2006) 187–197.

[29] J.W. Kim, I. Tchernyshyov, G.L. Semenza, C.V. Dang, HIF-1-mediated expression of pyruvate dehydrogenase kinase: A metabolic switch required for cellular adaptation to hypoxia, *Cell Metab.* **3** (2006) 177–185.

[30] M.I. Koukourakis, A. Giatromanolaki, E. Sivridis, K.C. Gatter, A.L. Harris, Pyruvate dehydrogenase and pyruvate dehydrogenase kinase expression in non small cell lung cancer and tumor-associated stroma, *Neoplasia* **7** (2005) 1–6.

[31] R.A. Gatenby, R.J. Gillies, Why do cancers have high aerobic glycolysis?, *Nat. Rev. Cancer* **4** (2004) 891–899.

[32] A.J. Levine, D.P. Lane (Eds.), The p53 family, Cold Spring Harbor Perspectives in Biology, Cold Spring Harbor Laboratory Press, Cold Spring Harbor, NY, USA, 2010, 360 pp., ISBN 978-0879698300.

[33] S.E. Kern, et al., Identification of p53 as a sequence-specific DNA-binding protein, *Science* **252** (1991) 1708–1711.

[34] D.P. Lane, p53, guardian of the genome, *Nature* **358** (1992) 15–16.

[35] P. May, E. May, Twenty years of p53 research: Structural and functional aspects of the p53 protein, *Oncogene* **18** (1999) 7621–7636; Corrigendum: *Oncogene* **19** (2000) 1734–1734.

[36] E. Toufektchan, F. Toledo, The guardian of the genome revisited: p53 downregulates genes required for telomere maintenance, DNA repair, and centromere structure, *Cancers (Basel)* **10** (2018), 135, https://doi.org/10.3390/cancers10050135.

[37] A.J. Levine, C.A. Finlay, P.W. Hinds, P53 is a tumor suppressor gene, *Cell* **S116** (2004) S67–S69.

[38] J.M. Nigro, et al., Mutations in the *p53* gene occur in diverse human tumour types, *Nature* **342** (1989) 705–708.

[39] A.L. Harris, Mutant p53—The commonest genetic abnormality in human cancer?, *J. Pathol.* **162** (1990) 5–6.

[40] A.J. Levine, J. Momand, C.A. Finlay, The p53 tumour suppressor gene, *Nature* **351** (1991) 453–456.

[41] M. Hollstein, D. Sidransky, B. Vogelstein, C.C. Harris, p53 mutations in human cancers, *Science* **253** (1991) 49–53.

[42] G. Matlashewski, P. Lamb, D. Pim, J. Peacock, L. Crawford, S. Benchimol, Isolation and characterization of a human p53 cDNA clone: Expression of the human p53 gene, *EMBO J.* **3** (1984) 3257–3262.

[43] D. Wolf, N. Harris, N. Goldfinger, V. Rotter, Isolation of a full-length mouse cDNA clone coding for an immunologically distinct p53 molecule, *Mol. Cell. Biol.* **5** (1985) 127–132.

[44] J.C. Bourdon, et al., p53 isoforms can regulate p53 transcriptional activity, *Genes Dev.* **19** (2005) 2122–2137.

[45] S. Surget, M.P. Khoury, J.-C. Bourdon, Uncovering the role of p53 splice variants in human malignancy: A clinical perspective, *Onco Targets Ther.* **7** (2014) 57–68, https://doi.org/10.2147/OTT.S53876.

[46] M. Isobe, B.S. Emanuel, D. Givol, M. Oren, C.M. Croce, Localization of gene for human p53 tumour antigen to band 17p13, *Nature* **320** (1986) 84–85.

[47] O.W. McBride, D. Merry, D. Givol, The gene for human p53 cellular tumor antigen is located on chromosome 17 short arm (17p13), *Proc. Natl. Acad. Sci. U. S. A.* **83** (1986) 130–134.

[48] D.P. Lane, L.V. Crawford, T antigen is bound to a host protein in SV40-transformed cells, *Nature* **278** (1979) 261–263.

[49] D.I.H. Linzer, A.J. Levine, Characterization of a 54K dalton cellular SV40 tumor antigen present in SV40-transformed cells and uninfected embryonal carcinoma cells, *Cell* **17** (1979) 43–52.

[50] A.B. DeLeo, G. Jay, E. Appella, G.C. Dubois, L.W. Law, L.J. Old, Detection of a transformation-related antigen in chemically induced sarcomas and other transformed cells of the mouse, *Proc. Natl. Acad. Sci. U. S. A.* **76** (1979) 2420–2424.

[51] J.A. DeCaprio, et al., SV40 large tumor antigen forms a specific complex with the product of the retinoblastoma susceptibility gene, *Cell* **54** (1988) 275–283.

[52] P.M. Chumakov, V.S. Iotsova, G.P. Georgiev, Isolation of a plasmid clone containing the mRNA sequence for mouse nonviral T-antigen (in Russian), *Dokl. Akad. Nauk S. S. S. R.* **267** (1982) 1272–1275.

[53] M. Oren, A.J. Levine, Molecular cloning of a cDNA specific for the murine p53 cellular tumor antigen, *Proc. Natl. Acad. Sci. U. S. A.* **80** (1983) 56–59.

[54] R. Zakut-Houri, M. Oren, B. Bienz, V. Lavie, S. Hazum, D. Givol, A single gene and a pseudogene for the cellular tumour antigen p53, *Nature* **306** (1983) 594–597.

[55] R. Zakut-Houri, B. Bienz-Tadmor, D. Givol, M. Oren, Human p53 cellular tumor antigen: cDNA sequence and expression in COS cells, *EMBO J.* **4** (1985) 1251–1255.

[56] C. Venot, M. Maratrat, C. Dureuil, E. Conseiller, L. Bracco, L. Debussche, The requirement for the p53 proline-rich functional domain for mediation of apoptosis is correlated with specific *PIG3* gene transactivation and with transcriptional repression, *EMBO J.* **17** (1998) 4668–4679.

[57] S. Larsen, T. Yokochi, E. Isogai, Y. Nakamura, T. Ozaki, A. Nakagawara, LMO3 interacts with p53 and inhibits its transcriptional activity, *Biochem. Biophys. Res. Commun.* **392** (2010) 252–257.

[58] K.L. Harms, X. Chen, The C terminus of p53 family proteins is a cell fate determinant, *Mol. Cell. Biol.* **25** (2005) 2014–2030.

[59] S. Bell, C. Klein, L. Müller, S. Hansen, J. Buchner, p53 contains large unstructured regions in its native state, *J. Mol. Biol.* **322** (2002) 917–927.

[60] N.J. MacLaine, T.R. Hupp, The regulation of p53 by phosphorylation: A model for how distinct signals integrate into the p53 pathway, *Aging (Albany NY)* **1** (2009) 490–502, https://doi.org/10.18632/aging.100047.

[61] N.J. MacLaine, T.R. Hupp, How phosphorylation controls p53, *Cell Cycle* **10** (2011) 916–921, https://doi.org/10.4161/cc.10.6.15076.

[62] A.R. Blanden, et al., Zinc shapes the folding landscape of p53 and establishes a pathway for reactivating structurally diverse cancer mutants, *eLife* **9** (2020), e61487, https://doi.org/10.7554/eLife.61487.

[63] J.-H. Ha, O. Prela, D.R. Carpizo, S.N. Loh, p53 and zinc: A malleable relationship, *Front. Mol. Biosci.* **9** (2022), 895887, https://doi.org/10.3389/fmolb.2022.895887.

[64] J. Zhu, S. Zhang, J. Jiang, X. Chen, Definition of the p53 functional domains necessary for inducing apoptosis, *J. Biol. Chem.* **275** (2000) 39927–39934.

[65] M.P. Khoury, J.-C. Bourdon, p53 isoforms: An intracellular microprocessor?, *Genes Cancer* **2** (2011) 453–465, https://doi.org/10.1177/1947601911408893.

[66] K.A. Avery-Kiejda, B. Morten, M.W. Wong-Brown, A. Mathe, R.J. Scott, The relative mRNA expression of p53 isoforms in breast cancer is associated with clinical features and outcome, *Carcinogenesis* **35** (2014) 586–596.

[67] L. Chin, et al., p53 deficiency rescues the adverse effects of telomere loss and cooperates with telomere dysfunction to accelerate carcinogenesis, *Cell* **97** (1999) 527–538.

[68] S. Tutton, P.M. Lieberman, A role of p53 in telomere protection, *Mol. Cell. Oncol.* **4** (2017), e1143078, https://doi.org/10.1080/23723556.2016.1143078.

[69] G. Babaei, et al., Crosslink between p53 and metastasis: Focus on epithelial–mesenchymal transition, cancer stem cell, angiogenesis, autophagy, and anoikis, *Mol. Biol. Rep.* **48** (2021) 7545–7557, https://doi.org/10.1007/s11033-021-06706-1.

[70] J.G. Teodoro, S.K. Evans, M.R. Green, Inhibition of tumor angiogenesis by p53: A new role for the guardian of the genome, *J. Mol. Med. (Berl.)* **85** (2007) 1175–1186, https://doi.org/10.1007/s00109-007-0221-2.

[71] S. Assadian, et al., p53 inhibits angiogenesis by inducing the production of Arresten, *Cancer Res.* **72** (2012) 1270–1279.

[72] A.K. Jain, et al., p53 regulates cell cycle and microRNAs to promote differentiation of human embryonic stem cells, *PLoS Biol.* **10** (2012), e1001268, https://doi.org/10.1371/journal.pbio.1001268.

[73] T. Maimets, I. Neganova, L. Armstrong, M. Lako, Activation of p53 by nutlin leads to rapid differentiation of human embryonic stem cells, *Oncogene* **27** (2008) 5277–5287.

[74] M. ter Huurne, T. Peng, G. Yi, G. van Mierlo, H. Marks, H.G. Stunnenberg, Critical role for *P53* in regulating the cell cycle of ground state embryonic stem cells, *Stem Cell Reports* **14** (2020) 175–183, https://doi.org/10.1016/j.stemcr.2020.01.001.

[75] B. Das, et al., HIF-2α suppresses p53 to enhance the stemness and regenerative potential of human embryonic stem cells, *Stem Cells* **30** (2012) 1685–1695, https://doi.org/10.1002/stem.1142.

[76] B.B. Lake, et al., Context-dependent enhancement of induced pluripotent stem cell reprogramming by silencing Puma, *Stem Cells* **30** (2012) 888–897, https://doi.org/10.1002/stem.1054.

[77] R.M. Marión, et al., A p53-mediated DNA damage response limits reprogramming to ensure iPS cell genomic integrity, *Nature* **460** (2009) 1149–1153.

[78] M.H. Yun, P.B. Gates, J.P. Brockes, Regulation of p53 is critical for vertebrate limb regeneration, *Proc. Natl. Acad. Sci. U. S. A.* **110** (2013) 17392–17397.

[79] R. Aloni-Grinstein, Y. Shetzer, T. Kaufman, V. Rotter, p53: The barrier to cancer stem cell formation, *FEBS Lett.* **588** (2014) 2580–2589.

[80] J.D. Oliner, K.W. Kinzler, P.S. Meltzer, D.L. George, B. Vogelstein, Amplification of a gene encoding a p53-associated protein in human sarcomas, *Nature* **358** (1992) 80–83.

[81] J. Momand, G.P. Zambetti, D.C. Olson, D. George, A.J. Levine, The mdm-2 oncogene product forms a complex with the p53 protein and inhibits p53-mediated transactivation, *Cell* **69** (1992) 1237–1245.

[82] R. Honda, H. Tanaka, H. Yasuda, Oncoprotein MDM2 is a ubiquitin ligase E3 for tumor suppressor p53, *FEBS Lett.* **420** (1997) 25–27.

[83] M. Li, et al., Deubiquitination of p53 by HAUSP is an important pathway for p53 stabilization, *Nature* **416** (2002) 648–653.

[84] A.K. Hock, A.M. Vigneron, S. Carter, R.L. Ludwig, K.H. Vousden, Regulation of p53 stability and function by the deubiquitinating enzyme USP42, *EMBO J.* **30** (2011) 4921–4930.

[85] C.J. Thut, J.A. Goodrich, R. Tijan, Repression of p53-mediated transcription by MDM2: A dual mechanism, *Genes Dev.* **11** (1997) 1974–1986.

[86] J.E. Purvis, K.W. Karhohs, C. Mock, E. Batchelor, A. Loewer, G. Lahav, p53 dynamics control cell fate, *Science* **336** (2012) 1440–1444.

[87] M. Wade, E.T. Wong, M. Tang, J.M. Stommel, G.M. Wahl, Hdmx modulates the outcome of p53 activation in human tumor cells, *J. Biol. Chem.* **281** (2006) 33036–33044.

[88] S.R. Grossman, et al., p300/MDM2 complexes participate in MDM2-mediated p53 degradation, *Mol. Cell* **2** (1998) 405–415.

[89] V. Kordinas, et al., Transcription of the tumor suppressor genes *p53* and *RB* in lymphocytes from patients with chronic kidney disease: Evidence of molecular senescence?, *Int. J. Nephrol.* **2012** (2012), 154397, https://doi.org/10.1155/2012/154397.

[90] B.A. Werness, A.J. Levine, P.M. Howley, Association of human papillomavirus types 16 and 18 E6 proteins with p53, *Science* **248** (1990) 76–79.

[91] K. Münger, B.A. Werness, N. Dyson, W.C. Phelps, E. Harlow, P.M. Howley, Complex formation of human papillomavirus E7 proteins with the retinoblastoma tumor suppressor gene product, *EMBO J.* **8** (1989) 4099–4105.

[92] M. Scheffner, J.M. Huibregtse, R.D. Vierstra, P.M. Howley, The HPV-16 E6 and E6-AP complex functions

as a ubiquitin-protein ligase in the ubiquitination of p53, *Cell* **75** (1993) 495–505.

[93] A.L. Talis, J.M. Huibregtse, P.M. Howley, The role of E6AP in the regulation of p53 protein levels in human papillomavirus (HPV)-positive and HPV-negative cells, *J. Biol. Chem.* **273** (1998) 6439–6445.

[94] S.S. Tungteakkhun, P.J. Duerksen-Hughes, Cellular binding partners of the human papillomavirus E6 protein, *Arch. Virol.* **153** (2008) 397–408.

[95] G.P. Dimri, M. Nakanishi, P.-Y. Desprez, J.R. Smith, J. Campisi, Inhibition of E2F activity by the cyclin-dependent protein kinase inhibitor p21 in cells expressing or lacking a functional retinoblastoma protein, *Mol. Cell. Biol.* **16** (1996) 2987–2997.

[96] J.O. Funk, S. Waga, J.B. Harry, E. Espling, B. Stillman, D.A. Galloway, Inhibition of CDK activity and PCNA-dependent DNA replication by p21 is blocked by interaction with the HPV-16 E7 oncoprotein, *Genes Dev.* **11** (1997) 2090–2100.

[97] L. Szekely, G. Selivanova, K.P. Magnusson, G. Klein, K.G. Wiman, EBNA-5, an Epstein–Barr virus-encoded nuclear antigen, binds to the retinoblastoma and p53 proteins, *Proc. Natl. Acad. Sci. U. S. A.* **90** (1993) 5455–5459.

[98] E. Kashuba, et al., Epstein-Barr virus-encoded EBNA-5 forms trimolecular protein complexes with MDM2 and p53 and inhibits the transactivating function of p53, *Int. J. Cancer* **128** (2011) 817–825.

[99] W. Chen, N.R. Cooper, Epstein-Barr virus nuclear antigen 2 and latent membrane protein independently transactivate p53 through induction of NF-κB activity, *J. Virol.* **70** (1996) 4849–4853.

[100] E. Moran, Interaction of adenoviral proteins with pRB and p53, *FASEB J.* **7** (1993) 880–885.

[101] A. Braithwaite, C. Nelson, A. Skulimowski, J. McGovern, D. Pigott, J. Jenkins, Transactivation of the p53 oncogene by E1a gene products, *Virology* **177** (1990) 595–605.

[102] T.K. Hale, A.W. Braithwaite, The adenovirus oncoprotein E1a stimulates binding of transcription factor ETF to transcriptionally activate the *p53* gene, *J. Biol. Chem.* **274** (1999) 23777–23786.

[103] M. Debbas, E. White, Wild-type p53 mediates apoptosis by E1A, which is inhibited by E1B, *Genes Dev.* **7** (1993) 546–554.

[104] X. Liu, R. Marmorstein, Structure of the retinoblastoma protein bound to adenovirus E1A reveals the molecular basis for viral oncoprotein inactivation of a tumor suppressor, *Genes Dev.* **21** (2007) 2711–2716.

[105] T. Nakajima, et al., Stabilization of p53 by adenovirus E1A occurs through its amino-terminal region by modification of the ubiquitin-proteasome pathway, *J. Biol. Chem.* **273** (1998) 20036–20045.

[106] P.A.J. Muller, K.H. Vousden, Mutant p53 in cancer: New functions and therapeutic opportunities, *Cancer Cell* **25** (2014) 304–317, https://doi.org/10.1016/j.ccr.2014.01.021.

[107] K.H. Khoo, C.S. Verma, D.P. Lane, Drugging the p53 pathway: Understanding the route to clinical efficacy, *Nat. Rev. Drug Discov.* **13** (2014) 217–236; Erratum: *Nat. Rev. Drug Discov.* **13** (2014) 314–314.

[108] J.L. Silva, et al., Recent synthetic approaches towards small molecule reactivators of p53, *Biomolecules* **10** (2020), 635, https://doi.org/10.3390/biom10040635.

[109] O. Hassin, M. Oren, Drugging p53 in cancer: One protein, many targets, *Nat. Rev. Drug Discov.* **22** (2023) 127–144.

[110] A.R. Sawkar, et al., Gaucher disease-associated glucocerebrosidases show mutation-dependent chemical chaperoning profiles, *Chem. Biol. (Cell Chem. Biol.)* **12** (2005) 1235–1244.

[111] V.J.N. Bykov, et al., Restoration of the tumor suppressor function to mutant p53 by a low-molecular-weight compound, *Nat. Med.* **8** (2002) 282–288.

[112] L.P. Rangel, et al., p53 reactivation with induction of massive apoptosis-1 (PRIMA-1) inhibits amyloid aggregation of mutant p53 in cancer cells, *J. Biol. Chem.* **294** (2019) 3670–3682.

[113] Q. Zhang, V.J.N. Bykov, K.G. Wiman, J. Zawacka-Pankau, APR-246 reactivates mutant p53 by targeting cysteines 124 and 277, *Cell Death Dis.* **9** (2018), 439, https://doi.org/10.1038/s41419-018-0463-7; Correction: *Cell Death Dis.* **10** (2019), 769, https://doi.org/10.1038/s41419-019-1997-z.

[114] L. Weinmann, et al., A novel p53 rescue compound induces p53-dependent growth arrest and sensitises glioma cells to Apo2L/TRAIL-induced apoptosis, *Cell Death Differ.* **15** (2008) 718–729, https://doi.org/10.1038/sj.cdd.4402301.

[115] M. Demma, et al., SCH529074, a small molecule activator of mutant p53, which binds p53 DNA binding domain (DBD), restores growth-suppressive function to mutant p53 and interrupts HDM2-mediated ubiquitination of wild type p53, *J. Biol. Chem.* **285** (2010) 10198–10212.

[116] J.J. Miller, et al., Bifunctional ligand design for modulating mutant p53 aggregation in cancer, *Chem. Sci.* **10** (2019) 10802–10814, https://doi.org/10.1039/C9SC04151F.

[117] T.D. Halazonetis, A.N. Kandil, Conformational shifts propagate from the oligomerization domain of p53 to its tetrameric DNA binding domain and restore DNA binding to select p53 mutants, *EMBO J.* **12** (1993) 5057–5064.

[118] F.P. Li, J.F. Fraumeni Jr., Soft-tissue sarcomas, breast cancer, and other neoplasms. A familial syndrome?, *Ann. Intern. Med.* **71** (1969) 747–752.

[119] J.M. Varley, Germline *TP53* mutations and Li-Fraumeni syndrome, *Hum. Mutat.* **21** (2003) 313–320.

[120] G.M. Clore, et al., Refined solution structure of the oligomerization domain of the tumour suppressor p53, *Nat. Struct. Biol.* **2** (1995) 321–333.

[121] P.D. Jeffrey, S. Gorina, N.P. Pavletich, Crystal structure of the tetramerization domain of the p53 tumor suppressor at 1.7 angstroms, *Science* **267** (1995) 1498–1502.

[122] G.M. Clore, High resolution solution NMR structure of the oligomerization domain of p53 by multi-dimensional NMR (sac structures), RCSB Protein Data Bank, 1999, https://doi.org/10.2210/pdb3sak/pdb.

[123] M.C. Pangborn, Isolation and purification of a serologically active phospholipid from beef heart, *J. Biol. Chem.* **143** (1942) 247–256.

[124] M. Schlame, L. Horvàth, L. Vìgh, Relationship between lipid saturation and lipid-protein interaction in liver mitochondria modified by catalytic hydrogenation with

reference to cardiolipin molecular species, *Biochem. J.* **265** (1990) 79–85.

[125] M. Schlame, S. Brody, K.Y. Hostetler, Mitochondrial cardiolipin in diverse eukaryotes. Comparison of biosynthetic reactions and molecular acyl species, *Eur. J. Biochem.* **212** (1993) 727–735.

[126] S. Matoba, et al., p53 regulates mitochondrial respiration, *Science* **312** (2006) 1650–1653.

[127] C. Wanka, et al., Synthesis of cytochrome *c* oxidase 2: A p53-dependent metabolic regulator that promotes respiratory function and protects glioma and colon cancer cells from hypoxia-induced cell death, *Oncogene* **31** (2012) 3764–3776.

[128] Y. Xiong, G.J. Hannon, H. Zhang, D. Casso, R. Kobayashi, D. Beach, p21 is a universal inhibitor of cyclin kinases, *Nature* **366** (1993) 701–704.

[129] J.W. Harper, et al., Inhibition of cyclin-dependent kinases by p21, *Mol. Biol. Cell* **6** (1995) 387–400.

[130] J.W. Harper, G.R. Adami, N. Wei, K. Keyomarsi, S.J. Elledge, The p21 Cdk-interacting protein Cip1 is a potent inhibitor of G1 cyclin-dependent kinases, *Cell* **75** (1993) 805–816.

[131] W.S. el-Deiry, et al., *WAF1*, a potential mediator of p53 tumor suppression, *Cell* **75** (1993) 817–825.

[132] D.J. Demetrick, et al., Chromosomal mapping of the genes for the human cell cycle proteins cyclin C (CCNC), cyclin E (CCNE), p21 (CDKN1) and KAP (CDKN3), *Cytogenet. Cell Genet.* **69** (1995) 190–192.

[133] A.L. Gartel, A.L. Tyner, The role of the cyclin-dependent kinase inhibitor p21 in apoptosis, *Mol. Cancer Ther.* **1** (2002) 639–649.

[134] K. Engeland, Cell cycle regulation: p53–p21–RB signaling, *Cell Death Differ.* **29** (2022) 946–960, https://doi.org/10.1038/s41418-022-00988-z.

[135] D. Dolezalova, et al., MicroRNAs regulate p21$^{Waf1/Cip1}$ protein expression and the DNA damage response in human embryonic stem cells, *Stem Cells* **30** (2012) 1362–1372.

[136] S. Waga, G.J. Hannon, D. Beach, B. Stillman, The p21 inhibitor of cyclin-dependent kinases controls DNA replication by interaction with PCNA, *Nature* **369** (1994) 574–578.

[137] V. Dulić, et al., p53-dependent inhibition of cyclin-dependent kinase activities in human fibroblasts during radiation-induced G1 arrest, *Cell* **76** (1994) 1013–1023.

[138] C. Deng, P. Zhang, J.W. Harper, S.J. Elledge, P. Leder, Mice lacking p21$^{CIP1/WAF1}$ undergo normal development, but are defective in G1 checkpoint control, *Cell* **82** (1995) 675–684.

[139] A. Hafner, J. Reyes, J. Stewart-Ornstein, M. Tsabar, A. Jambhekar, G. Lahav, Quantifying the central dogma in the p53 pathway in live single cells, *Cell Syst.* **10** (2020) 495–505, https://doi.org/10.1016/j.cels.2020.05.001.

[140] A.R. Barr, et al., DNA damage during S-phase mediates the proliferation-quiescence decision in the subsequent G1 via p21 expression, *Nat. Commun.* **8** (2017), 14728, https://doi.org/10.1038/ncomms14728.

[141] Z.-K. Yu, J.L.M. Gervais, H. Zhang, Human CUL-1 associates with the SKP1/SKP2 complex and regulates p21$^{CIP1/WAF1}$ and cyclin D proteins, *Proc. Natl. Acad. Sci. U. S. A.* **95** (1998) 11324–11329.

[142] G. Bornstein, J. Bloom, D. Sitry-Shevah, K. Nakayama, M. Pagano, A. Hershko, Role of the SCF^{Skp2} ubiquitin

ligase in the degradation of p21^{Cip1} in S phase, *J. Biol. Chem.* **278** (2003) 25752–25757.

[143] Y. Kim, N.G. Starostina, E.T. Kipreos, The CRL4^{Cdt2} ubiquitin ligase targets the degradation of p21^{Cip1} to control replication licensing, *Genes Dev.* **22** (2008) 2507–2519.

[144] T. Abbas, U. Sivaprasad, K. Terai, V. Amador, M. Pagano, A. Dutta, PCNA-dependent regulation of p21 ubiquitylation and degradation via the CRL4^{Cdt2} ubiquitin ligase complex, *Genes Dev.* **22** (2008) 2496–2506.

[145] N.N. Kreis, F. Louwen, J. Yuan, The multifaceted p21 (Cip1/Waf1/*CDKN1A*) in cell differentiation, migration and cancer therapy, *Cancers (Basel)* **11** (2019), 1220, https://doi.org/10.3390/cancers11091220.

[146] P. Leisibach, D. Schneiter, A. Soltermann, Y. Yamada, W. Weder, W. Jungraithmayr, Prognostic value of immunohistochemical markers in malignant thymic epithelial tumors, *J. Thorac. Dis.* **8** (2016) 2580–2591, https://doi.org/10.21037/jtd.2016.08.82.

[147] J. Zhang, D.T. Scadden, C.S. Crumpacker, Primitive hematopoietic cells resist HIV-1 infection via p21$^{Waf1/Cip1/Sdi1}$, *J. Clin. Invest.* **117** (2007) 473–481.

[148] H. Chen, et al., CD4$^+$ T cells from elite controllers resist HIV-1 infection by selective upregulation of p21, *J. Clin. Invest.* **121** (2007) 1549–1560.

[149] N. Vázquez, et al., Human immunodeficiency virus type 1-induced macrophage gene expression includes the p21 gene, a target for viral regulation, *J. Virol.* **79** (2005) 4479–4491.

[150] M.A. Subler, D.W. Martin, S. Deb, Inhibition of viral and cellular promoters by human wild-type p53, *J. Virol.* **66** (1992) 4757–4762.

[151] M.A. Subler, D.W. Martin, S. Deb, Activation of the human immunodeficiency virus type 1 long terminal repeat by transforming mutants of human p53, *J. Virol.* **68** (1994) 103–110.

[152] L. Duan, I. Ozaki, J.W. Oakes, J.P. Taylor, K. Khalili, R.J. Pomerantz, The tumor suppressor protein p53 strongly alters human immunodeficiency virus type 1 replication, *J. Virol.* **68** (1994) 4302–4313.

[153] R. Altschul, N. Theise, PopTest Oncology LLC/Palisades Therapeutics (Cliffside Park, NJ, USA), Palisades Therapeutics announces new anti-cancer drug-PT162, a p53-reactivating cell cycle checkpoint inhibitor, EINPresswire.com (January 3rd, 2023), https://www.einpresswire.com/article/609163965/palisades-therapeutics-announces-new-anti-cancer-drug-pt162-a-p53-reactivating-cell-cycle-checkpoint-inhibitor.

[154] B. Shi, et al., Inhibition of HIV early replication by the p53 and its downstream gene p21, *Virol. J.* **15** (2018), 53, https://doi.org/10.1186/s12985-018-0959-x.

[155] C.J. Li, C. Wang, D.J. Friedman, A.B. Pardee, Reciprocal modulations between p53 and Tat of human immunodeficiency virus type 1, *Proc. Natl. Acad. Sci. U. S. A.* **92** (1995) 5461–5464.

[156] F. Longo, M.A. Marchetti, L. Castagnoli, P.A. Battaglia, F. Gigliani, A novel approach to protein–protein interaction: Complex formation between the p53 tumor suppressor and the HIV Tat proteins, *Biochem. Biophys. Res. Commun.* **206** (1995) 326–334.

[157] Y. Ariumi, A. Kaida, M. Hatanaka, K. Shimotohno, Functional cross-talk of HIV-1 Tat with p53 through its C-terminal domain, *Biochem. Biophys. Res. Commun.* **287** (2001) 556–561.

[158] A.L. Greenway, et al., Human immunodeficiency virus type 1 Nef binds to tumor suppressor p53 and protects cells against p53-mediated apoptosis, *J. Virol.* **76** (2002) 2692–2702.

[159] B.E. Sawaya, K. Khalili, W.E. Mercer, L. Denisova, S. Amini, Cooperative actions of HIV-1 Vpr and p53 modulate viral gene transcription, *J. Biol. Chem.* **273** (1998) 20052–20057.

[160] I.H. Chowdhury, et al., HIV-1 Vpr activates cell cycle inhibitor p21/Waf1/Cip1: A potential mechanism of G2/M cell cycle arrest, *Virology* **305** (2003) 371–377.

[161] D. Genini, et al., HIV induces lymphocyte apoptosis by a p53-initiated, mitochondrial-mediated mechanism, *FASEB J.* **15** (2001) 5–6, https://doi.org/10.1096/fj.00-0336fje.

[162] W. Wu, et al., Drug 9AA reactivates p21/Waf1 and inhibits HIV-1 progeny formation, *Virol. J.* **5** (2008), 41, https://doi.org/10.1186/1743-422X-5-41.

[163] E. Clark, et al., Loss of G_1/S checkpoint in human immunodeficiency virus type 1-infected cells is associated with a lack of cyclin-dependent kinase inhibitor p21/Waf1, *J. Virol.* **74** (2000) 5040–5052.

[164] D.A. Withers, R.C. Harvey, J.B. Faust, O. Melnyk, K. Carey, T.C. Meeker, Characterization of a candidate *bcl-1* gene, *Mol. Cell. Biol.* **11** (1991) 4846–4853.

[165] T. Inaba, H. Matsushime, M. Valentine, M.F. Roussel, C.J. Sherr, A.T. Look, Genomic organization,

chromosomal localization, and independent expression of human cyclin D genes, *Genomics* **13** (1992) 565–574.

[166] Y. Xiong, J. Menninger, D. Beach, D.C. Ward, Molecular cloning and chromosomal mapping of *CCND* genes encoding human D-type cyclins, *Genomics* **13** (1992) 575–584.

[167] T. Motokura, et al., A novel cyclin encoded by a *bcl1*-linked candidate oncogene, *Nature* **350** (1991) 512–515.

[168] P. Neumeister, et al., *Cyclin D1* governs adhesion and motility of macrophages, *Mol. Biol. Cell* **14** (2003) 2005–2015.

[169] W. Holnthoner, et al., Fibroblast growth factor-2 induces Lef/Tcf-dependent transcription in human endothelial cells, *J. Biol. Chem.* **277** (2002) 45847–45853.

[170] T. Sakamaki, et al., Cyclin D1 determines mitochondrial function in vivo, *Mol. Cell. Biol.* **26** (2006) 5449–5469.

[171] V. Baldin, J. Lukas, M.J. Marcote, M. Pagano, G. Draetta, Cyclin D1 is a nuclear protein required for cell cycle progression in G_1, *Genes Dev.* **7** (1993) 812–821.

[172] E.A. Musgrove, C.E. Caldon, J. Barraclough, A. Stone, R.L. Sutherland, Cyclin D as a therapeutic target in cancer, *Nat. Rev. Cancer* **11** (2011) 558–572.

[173] R.M.L. Zwijsen, E. Wientjens, R. Klompmaker, J. van der Sman, R. Bernards, R.J.A.M. Michalides, CDK-independent activation of estrogen receptor by cyclin D1, *Cell* **88** (1997) 405–415.

[174] M. Fu, C. Wang, Z. Li, T. Sakamaki, R.G. Pestell, Minireview: Cyclin D1: Normal and abnormal functions, *Endocrinology* **145** (2004) 5439–5447.

[175] M. Fu, et al., Cyclin D1 inhibits peroxisome proliferator-activated receptor γ-mediated adipogenesis through histone deacetylase recruitment, *J. Biol. Chem.* **280** (2005) 16934–16941.

[176] A.T. Reutens, et al., Cyclin D1 binds the androgen receptor and regulates hormone-dependent signaling in a p300/CBP-associated factor (P/CAF)-dependent manner, *Mol. Endocrinol.* **15** (2001) 797–811.

[177] C. McMahon, T. Suthiphongchai, J. DiRenzo, M.E. Ewen, P/CAF associates with cyclin D1 and potentiates its activation of the estrogen receptor, *Proc. Natl. Acad. Sci. U. S. A.* **96** (1999) 5382–5387.

[178] D.S. Peeper, et al., Ras signalling linked to the cell-cycle machinery by the retinoblastoma protein, *Nature* **386** (1997) 177–181.

[179] D. Simoneschi, et al., CRL4^{AMBRA1} is a master regulator of D-type cyclins, *Nature* **592** (2021) 789–793.

[180] A.C. Chaikovsky, J. Sage, M. Pagano, D. Simoneschi, The long-lost ligase: CRL4^{AMBRA1} regulates the stability of D-type cyclins, *DNA Cell Biol.* **40** (2021) 1457–1461, https://doi.org/10.1089/dna.2021.0659.

[181] J. Jin, E.E. Arias, J. Chen, J.W. Harper, J.C. Walter, A family of diverse Cul4-Ddb1-interacting proteins includes Cdt2, which is required for S phase destruction of the replication factor Cdt1, *Mol. Cell* **23** (2006) 709–721, https://doi.org/10.1016/j.molcel.2006.08.010.

[182] J.R. Molina, A.A. Adjei, The Ras/Raf/MAPK pathway, *J. Thorac. Oncol.* **1** (2006) 7–9.

[183] J.A. McCubrey, et al., Roles of the Raf/MEK/ERK pathway in cell growth, malignant transformation and drug resistance, *Biochim. Biophys. Acta* **1773** (2007) 1263–1284.

[184] J.A. McCubrey, et al., Mutations and deregulation of Ras/Raf/MEK/ERK and PI3K/PTEN/Akt/mTOR cascades which alter therapy response, *Oncotarget* **3** (2012) 954–987, https://doi.org/10.18632/oncotarget.652.

[185] Y.-J. Guo, W.-W. Pan, S.-B. Liu, Z.-F. Shen, Y. Xu, L.-L. Hu, ERK/MAPK signalling pathway and tumorigenesis (Review), *Exp. Ther. Med.* **19** (2020) 1997–2007, https://doi.org/10.3892/etm.2020.8454.

[186] M. Dillon, A. Lopez, E. Lin, D. Sales, R. Perets, P. Jain, Progress on Ras/MAPK signaling research and targeting in blood and solid cancers, *Cancers (Basel)* **13** (2021), 5059, https://doi.org/10.3390/cancers13205059.

[187] P. Jansen-Dürr, et al., Differential modulation of cyclin gene expression by *MYC*, *Proc. Natl. Acad. Sci. U. S. A.* **90** (1993) 3685–3689.

[188] A. Philipp, et al., Repression of cyclin D1: A novel function of MYC, *Mol. Cell. Biol.* **14** (1994) 4032–4043.

[189] S.J. Taylor, D. Shalloway, Cell cycle-dependent activation of Ras, *Curr. Biol.* **6** (1996) 1621–1627.

[190] H. Aktas, H. Cai, G.M. Cooper, Ras links growth factor signaling to the cell cycle machinery via regulation of cyclin D1 and the Cdk inhibitor $p27^{KIP1}$, *Mol. Cell. Biol.* **17** (1997) 3850–3857.

[191] E. Kerkhoff, U.R. Rapp, Cell cycle targets of Ras/Raf signalling, *Oncogene* **17** (1998) 1457–1462.

[192] Y. Terada, S. Inoshita, O. Nakashima, M. Kuwahara, S. Sasaki, F. Marumo, Regulation of cyclin D1 expression and cell cycle progression by mitogen-activated protein kinase cascade, *Kidney Int.* **56** (1999) 1258–1261.

[193] J.-C. Chambard, R. Lefloch, J. Pouysségur, P. Lenormand, ERK implication in cell cycle regulation, *Biochim. Biophys. Acta* **1773** (2007) 1299–1310.

[194] S. Kampfer, et al., Protein kinase C isoforms involved in the transcriptional activation of cyclin D1 by transforming Ha-Ras, *J. Biol. Chem.* **276** (2001) 42834–42842.

[195] M. Shtutman, et al., The cyclin D1 gene is a target of the β-catenin/LEF-1 pathway, *Proc. Natl. Acad. Sci. U. S. A.* **96** (1999) 5522–5527.

[196] C. Albanese, et al., IKKα regulates mitogenic signaling through transcriptional induction of cyclin D1 via Tcf, *Mol. Biol. Cell* **14** (2003) 585–599.

[197] C. Albanese, et al., Transforming p21^{ras} mutants and c-Ets-2 activate the cyclin D1 promoter through distinguishable regions, *J. Biol. Chem.* **270** (1995) 23589–23597.

[198] J.R. Brown, et al., Fos family members induce cell cycle entry by activating cyclin D1, *Mol. Cell. Biol.* **18** (1998) 5609–5619.

[199] D. Joyce, et al., Integration of Rac-dependent regulation of cyclin D1 transcription through a nuclear factor-κB-dependent pathway, *J. Biol. Chem.* **274** (1999) 25245–25249.

[200] M. D'Amico, et al., The integrin-linked kinase regulates the cyclin D1 gene through glycogen synthase kinase 3β and cAMP-responsive element-binding protein-dependent pathways, *J. Biol. Chem.* **275** (2000) 32649–32657.

[201] J. Zhao, R. Pestell, J.-L. Guan, Transcriptional activation of cyclin D1 promoter by FAK contributes to

cell cycle progression, *Mol. Biol. Cell* **12** (2001) 4066–4077.

[202] M. Cheng, et al., The p21^{Cip1} and p27^{Kip1} CDK 'inhibitors' are essential activators of cyclin D-dependent kinases in murine fibroblasts, *EMBO J.* **18** (1999) 1571–1583.

[203] C.J. Sherr, J.M. Roberts, CDK inhibitors: Positive and negative regulators of G$_1$-phase progression, *Genes Dev.* **13** (1999) 1501–1512.

[204] I.B. Rosenwald, et al., Eukaryotic translation initiation factor 4E regulates expression of cyclin D1 at transcriptional and post-transcriptional levels, *J. Biol. Chem.* **270** (1995) 21176–21180.

[205] B. Culjkovic, I. Topisirovic, L. Skrabanek, M. Ruiz-Gutierrez, K.L.B. Borden, eIF4E promotes nuclear export of cyclin D1 mRNAs via an element in the 3′UTR, *J. Cell Biol.* **169** (2005) 245–256.

[206] A. Besson, S.F. Dowdy, J.M. Roberts, CDK inhibitors: Cell cycle regulators and beyond, *Dev. Cell* **14** (2008) 159–169, https://doi.org/10.1016/j.devcel.2008.01.013.

[207] J. Creff, A. Besson, Functional versatility of the CDK inhibitor p57^{Kip2}, *Front. Cell Dev. Biol.* **8** (2020), 584590, https://doi.org/10.3389/fcell.2020.584590.

[208] J.A. Diehl, M. Cheng, M.F. Roussel, C.J. Sherr, Glycogen synthase kinase-3β regulates cyclin D1 proteolysis and subcellular localization, *Genes Dev.* **12** (1998) 3499–3511.

[209] J.R. Alt, J.L. Cleveland, M. Hannink, J.A. Diehl, Phosphorylation-dependent regulation of cyclin D1 nuclear export and cyclin D1–dependent cellular transformation, *Genes Dev.* **14** (2000) 3102–3114.

[210] J.R. Alt, A.B. Gladden, J.A. Diehl, p21^{Cip1} promotes cyclin D1 nuclear accumulation via direct inhibition of nuclear export, *J. Biol. Chem.* **277** (2002) 8517–8523.

[211] S. Rocha, A.M. Martin, D.W. Meek, N.D. Perkins, p53 represses cyclin D1 transcription through down regulation of Bcl-3 and inducing increased association of the p52 NF-κB subunit with histone deacetylase 1, *Mol. Cell. Biol.* **23** (2003) 4713–4727.

[212] H. Liu, L. Zeng, Y. Yang, C. Guo, H. Wang, Bcl-3: A double-edged sword in immune cells and inflammation, *Front. Immunol.* **13** (2022), 847699, https://doi.org/10.3389/fimmu.2022.847699.

[213] K. Schumm, S. Rocha, J. Caamano, N.D. Perkins, Regulation of p53 tumour suppressor target gene expression by the p52 NF-κB subunit, *EMBO J.* **25** (2006) 4820–4832.

[214] S.D. Westerheide, M.W. Mayo, V. Anest, J.L. Hanson, A.S. Baldwin Jr., The putative oncoprotein Bcl-3 induces cyclin D1 to stimulate G_1 transition, *Mol. Cell. Biol.* **21** (2001) 8428–8436.

[215] E. Tashiro, A. Tsuchiya, M. Imoto, Functions of cyclin D1 as an oncogene and regulation of cyclin D1 expression, *Cancer Sci.* **98** (2007) 629–635, https://doi.org/10.1111/j.1349-7006.2007.00449.x.

[216] S. Qie, J.A. Diehl, Cyclin D1, cancer progression, and opportunities in cancer treatment, *J. Mol. Med. (Berl.)* **94** (2012) 1313–1326, https://doi.org/10.1007/s00109-016-1475-3.

[217] F.I. Montalto, F. De Amicis, Cyclin D1 in cancer: A molecular connection for cell cycle control, adhesion and invasion in tumor and stroma, *Cells* **9** (2020), 2648, https://doi.org/10.3390/cells9122648.

[218] R.J. Lee, et al., Cyclin D1 is required for transformation by activated Neu and is induced through an E2F-dependent signaling pathway, *Mol. Cell. Biol.* **20** (2000) 672–683.

[219] Q. Yu, Y. Geng, P. Sicinski, Specific protection against breast cancers by cyclin D1 ablation, *Nature* **411** (2001) 1017–1021.

[220] J. Hulit, et al., Cyclin D1 genetic heterozygosity regulates colonic epithelial cell differentiation and tumor number in *Apc^Min* mice, *Mol. Cell. Biol.* **24** (2004) 7598–7611.

[221] T.C. Wang, R.D. Cardiff, L. Zukerberg, E. Lees, A. Arnold, E.V. Schmidt, Mammary hyperplasia and carcinoma in MMTV-cyclin D1 transgenic mice, *Nature* **369** (1994) 669–671.

[222] C. Albanese, et al., Activation of the *cyclin D1* gene by the E1A-associated protein p300 through AP-1 inhibits cellular apoptosis, *J. Biol. Chem.* **274** (1999) 34186–34195.

[223] M.C. Casimiro, et al., ChIP sequencing of cyclin D1 reveals a transcriptional role in chromosomal instability in mice, *J. Clin. Invest.* **122** (2012) 833–843, https://doi.org/10.1172/JCI60256; Corrigendum: *J. Clin. Invest.* **123** (2013) 2332–2332, https://doi.org/10.1172/JCI70042.

[224] M.C. Casimiro, et al., Kinase-independent role of cyclin D1 in chromosomal instability and mammary tumorigenesis, *Oncotarget* **6** (2015) 8525–8538, https://doi.org/10.18632/oncotarget.3267.

[225] N.E. Brown, et al., Cyclin D1 activity regulates autophagy and senescence in the mammary epithelium, *Cancer Res.* **72** (2012) 6477–6489.

[226] M.C. Casimiro, et al., Cyclin D1 restrains oncogene-induced autophagy by regulating the AMPK–LKB1 signaling axis, *Cancer Res.* **77** (2017) 3391–3405.

[227] R.G. Pestell, New roles of cyclin D1, *Am. J. Pathol.* **183** (2013) 3–9, https://doi.org/10.1016/j.ajpath.2013.03.001.

[228] R.J. Lee, et al., pp60$^{v\text{-}src}$ induction of cyclin D1 requires collaborative interactions between the extracellular signal-regulated kinase, p38, and Jun kinase pathways. A role for cAMP response element-binding protein and activating transcription factor-2 in pp60$^{v\text{-}src}$ signaling in breast cancer cells, *J. Biol. Chem.* **274** (1999) 7341–7350.

[229] J.F. Bromberg, et al., *Stat3* as an oncogene, *Cell* **98** (1999) 295–303; Erratum: *Cell* **99** (1999) 239–239.

[230] I. Matsumura, et al., Transcriptional regulation of the cyclin D1 promoter by STAT5: Its involvement in cytokine-dependent growth of hematopoietic cells, *EMBO J.* **18** (1999) 1367–1377.

[231] M. Chesi, P.L. Bergsagel, L.A. Brents, C.M. Smith, D.S. Gerhard, W.M. Kuehl, Dysregulation of cyclin D1 by translocation into an IgH gamma switch region in two multiple myeloma cell lines, *Blood* **88** (1996) 674–681.

[232] J.A. Diehl, Cycling to cancer with cyclin D1, *Cancer Biol. Ther.* **1** (2002) 226–231, https://doi.org/10.4161/cbt.72.

[233] M. Shintani, et al., Overexpression of cyclin DI contributes to malignant properties of esophageal tumor cells by increasing VEGF production and decreasing Fas expression, *Anticancer Res.* **22** (2002) 639–647.

[234] F. Lu, A.B. Gladden, J.A. Diehl, An alternatively spliced cyclin D1 isoform, cyclin D1b, is a nuclear oncogene, *Cancer Res.* **63** (2003) 7056–7061.

[235] P. Jares, D. Colomer, E. Campo, Genetic and molecular pathogenesis of mantle cell lymphoma: Perspectives for new targeted therapeutics, *Nat. Rev. Cancer* **7** (2007) 750–762, https://doi.org/10.1038/nrc2230.

[236] G.R. Thomas, H. Nadiminti, J. Regalado, Molecular predictors of clinical outcome in patients with head and neck squamous cell carcinoma, *Int. J. Exp. Pathol.* **86** (2005) 347–363, https://doi.org/10.1111/j.0959-9673.2005.00447.x.

[237] M. Jin, et al., Cyclin D1, p16 and retinoblastoma gene product expression as a predictor for prognosis in non-small cell lung cancer at stages I and II, *Lung Cancer* **34** (2001) 207–218, https://doi.org/10.1016/S0169-5002(01)00225-2.

[238] H. Yamanouchi, et al., Expression of cyclin E and cyclin D1 in non-small cell lung cancers, *Lung Cancer* **31** (2001) 3–8, https://doi.org/10.1016/S0169-5002(00)00160-4.

[239] S. Gansauge, et al., Overexpression of cyclin D1 in human pancreatic carcinoma is associated with poor prognosis, *Cancer Res.* **57** (1997) 1634–1637.

[240] M. Hall, G. Peters, Genetic alterations of cyclins, cyclin-dependent kinases, and Cdk inhibitors in human cancer, *Adv. Cancer Res.* **68** (1996) 67–108.

[241] D.J. Simpson, et al., Aberrant expression of G_1/S regulators is a frequent event in sporadic pituitary adenomas, *Carcinogenesis* **22** (2001) 1149–1154.

[242] N.A. Hibberts, et al., Analysis of cyclin D1 (*CCND1*) allelic imbalance and overexpression in sporadic human

pituitary tumors, *Clin. Cancer Res.* **5** (1999) 2133–2139.

[243] V. Fantl, R. Smith, S. Brookes, C. Dickson, G. Peters, Chromosome 11q13 abnormalities in human breast cancer, *Cancer Surv.* **18** (1993) 77–94.

[244] D.M. Barnes, C.E. Gillett, Cyclin D1 in breast cancer, *Breast Cancer Res. Treat.* **52** (1998) 1–15.

[245] A. Arnold, A. Papanikolaou, Cyclin D1 in breast cancer pathogenesis, *J. Clin. Oncol.* **23** (2005) 4215–4224, https://doi.org/10.1200/JCO.2005.05.064.

[246] F.S. Kenny, et al., Overexpression of cyclin D1 messenger RNA predicts for poor prognosis in estrogen receptor-positive breast cancer, *Clin. Cancer Res.* **5** (1999) 2069–2076.

[247] M. Stendahl, Å. Kronblad, L. Rydén, S. Emdin, N.O. Bengtsson, G. Landberg, Cyclin D1 overexpression is a negative predictive factor for tamoxifen response in postmenopausal breast cancer patients, *Br. J. Cancer* **90** (2004) 1942–1948.

[248] V. Sandor, et al., P21-dependent G1 arrest with downregulation of cyclin D1 and upregulation of cyclin E by the histone deacetylase inhibitor FR901228, *Br. J. Cancer* **83** (2000) 817–825.

[249] J.F.R. Kerr, A.H. Wyllie, A.R. Currie, Apoptosis: A basic biological phenomenon with wide-ranging implications in tissue kinetics, *Br. J. Cancer* **26** (1972) 239–257.

[250] Z. Huang, The chemical biology of apoptosis: Exploring protein-protein interactions and the life and death of cells with small molecules, *Chem. Biol. (Cell Chem. Biol.)* **9** (2002) 1059–1072.

[251] R.S.Y. Wong, Apoptosis in cancer: From pathogenesis to treatment, *J. Exp. Clin. Cancer Res.* **30** (2011), 87, https://doi.org/10.1186/1756-9966-30-87.

[252] S. Elmore, Apoptosis: A review of programmed cell death, *Toxicol. Pathol.* **35** (2007) 495–516.

[253] G.C. Cavalcante, et al., A cell's fate: An overview of the molecular biology and genetics of apoptosis, *Int. J. Mol. Sci.* **20** (2019), 4133, https://doi.org/10.3390/ijms20174133.

[254] G. Chen, D.V. Goeddel, TNF-R1 signaling: A beautiful pathway, *Science* **296** (2002) 1634–1635.

[255] H. Wajant, The Fas signaling pathway: More than a paradigm, *Science* **296** (2002) 1635–1636.

[256] H. Li, H. Zhu, C.-j. Xu, J. Yuan, Cleavage of BID by caspase 8 mediates the mitochondrial damage in the Fas pathway of apoptosis, *Cell* **94** (1998) 491–501.

[257] S.B. Bratton, G.S. Salvesen, Regulation of the Apaf-1−caspase-9 apoptosome, *J. Cell Sci.* **123** (2010) 3209−3214, https://doi.org/10.1242/jcs.073643.

[258] T.C. Cheng, C. Hong, I.V. Akey, S. Yuan, C.W. Akey, A near atomic structure of the active human apoptosome, *eLife* **5** (2016), e17755, https://doi.org/10.7554/eLife.17755.

[259] R.J. Youle, A. Strasser, The BCL-2 protein family: Opposing activities that mediate cell death, *Nat. Rev. Mol. Cell Biol.* **9** (2008) 47–59.

[260] S. Uppuluri, L. Knipling, D.L. Sackett, J. Wolf, Localization of the colchicine-binding site of tubulin, *Proc. Natl. Acad. Sci. U. S. A.* **90** (1993) 11598–11602.

[261] J.M. Andreu, B. Perez-Ramirez, M.J. Gorbunoff, D. Ayala, S.N. Timasheff, Role of the colchicine ring A

and its methoxy groups in the binding to tubulin and microtubule inhibition, *Biochemistry* **37** (1998) 8356–8368.

[262] R. Bai, et al., Mapping the binding site of colchicinoids on β-tubulin. 2-Chloroacetyl-2-demethylthiocolchicine covalently reacts predominantly with cysteine 239 and secondarily with cysteine 354, *J. Biol. Chem.* **275** (2000) 40443–40452.

[263] R.B.G. Ravelli, et al., Insight into tubulin regulation from a complex with colchicine and a stathmin-like domain, *Nature* **428** (2004) 198–202.

[264] Y. Wang, et al., Structures of a diverse set of colchicine binding site inhibitors in complex with tubulin provide a rationale for drug discovery, *FEBS J.* **283** (2016) 102–111, https://doi.org/10.1111/febs.13555.

[265] E.C. McLoughlin, N.M. O'Boyle, Colchicine-binding site inhibitors from chemistry to clinic: A review, *Pharmaceuticals* **13** (2020), 8, https://doi.org/10.3390/ph13010008; Correction: *Pharmaceuticals* **13** (2020), 72, https://doi.org/10.3390/ph13040072.

[266] K.O. Alfarouk, et al., Glycolysis, tumor metabolism, cancer growth and dissemination. A new pH-based etiopathogenic perspective and therapeutic approach to an old cancer question, *Oncoscience* **1** (2014) 777–802, https://doi.org/10.18632/oncoscience.109; Erratum: *Oncoscience* **2** (2015) 317–317, https://doi.org/10.18632/oncoscience.158.

[267] R.M. Pascale, D.F. Calvisi, M.M. Simile, C.F. Feo, F. Feo, The Warburg effect 97 years after its discovery, *Cancers (Basel)* **12** (2020), 2819, https://doi.org/10.3390/cancers12102819.

[268] C. Liu, Y. Jin, Z. Fan, Mechanism of Warburg effect-induced chemoresistance in cancer, *Front. Oncol.* **11** (2021), 698023, https://doi.org/10.3389/fonc.2021.698023.

[269] A. Sapandowski, et al., Cardiolipin composition correlates with prostate cancer cell proliferation, *Mol. Cell. Biochem.* **410** (2015) 175–185, https://doi.org/10.1007/s11010-015-2549-1.

[270] S.T. Ahmadpour, K. Mahéo, S. Servais, L. Brisson, J.-F. Dumas, Cardiolipin, the mitochondrial signature lipid: Implication in cancer, *Int. J. Mol. Sci.* **21** (2020), 8031, https://doi.org/10.3390/ijms21218031.

[271] C. Di Carlo, et al., Integrated lipidomics and proteomics reveal cardiolipin alterations, upregulation of HADHA and long chain fatty acids in pancreatic cancer stem cells, *Sci. Rep.* **11** (2021), 13297, https://doi.org/10.1038/s41598-021-92752-5.

[272] A.C. Krieger, L.A. Macias, J.C. Goodman, J.S. Brodbelt, L.S. Eberlin, Mass spectrometry imaging reveals abnormalities in cardiolipin composition and distribution in astrocytoma tumor tissues, *Cancers (Basel)* **15** (2023), 2842, https://doi.org/10.3390/cancers15102842.

THE DRUG **PT162** (**NSC 796018**)

1. PT162 (NSC 796018)

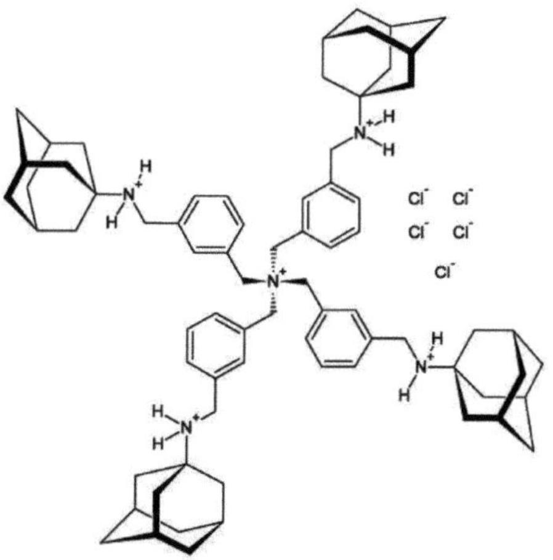

Fig. 1. The organic chemical structure formula of compound **1** [**PT162** (**NSC 796018**)]. Four adamantan-1-ammonium cages are included within.

1.1. The synthesis of salt-containing **PT162** (**PENTA**)

To find a potential complexation and/or stablization partner for retinazone [1,2], an attempt was made to synthesize a polyammonium polycation from the adamantane [3]-derived influenza A virus inhibitor [4] and *N*-methyl-D-aspartate (NMDA) subtype glutamate receptor antagonist [5] amantadine × HCl. For that purpose 1-aminoadamantane hydrochloride and an 1.5-fold molar excess of 1,3-bis(chloromethyl)benzene were dissolved in aqueous ethanol.

A solution of sodium hydroxide in water (3-fold molar excess) was added and the mixture was refluxed for 3 h. Successively acetone was added through the reflux condensor. After filtration, dilution with water, acidification with HCl and volume reduction, the reaction mixture was extracted with ethyl acetate to remove unreacted 1,3-bis(chloromethyl)benzene. Following additional volume reduction of the aqueous phase a crude product could be isolated by freezing. The crude product was dissolved in refluxing aqueous acetone and was hot filtrated. The filtrate was evaporated from the acetone and was acidified with HCl. Instantly, a white precipitate formed which represented the salt-containing **PT162** (**PENTA**).

1.2. The synthesis of pure **PT162** (**NSC 796018**)

Pure compound **1** [**PT162** (**NSC 796018**)] (Fig. 1) was synthesized from 1-aminoadamantane (amantadine) with 1,3-bis(chloromethyl)benzene (α,α'-dichloro-*m*-xylene) in refluxing absolute ethanol. Compound **1** [**PT162** (**NSC 796018**)] was a by-product of the synthesis obtained in 12.4% yield. The lipophilic main product was not isolated and removed by extraction with ethyl acetate. Crucial for successful synthesis of compound **1** was to utilize the free base 1-aminoadamantane instead of its commercial hydrochloride. Preceding synthesis, the free base 1-aminoadamantane was prepared from the hydrochloride by neutralization with NaOH, and this free base was used *in situ* for synthesis of compound **1** [**PT162** (**NSC 796018**)].

1.3. Structure elucidation of **PT162**

According to the structure elucidation by nuclear magnetic resonance (NMR) spectroscopy compound **1** [**PT162** (**NSC 796018**)] was obviously formed from

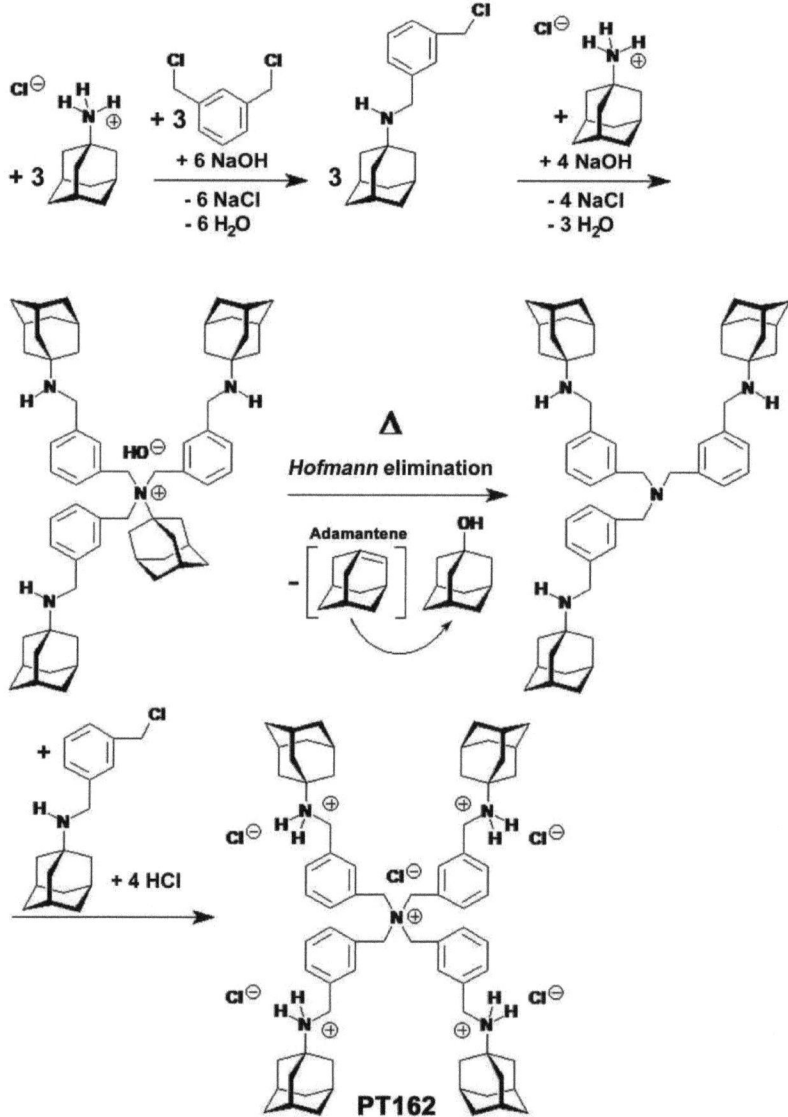

Fig. 2. The synthesis of the polyammonium polycation **PT162** from 1-aminoadamantane × HCl and 1,3-bis(chloromethyl)benzene. The intermediate *N*-[3-(chloromethyl)benzyl]-1-adamantanamine reacted with amantadine × HCl under influence of NaOH to *N,N,N*-tris{3-

[(tricyclo[3.3.1.1^{3,7}]decan-1-ylamino)methyl]benzyl}-1-adamantanammonium hydroxide, which in turn underwent *Hofmann* elimination [6] on heating at reflux under elimination of 1-adamantanol (produced from adamantene [7–9]). **PT162** resulted from quaternarization with another molecule *N*-[3-(chloromethyl)benzyl]-1-adamantanamine and acidification with hydrochloric acid (HCl).

the intermediate *N*-[3-(chloromethyl)benzyl]-1-adamantanamine (Fig. 2). The latter intermediate very probably quaternarized 1-aminoadamantane to give *N,N,N*-tris{3-[(tricyclo[3.3.1.1^{3,7}]decan-1-ylamino)methyl]benzyl}-1-adamantanammonium hydroxide (Fig. 2), which underwent *Hofmann* elimination [6] with 1-adamantanol being expelled. 1-Adamantanol is produced from adamantene, a known reaction intermediate [7–9]. The resulting tris{3-[(tricyclo[3.3.1.1^{3,7}]decan-1-ammonio)methyl]benzyl}amine in turn was quaternarized by *N*-[3-(chloromethyl)benzyl]-1-adamantanamine to yield, after acidification with HCl, tetrakis{3-[(tricyclo[3.3.1.1^{3,7}]decan-1-ammonio)methyl] benzyl}ammonium pentachloride {compound **1 [PT162 (NSC 796018)]**} (Fig. 2). The structure of salt-containing **PT162 (PENTA)** was secured by analysis of its ^{1}H- (Fig. 3) and ^{13}C-NMR (Fig. 4) spectra recorded in DMSO-d_6. The proton NMR of the aliphatic part of salt-containing **PT162 (PENTA)** was analysed for (Fig. 3): δ 1.62 (3 H, d; $^2J_{gem}$ = −12.1 Hz; δ-CH$_{axial}$), 1.69 (3 H, d; $^2J_{gem}$ = −12.4 Hz; δ-CH$_{equatorial}$), 2.02 (6 H, s; β-CH$_2$), 2.15 (3 H, s; γ-CH), 4.10 (2 H, t; $^3J_{vicinal}$ = 6.3 Hz; 8-CH$_2$), 4.78 (2 H, s; 7-CH$_2$). The proton NMR of the aromatic part of salt-containing **PT162 (PENTA)** was analysed for: δ 7.42–7.49 (2 H, m; H-4, H-6), 7.65 (1 H, d; $^3J_{ortho}$ = 7.1 Hz; H-5), 7.69 (1 H, s; H-2). The three axial δ-protons of the adamantane cage were split from the corresponding three equatorial δ-protons. A broad ammonium resonance was found at δ 9.24 (2 H, br s; 8-NH$_2^+$ ammonium). The aliphatic resonances contained an adamantane part,

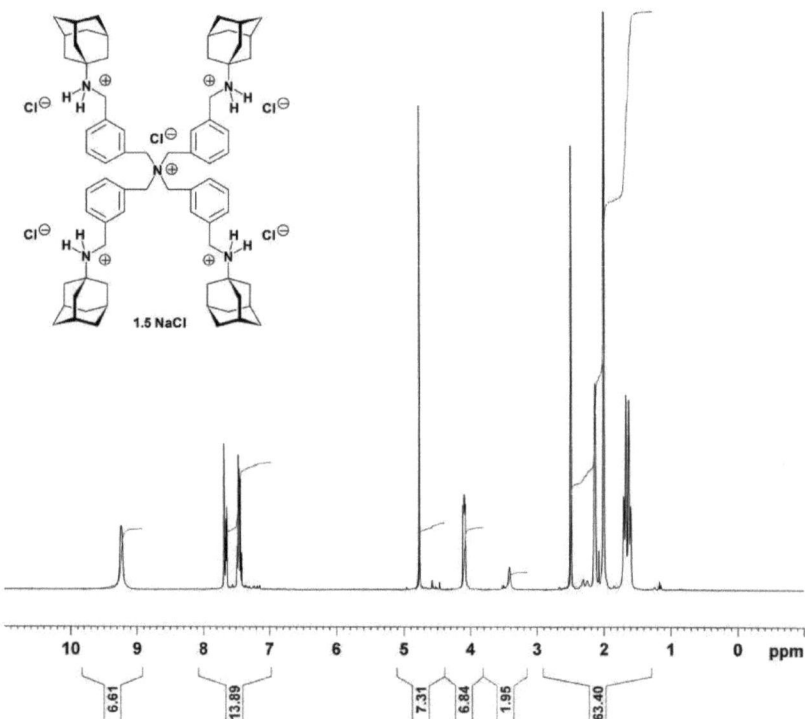

Fig. 3. The 400.13 MHz ^{1}H-NMR spectrum (in DMSO-d_6) of the salt-containing polyammonium polycation tetrakis{3-[(tricyclo[3.3.1.1^{3,7}]decan-1-ammonio)methyl]benzyl}ammonium pentachloride × 1.5 (sodium chloride) = salt-containing **PT162** (**PENTA**).

two methylene groups and an ammonium resonance in the integrated proton ratio 15 : 2 : 2 : 2. This pointed to a symmetric ammonium molecule with two different *m*-xylylene methylene groups which were derived from 1,3-bis(chloromethyl)benzene (*m*-xylylene dichloride). Obviously, the ammonium resonance originated from an (1-adamantyl-NH$_2$-*R*)$^+$ system. Therefore, only two reasonable possibilities for the structure of compound **1** (**PT162**) remained. The first would be di{3-[(tricyclo[3.3.1.1^{3,7}]decan-

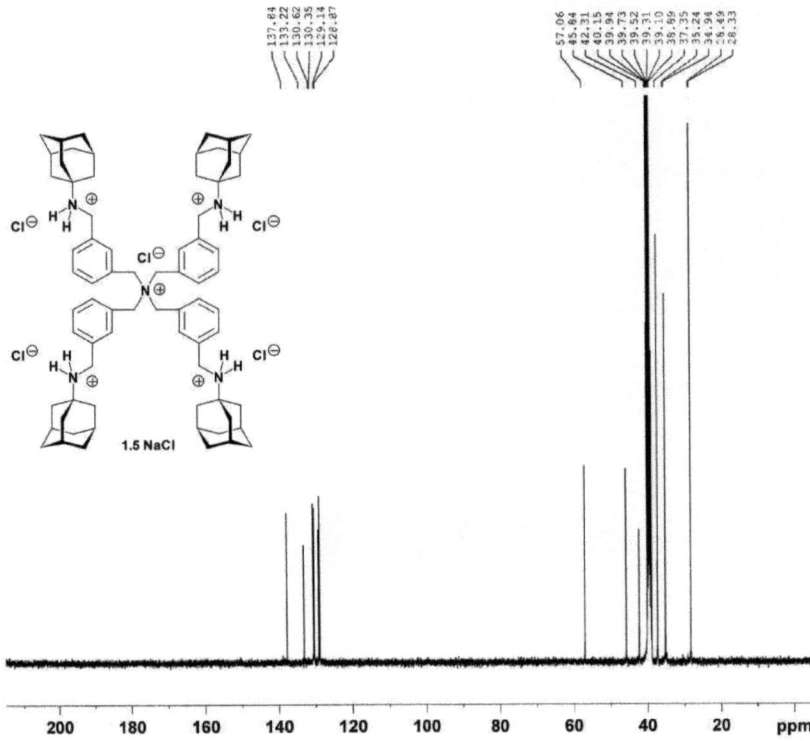

Fig. 4. The 100.62 MHz ^{13}C-NMR spectrum (in DMSO-d_6) of the salt-containing polyammonium polycation tetrakis{3-[(tricyclo[3.3.1.1^{3,7}] decan-1-ammonio)methyl]benzyl}ammonium pentachloride × 1.5 (sodium chloride) = salt-containing **PT162 (PENTA)**.

1-ammonio)methyl]benzyl}ether dichloride (Fig. 5), the second being expressed by the already given formula (Fig. 1). The former structure could be ruled out for the following reasons: (i) the oxygen elemental analysis of salt-containing **PT162 (PENTA)** showed only trace amounts of oxygen ($w \leq 0.82\%$) resulting from the ethanol and acetone traces contained in salt-containing **PT162 (PENTA)**, (ii) the absence of a commonly very strong dibenzyl ether band in the FT–IR spectrum (Fig. 6) expected at $\tilde{\nu}$ 1090 cm^{-1} for dibenzyl

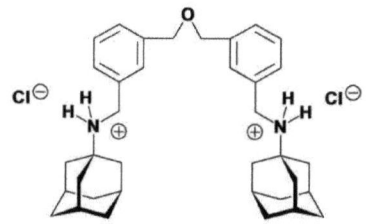

Fig. 5. The structure of the dibenzyl ether derivative di{3-[(tricyclo[3.3.1.1^{3,7}]decan-1-ammonio)methyl]benzyl}ether dichloride. This hypothetical structure was considered as alternative reaction product in the synthesis of **PT162**.

ether [10], (iii) the downfield methylene δ 4.78 (2 H, s; 7-CH$_2$) did not match the typical dibenzyl ether chemical shift found at δ 4.54 ppm (in CDCl$_3$) [11], and (iv) the analysis of the carbon-13 NMR spectrum of salt-containing **PT162** (**PENTA**) (Fig. 4). The ^{13}C-NMR of the aliphatic part of salt-containing **PT162** (**PENTA**) was analysed for: δ 28.50 (γ-CH), 35.25 (δ-CH$_2$), 37.35 (β-CH$_2$), 42.31 (8-CH$_2$), 45.84 (7-CH$_2$), 57.06 (α-C). The ^{13}C-NMR of the aromatic part of salt-containing **PT162** (**PENTA**) was analysed for: δ 128.87 (C-4)*, 129.14 (C-6)*, 130.36 (C-2)*, 130.62 (C-5)*, 133.22 (C-3), 137.84 (C-1). The starred assignments are tentative and interchangeable (they could not be assigned unequivocally to the individual carbons). Clearly the structure proof could be gained by looking at the downfield methylene δ 45.84 (7-CH$_2$) which did not fit the typical dibenzyl ether α-CH$_2$ chemical shift found at δ 72.10 ppm (in CDCl$_3$) [11]. The 100.62 MHz ^{13}C-<u>D</u>istortionless <u>E</u>nhancement by <u>P</u>olarization <u>T</u>ransfer Including Detection of <u>Q</u>uaternary Nuclei (DEPTQ) [12,13] (DEPTQ ^{13}C-NMR) subspectrum (in DMSO-d_6) of salt-containing **PT162** (**PENTA**) (Fig. 7) secured the given CH$_2$ assignments, and proved that the resonance at δ 57.06 ppm originated from a quaternary carbon. The assignments were further verified by analysis of the gradient-selected <u>C</u>orrelation <u>S</u>pectroscop<u>y</u> (gs-COSY) two-dimensional ^{1}H–^{1}H-correlation spectrum [13] (Fig. 8), the gradient-selected <u>H</u>eteronuclear <u>M</u>ultiple <u>Q</u>uantum <u>C</u>oherence (gs-

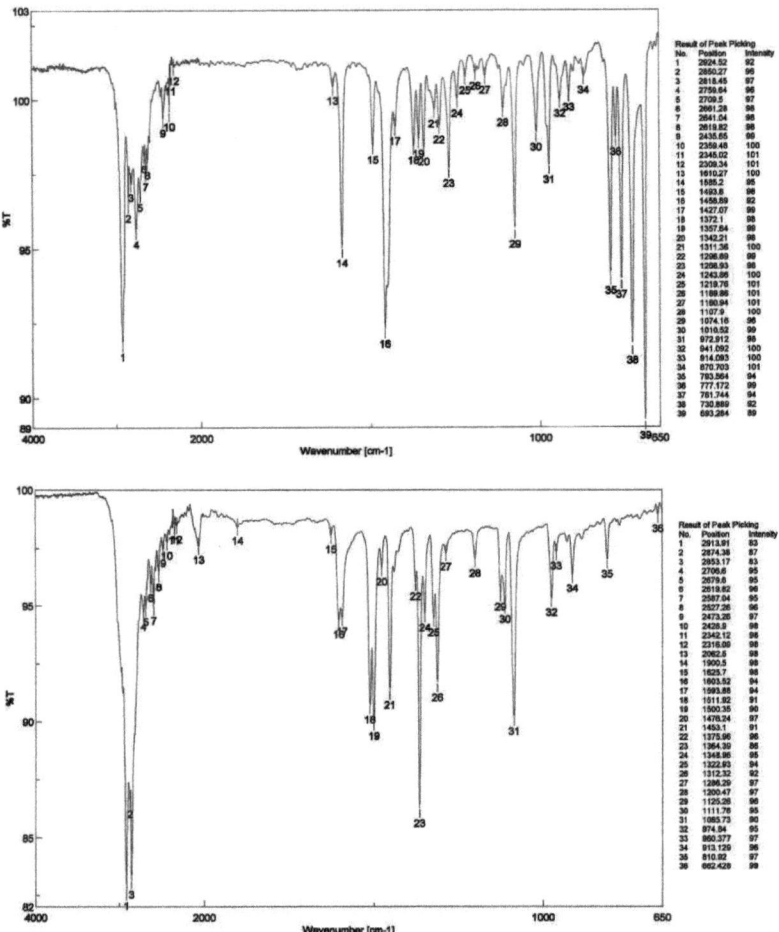

Fig. 6. The *Fourier*–transform infrared (FT–IR) absorption spectra of the salt-containing tetrakis{3-[(tricyclo[3.3.1.1^{3,7}]decan-1-ammonio)methyl] benzyl}ammonium pentachloride × 1.5 (sodium chloride) = salt-containing **PT162** (**PENTA**) (top), and of the reference substance amantadine hydrochloride (1-adamantanammonium chloride) (bottom), both recorded with neat substance.

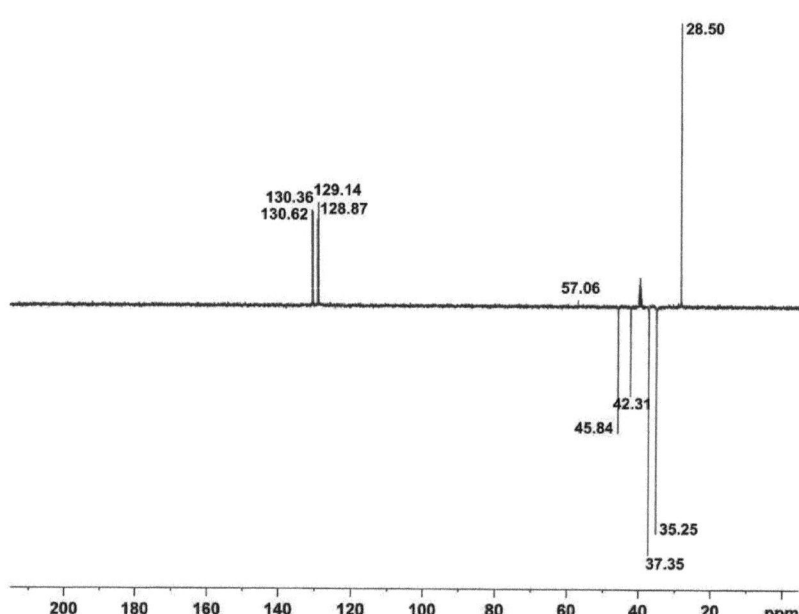

Fig. 7. The 100.62 MHz ^{13}C-$\underline{D}$istortionless $\underline{E}$nhancement by $\underline{P}$olarization $\underline{T}$ransfer Including Detection of $\underline{Q}$uaternary Nuclei (DEPTQ) [12,13] (DEPTQ ^{13}C-NMR) spectrum (in DMSO-d_6) of the salt-containing polyammonium polycation tetrakis{3-[(tricyclo[3.3.1.1^{3,7}]decan-1-ammonio)methyl]benzyl}ammonium pentachloride × 1.5 (sodium chloride) = salt-containing **PT162** (**PENTA**). Quaternary carbons (C), methine (CH) and methyl (CH$_3$) group moieties are of positive phase, methylene (CH$_2$) group moieties are of negative phase. The quaternary carbon δ 57.06 ppm (α-C) is weak in intensity. The aromatic quaternary carbons δ 133.22 ppm (C-3) and 137.84 ppm (C-1) could not being detected.

HMQC) [13] (Fig. 9), and the gradient-selected $\underline{H}$eteronuclear $\underline{M}$ultiple $\underline{B}$ond $\underline{C}$orrelation (gs-HMBC) [13] (Fig. 10) two-dimensional ^{1}H–^{13}C-correlation spectra of salt-containing **PT162** (**PENTA**).

Conclusively, the second structure possibility, the true formula, must be depicted by **PT162** (Fig. 1), because all

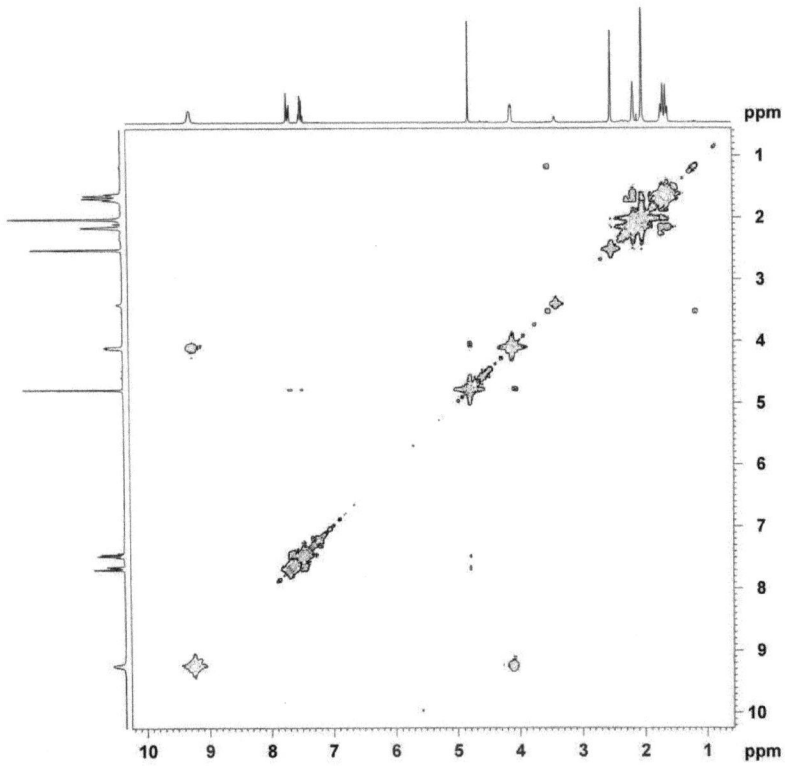

Fig. 8. The 400.13 MHz gradient-selected <u>C</u>orrelation <u>S</u>pectroscopy (gs-COSY) two-dimensional ^1H–^1H-correlation spectrum [13] (in DMSO-d_6) of the salt-containing polyammonium polycation tetrakis{3-[(tricyclo[3.3.1.1^{3,7}]decan-1-ammonio)methyl]benzyl}ammonium penta-chloride × 1.5 (sodium chloride) = salt-containing **PT162** (**PENTA**).

other possibilities would not agree with the unequivocal NMR data. Finally, the FT–IR spectrum of salt-containing **PT162** (**PENTA**) was compared to the corresponding spectrum of amantadine hydrochloride (Fig. 6). Certain characteristics shared by both spectra could be recognized. The strong absorption band in salt-containing **PT162** (**PENTA**) at $\tilde{v}$ 2925/2850 cm^{-1} was created by aliphatic v(C–H) stretching vibrations. In amantadine hydrochloride this absorption could

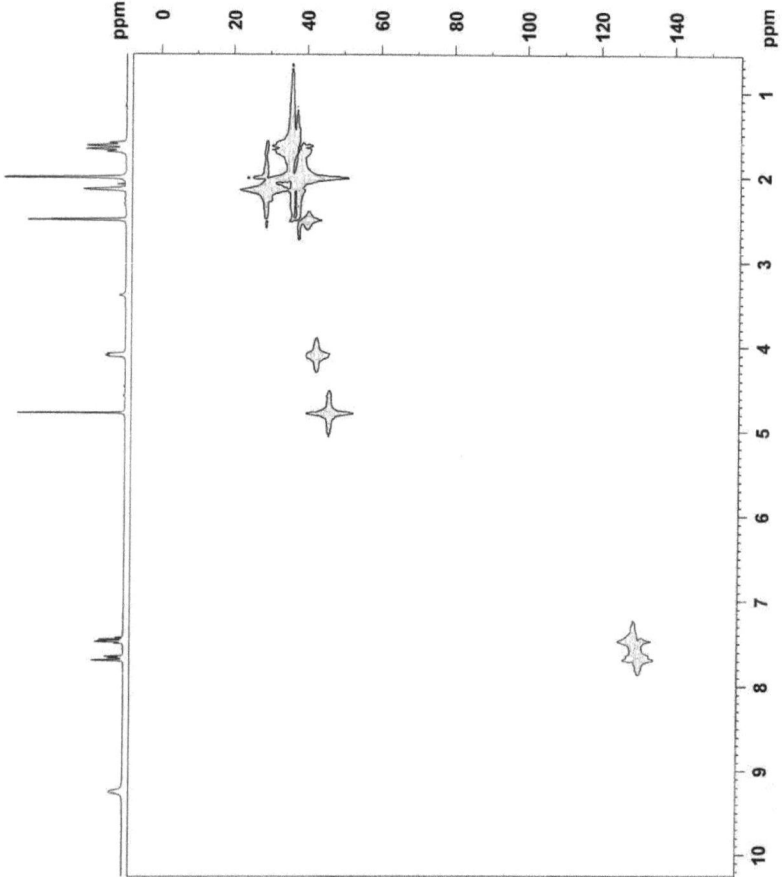

Fig. 9. The 400.13/100.62 MHz gradient-selected <u>H</u>eteronuclear <u>M</u>ultiple <u>Q</u>uantum <u>C</u>oherence (gs-HMQC) two-dimensional ^{1}H–^{13}C-correlation spectrum [13] (in DMSO-d_6) of the salt-containing polyammonium polycation tetrakis{3-[(tricyclo[3.3.1.1^{3,7}]decan-1-ammonio)methyl] benzyl}ammonium pentachloride × 1.5 (sodium chloride) = salt-containing **PT162** (**PENTA**).

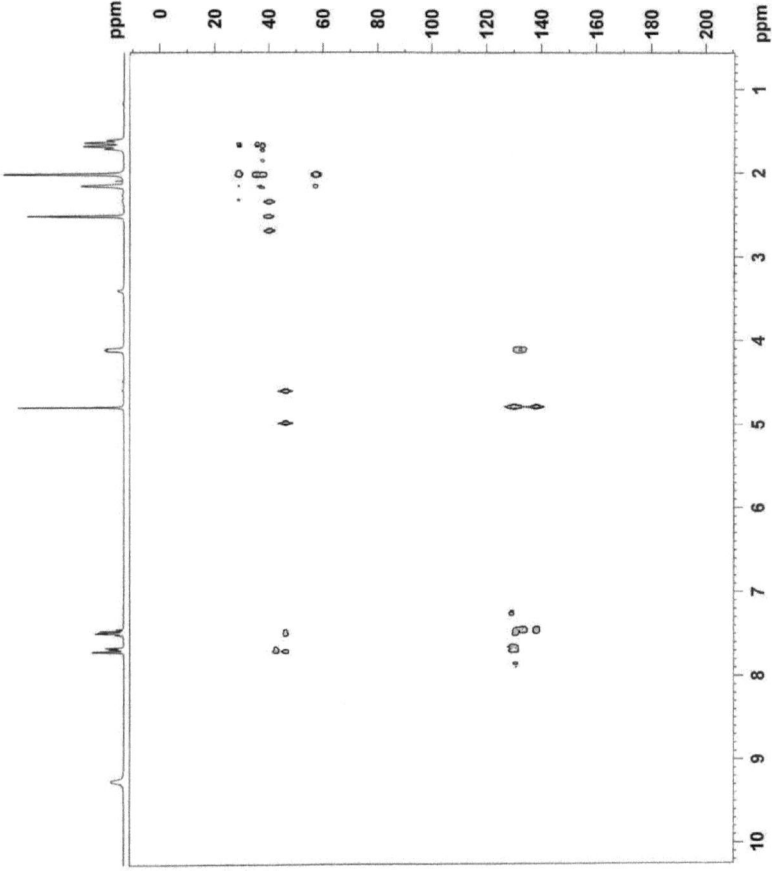

Fig. 10. The 400.13/100.62 MHz gradient-selected <u>H</u>eteronuclear <u>M</u>ultiple <u>B</u>ond <u>C</u>orrelation (gs-HMBC) two-dimensional ^{1}H–^{13}C-correlation spectrum [13] (in DMSO-d_6) of the salt-containing polyammonium polycation tetrakis{3-[(tricyclo[3.3.1.1^{3,7}]decan-1-ammonio)methyl] benzyl}ammonium pentachloride × 1.5 (sodium chloride) = salt-containing **PT162 (PENTA)**.

Fig. 11 (next page). The 700.43 MHz ^{1}H-NMR spectrum (in DMSO-d_6) of the pure polyammonium polycation tetrakis{3-[(tricyclo[3.3.1.1^{3,7}] decan-1-ammonio)methyl]benzyl}ammonium pentachloride = pure (salt-free) compound **1** [**PT162 (NSC 796018)**].

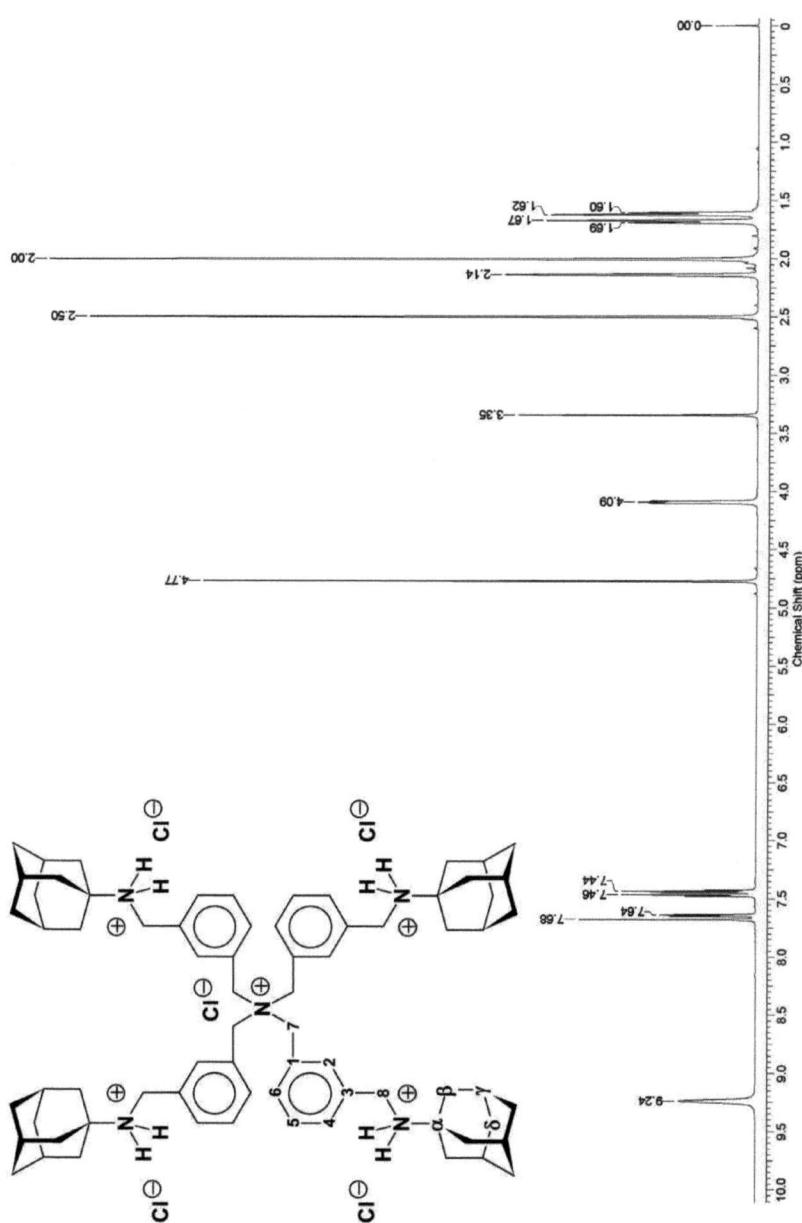

be found at $\tilde{v}$ 2914/2853 cm^{-1}. Aliphatic progression bands associated to these peaks could be found in both spectra. These absorptions mainly could be ascribed to the adamantane cages present in both compounds. Typical bands were found at $\tilde{v}$ 1610/1585/1459/1074 cm^{-1} [salt-containing **PT162** (**PENTA**)], in amantadine hydrochloride at $\tilde{v}$ 1626/1594/1500/1086 cm^{-1}. They probably originate from the 1-adamantanammonium structure shared by both compounds. In addition, salt-containing **PT162** (**PENTA**) clearly showed the *m*-xylylene aromatic linker resonances at $\tilde{v}$ 794/762/731/693 cm^{-1} which are not seen with amantadine hydrochloride.

The elemental analysis of salt-containing **PT162** (**PENTA**) revealed its sodium chloride content by calculating within ±0.3% for carbon and hydrogen. The NaCl obviously was co-precipitated in the final isolation step, which is not surprising when considering the polyammonium chloride character of **PT162**. The nitrogen value was found to be 1.13% lower than calculated for $C_{72}H_{100}N_5Cl_5 \times 1.5$ NaCl. The reason for this deficit could be the $[N(CH_2R)_4]^+$ tetrasubstituted ammonium structure of the central ammonium nitrogen. Compounds of this type are known to cause combustion problems [14]. It could be speculated that the sodium content (NaCl) in salt-containing **PT162** (**PENTA**) led to formation of only partially combustible sodium nitrate (NaNO$_3$). Mutually both effects could be responsible for the wrong nitrogen analysis of salt-containing **PT162** (**PENTA**). Since the other analytical data of salt-containing **PT162** (**PENTA**) are all very conclusive, the unsatisfactory nitrogen analysis should not be overrated. Taken together, the structure of salt-containing **PT162** (**PENTA**) could be demonstrated without doubt, especially when evaluating the unequivocal NMR data.

The structure of pure (salt-free) compound **1** [**PT162** (**NSC 796018**)] was secured by ^{1}H-NMR (Fig. 11) and ^{13}C-DEPTQ (data not shown) spectroscopy experiments, as well as elemental analysis and FT–IR spectroscopy. By ^{1}H-NMR, through the integration of the proton resonance peaks, and by ^{13}C-NMR, the highly symmetric structure of compound **1** [**PT162** (**NSC 796018**)] was proved. Compound **1** [**PT162** (**NSC 796018**)] represents a pentaammonium cation with a quaternary center and four secondary amine functions. The four functional bridges are *m*-xylylene linkers which connect the central quaternary ammonium cation chloride with four *N*-substituted 1-adamantanammonium chloride moieties. The resulting chemical structure of compound **1** is given (Fig. 1). Compound **1** was registered by the National Cancer Institute (NCI) as **NSC 796018**.

2. References

[1]   A.J. Kesel, Broad-spectrum antiviral activity including human immunodeficiency and hepatitis C viruses mediated by a novel retinoid thiosemicarbazone derivative, *Eur. J. Med. Chem.* **46** (2011) 1656–1664.

[2]   A.J. Kesel, et al., Retinazone inhibits certain blood-borne human viruses including Ebola virus Zaire, *Antivir. Chem. Chemother.* **23** (2014) 197–215.

[3]   S. Landa, V. Macháček, Sur l'adamantane, nouvel hydrocarbure extrait du naphte, *Coll. Czech. Chem. Commun.* **5** (1933) 1–5.

[4]   W.L. Davies, et al., Antiviral activity of 1-adamantanamine (amantadine), *Science* **144** (1964) 862–863.

[5]   W. Danysz, C.G. Parsons, J. Kornhuber, W.J. Schmidt, G. Quack, Aminoadamantanes as NMDA receptor

antagonists and antiparkinsonian agents – Preclinical studies, *Neurosci. Biobehav. Rev.* **21** (1997) 455–468.

[6] A.W. Hofmann, Einwirkung der Wärme auf die Ammoniumbasen, *Ber. dtsch. chem. Ges.* **14** (1881) 659–669.

[7] J.E. Gano, L. Eizenberg, Short-lived intermediates. IV. Adamantene, *J. Am. Chem. Soc.* **95** (1973) 972–974.

[8] N. Bian, M. Jones Jr., More on adamantene, *J. Am. Chem. Soc.* **117** (1995) 8957–8961.

[9] E.L. Tae, Z. Zhu, M.S. Platz, A matrix isolation, laser flash photolysis, and computational study of adamantene, *J. Phys. Chem. A* **105** (2001) 3803–3807.

[10] J.Y. Baek, S.J. Lee, B.H. Han, Direct synthesis of symmetric ethers from carbonyl compounds using $SbI_3/PhSiH_3$, *J. Korean Chem. Soc.* **48** (2004) 220–224.

[11] T. Nishiyama, H. Kameyama, H. Maekawa, K. Watanuki, Ether synthesis using trifluoromethane-sulfonic anhydride or triflates under mild reaction conditions, *Can. J. Chem.* **77** (1999) 258–262.

[12] R. Burger, P. Bigler, DEPTQ: Distorsionless enhancement by polarization transfer including the detection of quaternary nuclei, *J. Magn. Res.* **135** (1998) 529–534.

[13] S. Berger, S. Braun, 200 and more NMR experiments. A practical course, 1st ed., Wiley-VCH Verlag GmbH & Co. KGaA, Weinheim, 2004, 854 pp., ISBN 978-3527310678.

[14] E. Kozłowski, M. Biziuk, A new method for simultaneous determination of nitrogen, hydrogen and halogen in organic compounds, *Mikrochim. Acta (Wien)* **72** (1979) 1–17, https://doi.org/10.1007/BF01198043.

CHAPTER TWO

THE DRUG **PT166 (NSC 750423)**

1. PT166 (NSC 750423)

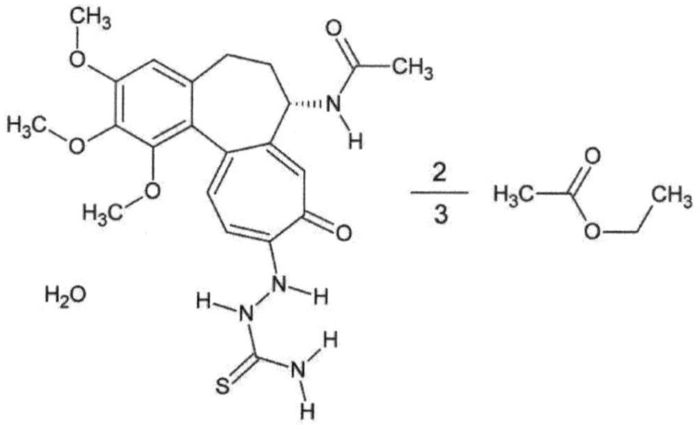

Fig. 12. The organic chemical structure formula of compound **2** [**PT166** (**NSC 750423**)]. It contains a water of crystallization and ⅔ (ethyl acetate).

1.1. The synthesis of drug **PT166 (NSC 750423)**

Compound **2** [**PT166** (**NSC 750423**)] was synthesized from (–)-colchicine sesquihydrate (× 1½ H_2O) and thiosemicarbazide under catalysis of sodium hydroxide (NaOH) in refluxing 90% (*v*/*v*) aqueous ethanol. The structure (Fig. 1) of compound **2** [**PT166** (**NSC 750423**)] was secured by X-ray crystallography (see Chapter Two, Section 1.3.), ^{1}H-NMR (Fig. 14) and ^{13}C-NMR spectroscopy (data not shown) experiments, as well as elemental analysis and FT–IR spectroscopy (Fig. 16). The thiosemicarbazide moiety is

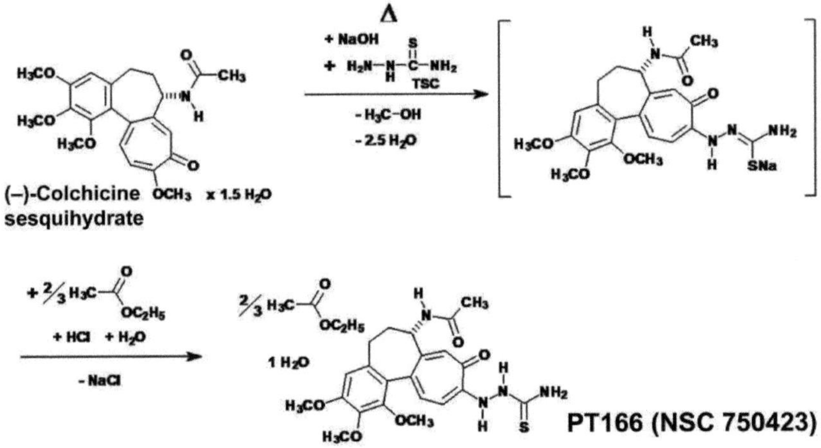

Fig. 13. The synthesis of the modified colchic(in)oid 10-(2-carbamothioylhydrazinyl)-10-demethoxycolchicine monohydrate × ⅔ (ethyl acetate) {compound **2** [**PT166 (NSC 750423)**]} by NaOH-catalyzed amidation (amino-de-alkoxylation) of the vinylogous (tropolonic) carboxylic acid methyl ester (−)-colchicine. Methanol was split off by thiosemicarbazide (TSC) from (−)-colchicine during short refluxing. Subsequently, the product compound **2** [**PT166 (NSC 750423)**] was liberated from a monosodium salt intermediate by acidification with hydrochloric acid and extraction with ethyl acetate. The term colchic(in)oid is now well accepted and documented in literature [1].

attached at the former position of the 10-methoxy group in colchicine. The point of connection is the terminal nitrogen of the hydrazinyl moiety of thiosemicarbazide. Compound **2** [**PT166 (NSC 750423)**] was registered by National Cancer Institute (NCI) as **NSC 750423**.

Equimolar quantities of (−)-colchicine and thiosemicarbazide were dissolved in 90% (*v/v*) aqueous ethanol by refluxing for 5 min. After adding a slight excess of sodium hydroxide dissolved in water, the deep orange-red solution was refluxed for 5 min. The cold deep orange-red solution, after pre-cooling, was nearly neutralized by dropwise addition of hydrochloric acid. Afterwards, the volume of the solution was reduced *in vacuo*. The reddish-brown solution was then mixed with water, and was acidified with aqueous hydrochloric acid. The oily emulsion was extracted with ethyl acetate (EtOAc). The separated aqueous layer (pH 2) was additionally extracted with a second volume of EtOAc. After neutralization of this aqueous phase with sodium hydrogen carbonate, the aqueous phase (pH 7–8) was extracted twice with EtOAc each. The EtOAc phases were combined and washed twice with water. The washed EtOAc phase, which already precipitated, was mixed with acetone and frozen at −25 °C. If precipitation did not start spontaneously, the volume of the solution was reduced *in vacuo* until coagulation started. The evolved yellow crystalline precipitate of compound **2** [**PT166** (**NSC 750423**)] was filtered and dried. From the combined aqueous phases by cooling a second crop of compound **2** [**PT166** (**NSC 750423**)] could be obtained. The underlying molecular reactions for this synthesis are pictured (Fig. 13).

Compound **2** [**PT166** (**NSC 750423**)] was quite pure as judged by ^{1}H-NMR spectroscopy. The representative ^{1}H-NMR spectrum of compound **2** [**PT166** (**NSC 750423**)] in DMSO-d_6 is pictured (Fig. 14).

1.2. The nuclear magnetic resonance spectra of **PT166**

It is known that colchic(in)oids have the tendency to retain solvents, like water [2] and/or ethyl acetate [3], very firmly. Natural (−)-colchicine itself retained chloroform [4–6], dibromomethane/diiodomethane [7], or water as dihydrate [7,8] or sesquihydrate [6,9]. Therefore, it could be understood that compound **2** [**PT166** (**NSC 750423**)] was obtained as monohydrate × ⅔ (ethyl acetate) binary solvate, as judged by ^{1}H-NMR and elemental analysis.

The ^{1}H-NMR resonances of the colchic(in)oid **62** were assigned with help of literature [10–13], especially [11] which

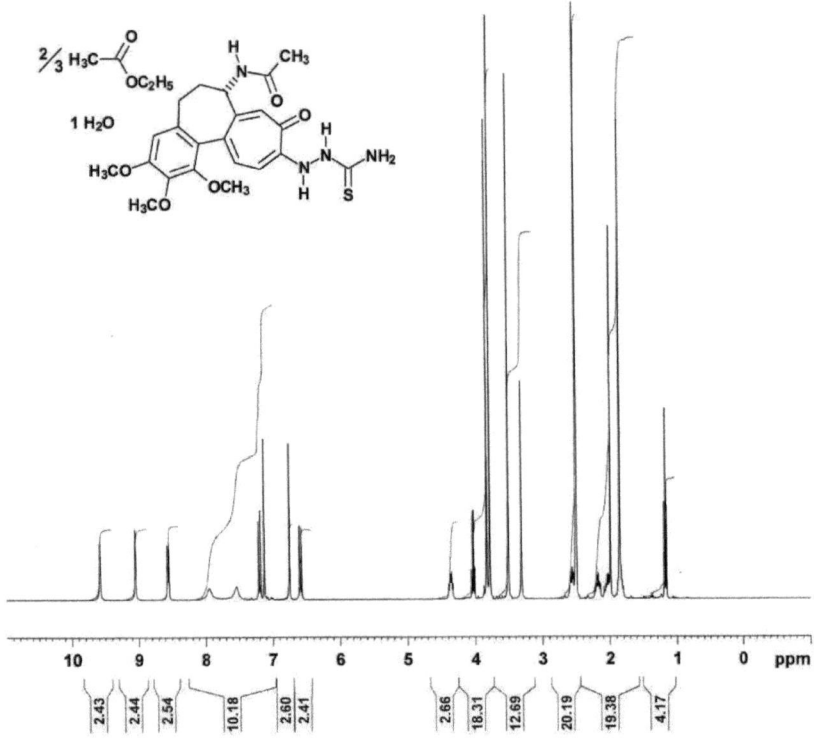

Fig. 14. The 400.13 MHz ¹H-NMR spectrum (in DMSO-d_6) of the colchic(in)oid   10-(2-carbamothioylhydrazinyl)-10-demethoxycolchicine monohydrate × ⅔ (ethyl acetate) = compound **2** [**PT166** (**NSC 750423**)]. Downfield of δ 11 ppm no resonances were detected.

gave a complete assignment of the protons in the ¹H-NMR spectrum of (–)-colchicine (in CDCl₃). Compound **2** [**PT166** (**NSC 750423**)] represents a completely new compound, never synthesized before [according to Chemical Abstracts Service (CAS) SciFinder®]. Therefore, the proton NMR spectrum (Fig. 14) of compound **2** [**PT166** (**NSC 750423**)] was interpreted by own effort to the point it was possible without doubt.

Aliphatic proton resonances of compound **2** [**PT166** (**NSC 750423**)] dissolved in DMSO-d_6 could be differentiated as: δ 1.18 (1.5 H, t; ^3J = 7.1 Hz; O–CH$_2$–CH$_3$ ethyl acetate), 1.85 (1 H, m; H$_A$-6), 1.86 (3 H, s; 17-CH$_3$), 1.99 (1.5 H, s; ROOC–CH$_3$ ethyl acetate), 2.05 (1 H, m; H$_B$-6), 2.19 (1 H, m; H$_A$-5), 2.57 (1 H, m; H$_B$-5), 3.51 (3 H, s; 13-OCH$_3$)*, 3.79 (3 H, s; 15-OCH$_3$)*, 3.83 (3 H, s; 14-OCH$_3$)*, 4.03 (1 H, q; ^3J = 7.1 Hz; O–CH$_2$–CH$_3$ ethyl acetate), 4.37 (1 H, m; H-7). The three starred assignments (*) are tentative and interchangeable [they could not be assigned unequivocally to the individual methoxyl protons, because their chemical shifts did nearly coincide (Fig. 14)]. The gradient-selected Correlation Spectroscopy (gs-COSY) two-dimensional ^{1}H–^{1}H-correlation spectrum [14] proton–proton couplings (data not shown) in connection with the gradient-selected Heteronuclear Multiple Quantum Coherence (gs-HMQC) [14] ^{13}C–^{1}H couplings (data not shown) gave the required informations to assign the proton resonances of compound **2** [**PT166** (NSC **750423**)].

Aromatic or troponic protons in compound **2** [**PT166** (NSC **750423**)] were identified as: δ 6.60 (1 H, d; ^3J = 11.1 Hz; H-11), 6.76 (1 H, s; H-4), 7.14 (1 H, s; H-8), 7.20 (1 H, d; ^3J = 10.9 Hz; H-12). The acetamide N–H, which coupled to H-7, could be recognized at δ 8.56 (1 H, d; ^3J = 7.6 Hz; N–H acetamide). Exchangeable protons of the thiosemicarbazide moiety, detectable in DMSO-d_6, could be unequivocally assigned as: δ 7.56 (1 H, br s; H$_2$N–C=S amino, 4'-H$_A$), 7.96 (1 H, br s; H$_2$N–C=S amino, 4'-H$_B$), 9.06 (1 H, s; 1'-N–H), 9.59 (1 H, s; 2'-N–H). In the gradient-selected Correlation Spectroscopy (gs-COSY) two-dimensional ^{1}H–^{1}H-correlation spectrum [14] (data not shown) of compound **2** [**PT166** (NSC **750423**)] (in DMSO-d_6) no W-shaped long-range ^4J (^{1}H–^{1}H) coupling, known as zig-zag (W) coupling, was found. This differentiates compound **2** [**PT166** (NSC **750423**)] from the thiosemicarbazones (*E*)-4-(dimethylamino)benzaldehyde thiosemicarbazone [15] and (*E*)-4-bromo-2-fluorobenzaldehyde thiosemicarbazone [15], where such a

"W" coupling was observed [15]. This pointed to sterical fixation as prerequisite for observable W couplings in (*E*)-4-(dimethylamino)benzaldehyde thiosemicarbazone and (*E*)-4-bromo-2-fluorobenzaldehyde thiosemicarbazone, which obviously is not realized in compound **2** [**PT166** (**NSC 750423**)]. This proved that compound **2** [**PT166** (**NSC 750423**)] is not a thiosemicarbazone. Furthermore, the protons of the tropone (ring C) could be unequivocally assigned, and their coupling constants secured that no benzilic-type rearrangement happened to the tropolone, a reaction seen with colchic(in)oids under certain (alkaline) conditions, leading occasionally to the rearrangement products allocolchicine (colchicic acid methyl ester) [16,17] or colchicic acid (allocolchiceine) [18], both being aromatic in ring C. Under the reaction conditions employed for the synthesis of compound **2** [**PT166** (**NSC 750423**)], the allocolchiceine sodium salt (Fig. 15) could be expected as a side product, but was not observed. This benzilic-type rearrangement (Fig. 15) was elucidated by *Šantavý* [17] and *Fernholz* [18].

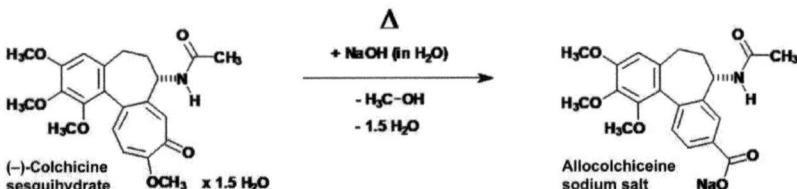

Figure 15. The possible side product in the synthesis of compound **2** [**PT166** (**NSC 750423**)], the allocolchiceine (syn. colchinoic acid, colchicinoic acid, colchicic acid) monosodium salt, originating from hydrolytic ring C contraction by a benzilic-type rearrangement.

The ^{13}C-NMR spectrum of compound **2** [**PT166** (**NSC 750423**)] in DMSO-d_6 was interpreted with help of literature data on (–)-colchicine [11] and (–)-colchiceine [19]. In addition, own experimental observations were applied in the following aliphatic carbon assignments: δ 14.05 (O–CH$_2$–CH_3 ethyl acetate), 20.72 (ROOC–CH_3 ethyl acetate), 22.49 (C-17, CH$_3$ acetamide), 29.33 (C-5), 36.34 (C-6), 51.38 (C-7), 55.84 (14-OCH$_3$)**, 59.72 (O–CH_2–CH$_3$ ethyl acetate), 60.62 (13-OCH$_3$, 15-OCH$_3$)**. The two double-starred assignments (**) are tentative and interchangeable (they could not be assigned unequivocally to the individual carbons). The aromatic and troponic carbon resonances, the carbonyl and the thiocarbonyl resonances, were detected as: δ 107.61 (C-4), 108.27 (C-11), 126.23 (C-8), 131.57 (C-1a), 134.26 (C-4a), 137.21 (C-12), 140.71 (C-3)***, 150.34 (C-1)***, 150.40 (C-10), 150.46 (C-12a), 152.61 (C-2)***, 152.73 (C-7a), 168.39 (C-16, HN–C=O amide), 170.30 (C=O ester carbonyl, ethyl acetate), 174.81 (C-9, C=O carbonyl), 181.86 (C-3', C=S thiocarbonyl). The three triple-starred resonances (***) could not being assigned unequivocally to their individual carbon.

By these analyses it was found that the amidation product of (–)-colchicine, the substituted thiosemicarbazide compound **2** [**PT166 (NSC 750423)**], was not cyclic with regard to the thiosemicarbazide unit at ring C of compound **2** [**PT166 (NSC 750423)**]. This was quite surprising, since the reaction product of (–)-colchicine with thiourea was cyclic with respect to the thiourea substitution in ring C [20,21], which seemed surprising in turn, because the tropolonic C-9 carbonyl group in (–)-colchicine did not react with common carbonyl reagents like hydroxylamine or semicarbazide [22,23]. The reason for the latter irregularity could be the special tropylium oxide resonance type of tropones and tropolones [24–28]. Therefore, the synthesis of compound **2** [**PT166 (NSC 750423)**] clearly obeyed the common rules for chemical reactivity of tropolones, whereas the synthesis of the cyclic thiourea congener [20,21] of compound **2** [**PT166**

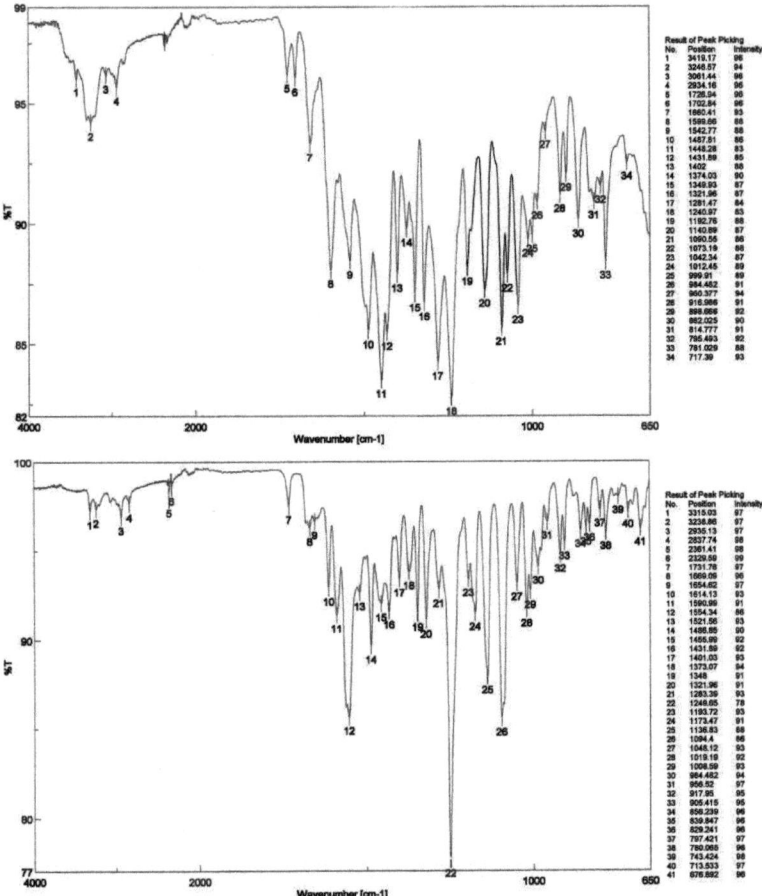

Fig. 16. The *Fourier*–transform infrared (FT–IR) absorption spectra of the colchic(in)oid   10-(2-carbamothioylhydrazinyl)-10-demethoxycolchicine monohydrate × ⅔ (ethyl acetate) = compound **2** [**PT166 (NSC 750423)**] (top), and of the reference substance (−)-colchicine sesquihydrate [(−)-colchicine × 1½ H₂O] (bottom), both recorded with neat substance.

(**NSC 750423**)] did not follow the common chemical reactivity experience for tropolones.

The *Fourier*–transform infrared (FT–IR) absorption spectra of the colchic(in)oid 10-(2-carbamothioylhydrazinyl)-10-demethoxycolchicine monohydrate × ⅔ (ethyl acetate) = compound **2** [**PT166 (NSC 750423)**] (top), and the reference substance (−)-colchicine sesquihydrate [(−)-colchicine × 1½ H₂O] (bottom) are pictured (Fig. 16) for comparison.

Interestingly, the natural colchic(in)oids (−)-colchicine, and the partialsynthetic (−)-colchicine derivative *N*-acetylcolchinol methyl ether (Fig. 17), occur in pure atropisomeric forms (Fig. 17), as was elucidated by *Brossi et al.* [29,30]. The natural forms have the (a*S*,7*S*)-absolute configuration (Fig. 17). The correct assignment of the absolute configuration of (−)-colchicine was given as (a*S*,7*S*) by *Brossi et al.* [30] according to the *Cahn–Ingold–Prelog* (*CIP*) rules. The wrong (a*R*,7*S*)-absolute configuration was firstly postulated in 1981 during studies on tubulin binding by (−)-colchicine [31], and later in 1999 by *Berg & Bladh* [32]. The absolute configuration at C-7 was established earlier as (7*S*) [33] by chemical degradation of natural (−)-colchicine to *N*-acetyl-L-glutamic acid.

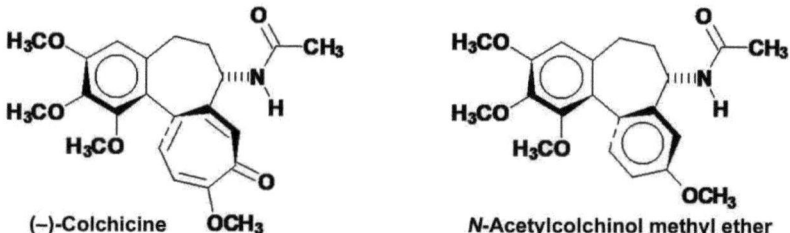

(−)-Colchicine   *N*-Acetylcolchinol methyl ether

Figure 17. The atropisomerism of natural (−)-colchicine and its degradation product *N*-acetylcolchinol methyl ether. Both exhibit the (a*S*,7*S*)-absolute configuration, as was proved by *Brossi et al.* [29,30].

Taken together, the structure of the modified colchic(in)oid compound **2** [**PT166** (**NSC 750423**)] could be proved with considerable evidence, and biological effects, especially antineoplastic properties, are expected from biological testing of compound **2** [**PT166** (**NSC 750423**)]. Renewed interest in colchic(in)oid research is indicated by reports on conjugating (−)-colchicine to vitamin B_{12} (cobalamin) [34] or paclitaxel (taxol) [35]. These colchic(in)oid conjugates were suggested for the chemotherapy of various neoplastic conditions.

1.3. The X-ray crystallographic crystal and molecular structure determination of compound 2 (PT166)

PT166 was crystallized from ethyl acetate and a single crystal was selected for X-ray crystallographic determination (at $\vartheta = 100$ K) of the crystal and molecular structure of compound **2** (**PT166**) (Fig. 18, Fig. 19, Fig. 20, Fig. 21, Fig. 22). Compound **2** (**PT166**) crystallized in the monoclinic space group $P2_1$ with ethyl acetate and water of crystallization $[C_{22}H_{26}N_4O_5S \times 1.5\ H_2O \times 0.5\ (C_4H_8O_2)]$ $(Z = 4)$ (Fig. 18). The crystal packing (Fig. 20) with indicated hydrogen bonds (Fig. 21) in the unit cell $(Z = 2)$ of compound **2** (**PT166**) is depicted. It should be noted that the molecule **PT166** is helical stereogenic and shows the [*M(inus)*]-helicity as *N*-[(a*S*,7*S*)-10-(2-carbamothioylhydrazinyl)-1,2,3-trimethoxy-9-oxo-5,6,7,9-tetrahydrobenzo[*a*]heptalen-7-yl]acetamide (Fig. 22). The helical axis atropisomerism view of one independent, isolated molecule of compound **2** (**PT166**) as found in the single crystal is depicted (Fig. 22). This stands in contradiction to a report that claimed the [*P(lus)*]-helicity (a*R*) for (−)-colchicine [32]. The classification of (*M*)-helicity for compound **2** (**PT166**) followed the *Cahn–Ingold–Prelog* (CIP) rules for assignment of molecular helicity [36,37]. The (*M*)-helicity of (−)-colchicine was previously assigned correctly by *Brossi et al.* [30]. The X-ray crystallographic structure was deposited at The Cambridge Crystallographic Data Centre (CCDC) and assigned the deposition № **CCDC 1839505** (ID: **RIVGOW**). The crystal data of the X-ray crystallographic determination of the crystal and molecular structure of compound **2** (**PT166**) are tabulated (Table 1).

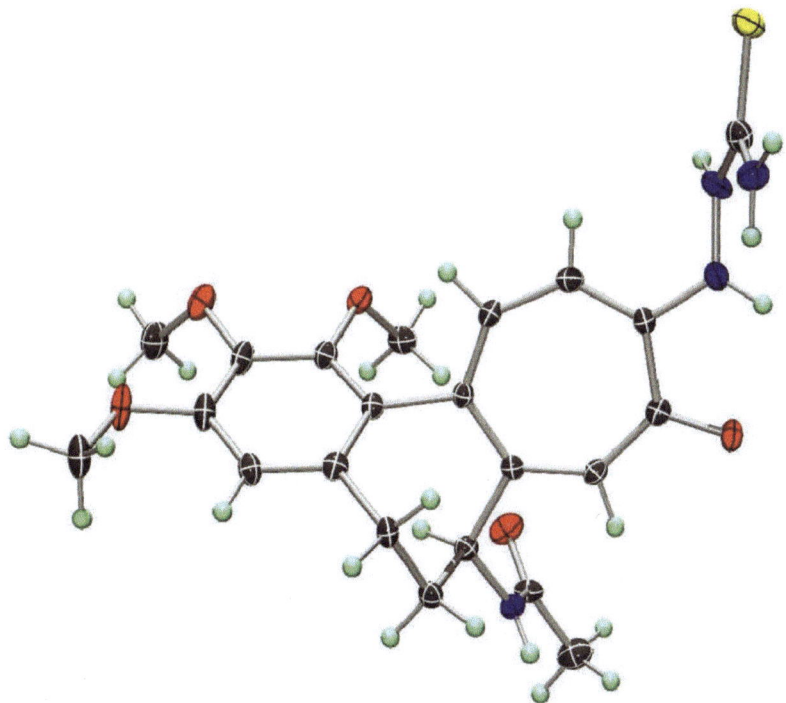

Fig. 18. The molecular view of one independent, isolated molecule of compound **2** (**PT166**) as found in the single crystal. Compound **2** (**PT166**) crystallized in the monoclinic space group $P2_1$ as sesquihydrate hemi(ethyl acetate) solvate ($C_{24}H_{33}N_4O_{7.50}S$) [$C_{22}H_{26}N_4O_5S$ × 1.5 H_2O × 0.5 ($C_4H_8O_2$)] ($Z = 4$). Compound **2** (**PT166**) is helical stereogenic and shows the (*M*)-helicity. The plane of the thiourea moiety in the 10-(thiosemicarbazide) substituent shows +119.1° torsion angle towards the 2-aminotropone plane. The structure was deposited at the Cambridge Crystallographic Data Centre (CCDC) under № **CCDC 1839505**.

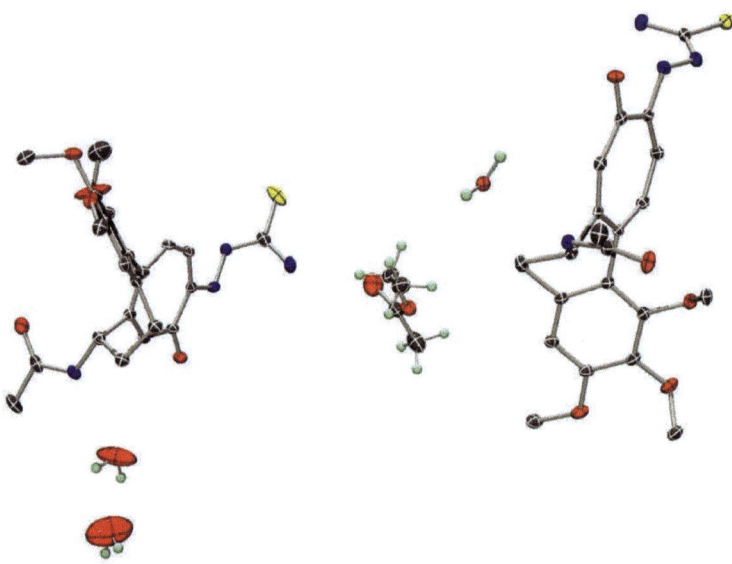

Fig. 19. One formula unit ($Z = 2$) in the monoclinic (space group $P2_1$) unit cell of compound **2** (**PT166**) ($C_{24}H_{33}N_4O_{7.50}S$) crystallized as hydrate (ethyl acetate) solvate ($2\ C_{22}H_{26}N_4O_5S \times 3\ H_2O \times C_4H_8O_2$) $C_{48}H_{66}N_8O_{15}S_2$ ($M = 1059.23$ g/mol) as found in the single crystal.

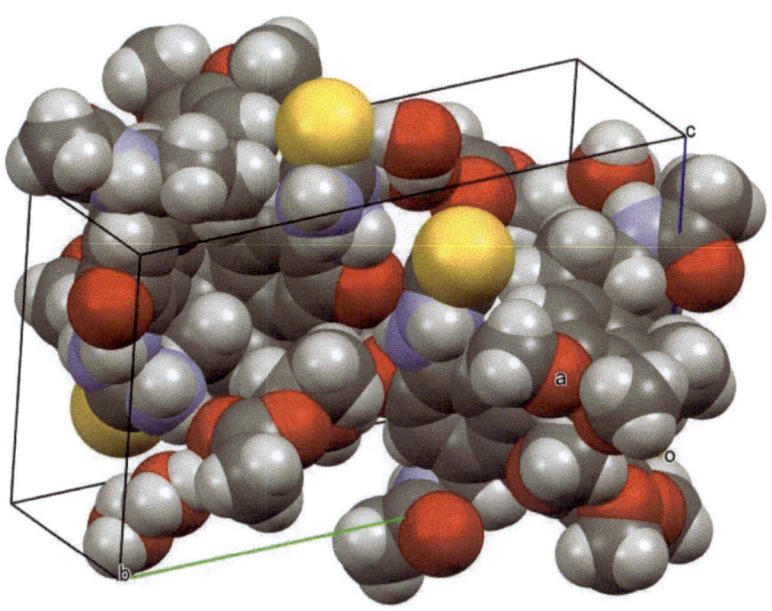

Fig. 20. Crystal packing in the monoclinic (space group $P2_1$) unit cell ($Z = 2$) of compound **2** (**PT166**) crystallized as hydrate (ethyl acetate) solvate ($2\ C_{22}H_{26}N_4O_5S \times 3\ H_2O \times C_4H_8O_2$) $C_{48}H_{66}N_8O_{15}S_2$ ($M = 1059.23$ g/mol). Unit cell dimensions (a, b, c are indicated from the origin o): $a = 9.1886(5)$ Å, $b = 20.9047(10)$ Å, $c = 13.9841(7)$ Å, $\alpha = 90.00°$, $\beta = 106.153(2)°$, $\gamma = 90.00°$, $V = 2580.1(2)$ Å^3.

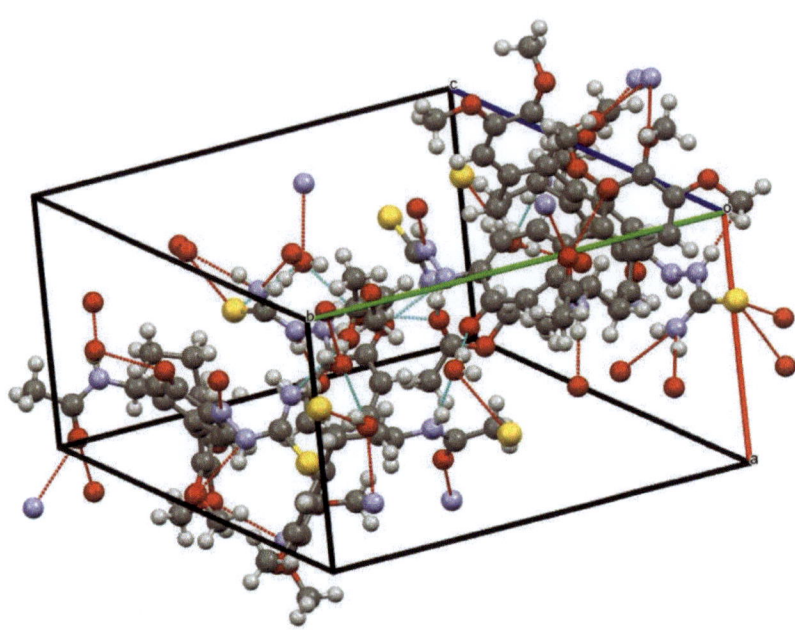

Fig. 21. Crystal packing showing the hydrogen bonds (H bonds, shown as colored dashed lines) in the monoclinic (space group $P2_1$) unit cell ($Z = 2$) of compound **2** (**PT166**) crystallized as hydrate (ethyl acetate) solvate (2 $C_{22}H_{26}N_4O_5S \times 3\ H_2O \times C_4H_8O_2$) $C_{48}H_{66}N_8O_{15}S_2$ ($M = 1059.23$ g/mol). Unit cell dimensions (a, b, c are indicated from the origin o): $a = 9.1886(5)$ Å, $b = 20.9047(10)$ Å, $c = 13.9841(7)$ Å, $\alpha = 90.00°$, $\beta = 106.153(2)°$, $\gamma = 90.00°$, $V = 2580.1(2)$ Å^3.

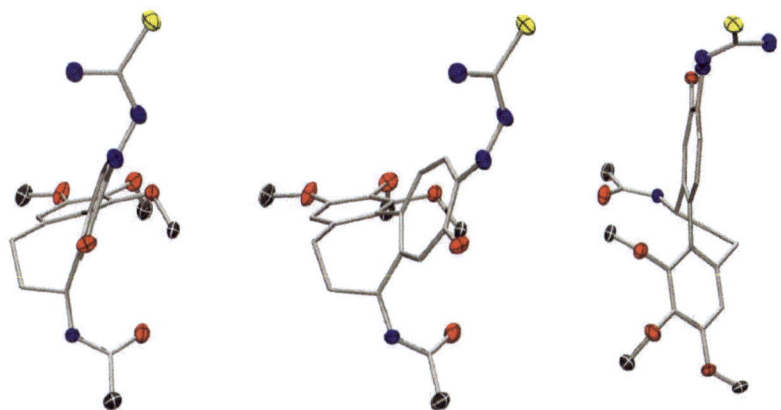

Fig. 22. The helical axis atropisomerism view of one independent, isolated molecule of compound **2** (**PT166**) as found in the single crystal. Compound **2** (**PT166**), the substance *N*-[(a*S*,7*S*)-10-(2-carbamothioylhydrazinyl)-1,2,3-trimethoxy-9-oxo-5,6,7,9-tetrahydrobenzo[*a*]heptalen-7-yl]acetamide, is helical stereogenic and shows the [*M(inus)*]-helicity. Priority rules [36,37] show the helical axis turn in (*S*).

Table 1. Tabulation of the summarized crystallographic data of the X-ray crystallographic determination of the crystal and molecular structure of compound **2** (**PT166**) crystallized as sesquihydrate hemi(ethyl acetate) solvate ($C_{24}H_{33}N_4O_{7.50}S$) [$C_{22}H_{26}N_4O_5S \times 1.5\ H_2O \times 0.5\ (C_4H_8O_2)$].

Data	**PT166** (cu144, colch-TSC)
Empirical formula	$C_{48}H_{66}N_8O_{15}S_2$
Formula weight, M_r (g·mol^{-1})	1059.23
Temperature, T (K)	100(2)
Radiation, λ (Å)	Mo$_{K\alpha}$ 0.71073
Crystal system	Monoclinic
Space group	$P2_1$

Table 1 continued at next page.

Unit cell dimensions	
a (Å)	9.1886(5)
b (Å)	20.9047(10)
c (Å)	13.9841(7)
α (°)	90.00
β (°)	106.153(2)
γ (°)	90.00
Unit cell volume, V (Å^3)	2580.1(2)
Formula units *per* unit cell, Z	2
Calculated density, ρ_{calc} (Mg·m^{-3})	1.363
Absorption coefficient, μ (mm^{-1})	0.178
$F(000)$	1124
Theta (ϑ) range for collection	1.80 to 26.05°
Reflections collected	49598
Independent reflections	9686
Minimum / maximum transmission, T_{min} / T_{max}	0.9193 / 0.9929
Absorption correction	Multi-scan, *SADABS* 2008/1 (Sheldrick, 2008)
Refinement method	Full-matrix least-squares on F^2

Table 1 continued at next page.

Data / parameters / restraints	9686 / 693 / 5
Goodness−of−fit on F^2	1.021
Flack parameter, x_{Flack}	0.09(6)
Final R indices [$I > 2\sigma(I)$]	$R_1 = 0.0506$, $wR^2 = 0.1269$
R indices (all data)	$R_1 = 0.0594$, $wR^2 = 0.1325$
Maximum / minimum residual electron density, $\Delta\rho_{max} / \Delta\rho_{min}$ (e·Å^{-3})	0.747 / −0.496

Summary of the crystal data for compound **2** (**PT166**): $C_{24}H_{33}N_4O_{7.50}S$ [$C_{22}H_{26}N_4O_5S \times 1½ \; H_2O \times ½ \; (C_4H_8O_2)$], $M_r = 529.60$ g/mol, colorless plate, $0.48 \times 0.31 \times 0.04$ mm^3, monoclinic space group $P2_1$, $a = 9.1886(5)$ Å, $b = 20.9047(10)$ Å, $c = 13.9841(7)$ Å, $\beta = 106.153(2)°$, $V = 2580.1(2)$ Å^3, $Z = 4$, $\rho_{calcd} = 1.363$ g·cm^{-3}, $\mu = 0.178$ mm^{-1}, $F(000) = 1124$, $T = 100(2)$ K, $x_{Flack} = 0.09(6)$, $R_1 = 0.0594$, $wR^2 = 0.1325$, 9686 independent reflections [$2\vartheta \leq 52.1°$] and 693 parameters. Computer programs utilized: *APEX2* ver. 2008.3 (Bruker AXS, 2008), *Saint+* ver. 7.53A (Bruker AXS, 2008), *SHELXS97* (Sheldrick, 2008), *SHELXL97* (Sheldrick, 2008), *XP* ver. 5.1 (Bruker AXS, 1998).

2. References

[1] N. Sharifi, et al., A bifunctional colchicinoid that binds to the androgen receptor, *Mol. Cancer Ther.* **6** (2007) 2328–2336.

[2] M.F. Mackay, J.D. Morrison, J.M. Gulbis, Crystal structure of triclinic colchiceine hemihydrate, *Aust. J. Phys.* **38** (1985) 413–420.

[3]   J.V. Silverton, The structure of colchiceine ethyl acetate–water solvate, *Acta Crystallogr. B* **35** (1979) 2800–2803.

[4]   S. Zeisel, Über Colchicin und Colchiceïn, *Monatsh. Chem.* **4** (1883) 162–164.

[5]   S. Zeisel, Über das Colchicin. I. Abhandlung, *Monatsh. Chem.* **7** (1886) 557–596.

[6]   J.W. Cook, J.D. Loudon, Colchicine, In: R.H.F. Manske, H.L. Holmes (Eds.), The alkaloids: Chemistry and physiology, Vol. II, Academic Press Inc., New York, 1952, p. 265.

[7]   M.V. King, J.L. de Vries, R. Pepinsky, An X-ray diffraction determination of the chemical structure of colchicine, *Acta Crystallogr.* **5** (1952) 437–440.

[8]   L. Lessinger, T.N. Margulis, The crystal structure of colchicine. A new application of magic integers to multiple-solution direct methods, *Acta Crystallogr. B* **34** (1978) 578–584.

[9]   H.W.B. Clewer, S.J. Green, F. Tutin, The constituents of *Gloriosa superba*, *J. Chem. Soc., Trans.* **107** (1915) 835–846.

[10] F. Clerici, S. Mottadelli, L.M. Rossi, ^{1}H- and ^{13}C-NMR spectra of thiocolchicine and derivatives: A complete analysis, *J. Nat. Prod.* **58** (1995) 259–263.

[11] D. Meksuriyen, L.-J. Lin, G.A. Cordell, S. Mukhopadhyay, S.K. Banerjee, NMR studies of colchicine and its photoisomers, β- and γ-lumicolchicines, *J. Nat. Prod.* **51** (1988) 88–93.

[12] M.A. Iorio, A. Brossi, J.V. Silverton, 7-Oxo-deacetamidocolchiceine   and   7-benzylimino-

deacetamido-colchiceine: Two novel products from the base catalysed reaction of (–)-*N*-benzylidene-deacetylcolchiceine, *Helv. Chim. Acta* **61** (1978) 1213–1220.

[13] C.D. Hufford, H.-G. Capraro, A. Brossi, ^{13}C- and ^{1}H-NMR. Assignments for colchicine derivatives, *Helv. Chim. Acta* **63** (1980) 50–56.

[14] S. Berger, S. Braun, 200 and more NMR experiments. A practical course, 1st ed., Wiley-VCH Verlag GmbH & Co. KGaA, Weinheim, 2004, 854 pp., ISBN 978-3527310678.

[15] A.J. Kesel, Broad-spectrum antiviral activity including human immunodeficiency and hepatitis C viruses mediated by a novel retinoid thiosemicarbazone derivative, *Eur. J. Med. Chem.* **46** (2011) 1656–1664.

[16] R.M. Horowitz, G.E. Ullyot, Colchicine. Some reactions of ring C, *J. Am. Chem. Soc.* **74** (1952) 587–592.

[17] Fr. Šantavý, Préparation de l'acide colchicique à partir de la colchicine, *Helv. Chim. Acta* **31** (1948) 821–826.

[18] H. Fernholz, Über die Umlagerung des Colchicins mit Natriumalkoholat und die Struktur des Ringes C, *Justus Liebigs Ann. Chem.* **568** (1950) 63–72.

[19] C.D. Hufford, C.C. Collins, A.M. Clark, Microbial transformations and ^{13}C-NMR analysis of colchicine, *J. Pharm. Sci.* **68** (1979) 1239–1243.

[20] T. Nozoe, T. Ikemi, S. Itô, Some derivatives from colchicine, *Proc. Japan Acad. (Nippon-gakushiin-kiyô, Tokyo)* **30** (1954) 609–613.

[21] T. Nozoe, T. Ikemi, S. Itô, Derivatives of colchicine, *Sci. Rep. Tôhoku Univ. Ser. 1 (Tôhoku-daigaku-rika-hôkoku, dai 1-shû, kagaku, Sendai)* **38** (1954) 117–129.

[22] A. Windaus, H. Schiele, Die Konstitution des Colchicins, *Nachr. Ges. Wiss. Göttingen Math.-Phys. Kl. 1923* (1924) 17–36.

[23] J.W. Cook, J.D. Loudon, Colchicine, In: R.H.F. Manske, H.L. Holmes (Eds.), The alkaloids: Chemistry and physiology, Vol. II, Academic Press Inc., New York, 1952, p. 273.

[24] J.W. Cook, J.D. Loudon, The tropolones, *Quart. Rev. Chem. Soc. (London)* **5** (1951) 99–130.

[25] P.L. Pauson, Tropones and tropolones, *Chem. Rev.* **55** (1955) 9–136.

[26] H.J. Dauben Jr., H.J. Ringold, Synthesis of tropone, *J. Am. Chem. Soc.* **73** (1951) 876–876.

[27] W. von E. Doering, F.L. Detert, Cycloheptatrienylium oxide, *J. Am. Chem. Soc.* **73** (1951) 876–877.

[28] R.L. Redington, C.W. Bock, MO study of singlets, triplets, and tunneling in tropolone. 1. Geometries, tunneling, and vibrations in the ground electronic state, *J. Phys. Chem.* **95** (1991) 10284–10294.

[29] A. Brossi, et al., Colchicine and its analogues: Recent findings, *Med. Res. Rev.* **8** (1988) 77–94.

[30] A. Brossi, et al., aS,7S-absolute configuration of natural (–)-colchicine and allo-congeners, *FEBS Lett.* **262** (1990) 5–7.

[31] H.W. Detrich III, R.C. Williams Jr., T.L. Macdonald, L. Wilson, D. Puett, Changes in the circular dichroic

spectrum of colchicine associated with its binding to tubulin, *Biochemistry* **20** (1981) 5999–6005.

[32] U. Berg, H. Bladh, The absolute configuration of colchicine by correct application of the *CIP* rules, *Helv. Chim. Acta* **82** (1999) 323–325.

[33] H. Corrodi, E. Hardegger, Die Konfiguration des Colchicins und verwandter Verbindungen, *Helv. Chim. Acta* **38** (1955) 2030–2033.

[34] J.D. Bagnato, A.L. Eilers, R.A. Horton, C.B. Grissom, Synthesis and characterization of a cobalamin– colchicine conjugate as a novel tumor-targeted cytotoxin, *J. Org. Chem.* **69** (2004) 8987–8996.

[35] K. Bombuwala, et al., Colchitaxel, a coupled compound made from microtubule inhibitors colchicine and paclitaxel, *Beilstein J. Org. Chem.* **2** (2006), 13, https://doi.org/10.1186/1860-5397-2-13.

[36] R.S. Cahn, C. Ingold, V. Prelog, Spezifikation der molekularen Chiralität, *Angew. Chem.* **78** (1966) 413–447.

[37] R.S. Cahn, C. Ingold, V. Prelog, Specification of Molecular Chirality, *Angew. Chem. Int. Ed. Engl.* **5** (1966) 385–415.

CHAPTER THREE

THE DRUG **PT167** (NSC 799315)

1. PT167 (NSC 799315)

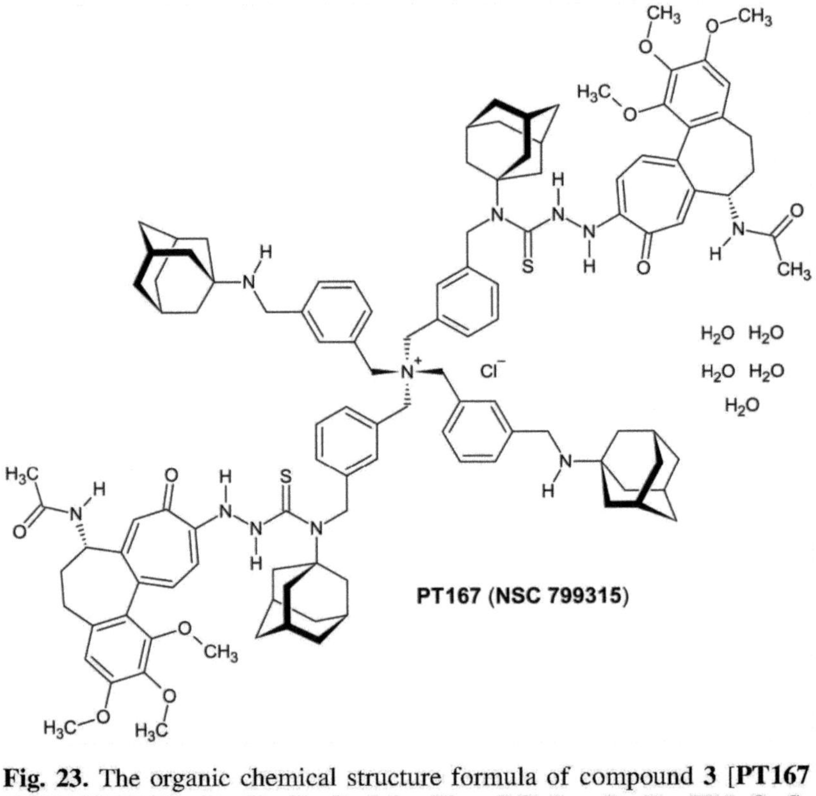

PT167 (NSC 799315)

Fig. 23. The organic chemical structure formula of compound **3** [**PT167 (NSC 799315)**] = $C_{116}H_{142}N_{11}O_{10}S_2^+ \times Cl^- \times 5\ H_2O = C_{116}H_{152}ClN_{11}O_{15}S_2$ (*M* = 2040.10 g/mol). The compound **3** [**PT167 (NSC 799315)**] contains one chloride anion (Cl^-) and five water of crystallization ($\times$ 5 H_2O).

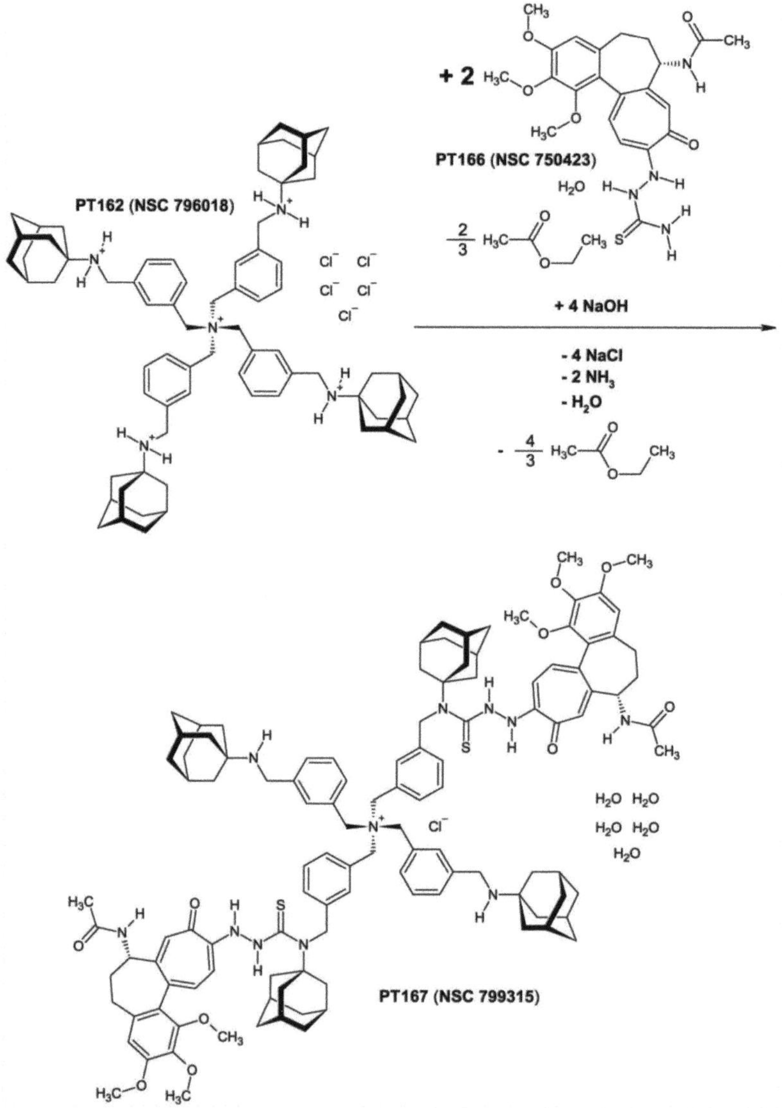

Fig. 24. The synthesis of compound **3** [**PT167 (NSC 799315)**] = $C_{116}H_{142}N_{11}O_{10}S_2^+ \times Cl^- \times 5\ H_2O = C_{116}H_{152}ClN_{11}O_{15}S_2$ (M = 2040.10 g/mol) by *trans*-(thio)amidation [1,2] catalysed by sodium hydroxide (NaOH) at room temperature from compound **1** [**PT162 (NSC 796018)**] and compound **2** [**PT166 (NSC 750423)**].

1.1. The synthesis of drug **PT167** (**NSC 799315**)

Compound **3** [**PT167** (**NSC 799315**)] (Fig. 23) was synthesized from compound **1** [**PT162** (**NSC 796018**)] and compound **2** [**PT166** (**NSC 750423**)] by *trans*-(thio)amidation catalysed by sodium hydroxide (NaOH) at room temperature. A similar *trans*-(thio)amidation originating from a thiosemicarbazide or thiosemicarbazone moiety was observed previously in the synthesis of retinazone, a retinoid thiosemicarbazone derivative [1,2]. As a result compound **2** [**PT166** (**NSC 750423**)] was connected to compound **1** [**PT162** (**NSC 796018**)] through a thioamide-bonding at an adamantanamine nitrogen (Fig. 24). The molecular stoichiometry of compound **3** [**PT167** (**NSC 799315**)] was determined by ^{1}H-NMR (Fig. 25) spectroscopy experiments, as well as elemental analysis. Compound **1** recieved two molecules of compound **2** by *trans*-amidation to yield compound **3**. The ^{1}H-NMR spectrum of compound **3** (Fig. 25) exhibits a peculiar resonance compression [the adamantane resonances 2.00 (24 H; β-CH$_2$), 2.14 (12 H; γ-CH) could not being detected] induced by the large (macro)molecular structure of compound **3** [**PT167** (**NSC 799315**)]. This points to intramolecular (hydrophobic) interation between the β-methylene and γ-methine structural elements of the compound **1** [**PT162** (**NSC 796018**)]-derived adamantanamine cages with the tropone ring (especially H-11) of the colchic(in)oid

Fig. 25 (next page). The 700.43 MHz ^{1}H-NMR spectrum of compound **3** [**PT167** (**NSC 799315**)] = $C_{116}H_{142}N_{11}O_{10}S_2{}^+ \times Cl^- \times 5\ H_2O$ = $C_{116}H_{152}ClN_{11}O_{15}S_2$ (M = 2040.10 g/mol) dissolved in DMSO-d_6. Yellow marked is the solvent DMSO-d_6 residual resonance [DMSO-d_5h_1 quintet at δ 2.50 ppm, $^2J_{\text{gem}}$ (^{2}H–^{1}H) = 1.9 Hz] [DMSO]. The water broad singlet resonance is found at δ 3.32 ppm. Traces of the utilized synthesis solvents ethanol (triplet, δ 1.05 ppm; quartet, δ 3.44 ppm) and acetone (singlet, δ 2.09 ppm) can be detected.

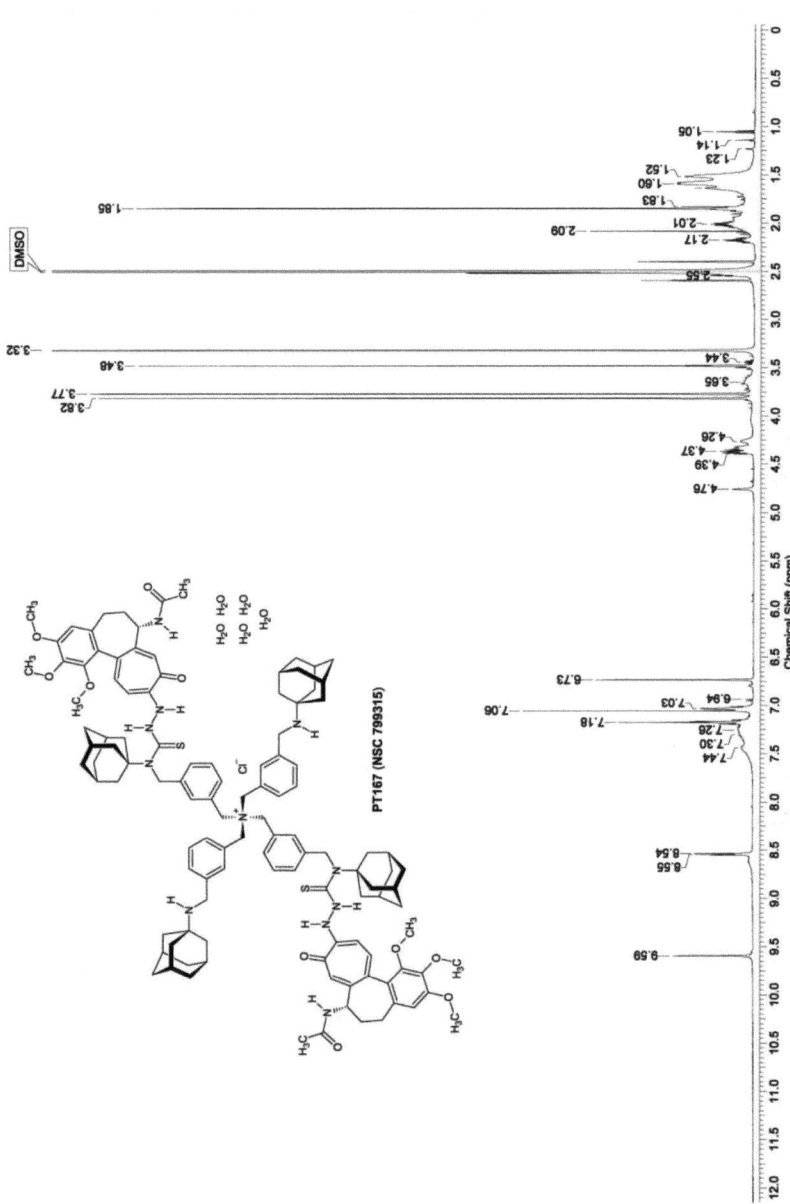

PT167 (NSC 799315)

part of compound **3** [**PT167** (**NSC799315**)]. An intramolecular interaction between the β-methylene and γ-methine structural elements of the adamantanamine cages with H-11 of the 10-(thiosemicarbazide)-substituted tropone ring in compound **3** [**PT167** (**NSC 799315**)] could be demonstrated by molecular modeling (Fig. 26). The resulting overall chemical structure of compound **3** is given (Fig. 23). Compound **3** (**PT167**) was registered by the National Cancer Institute (NCI) as **NSC 799315**.

1.2. The proton nuclear magnetic resonance spectrum (^{1}H-NMR) of **PT167** (**NSC 799315**)

Evidence for the formulation of compound **3** [**PT167** (**NSC 799315**)] as the macromolecular entity [(bis{3-[(tricyclo[3.3.1.1^{3,7}]decan-1-ylamino)methyl]benzyl}ammon-io)bis(methanediylbenzene-3,1-diylmethanediyl)]di-2-[(aS,7S)-7-(acetylamino)-1,2,3-trimethoxy-9-oxo-5,6,7,9-tetrahydrobenzo[a]heptalen-10-yl]-N-(tricyclo[3.3.1.1^{3,7}]decan-1-yl)hydrazinecarbothioamide chloride pentahydrate stems from the proton NMR (^{1}H-NMR) spectrum of compound **3** [**PT167** (**NSC 799315**)] dissolved in deuterated dimethyl sulfoxide (DMSO-d_6) (Fig. 25). The proton resonances were measured as chemical shifts δ (ppm): δ 1.48–1.68 (24 H, br m; δ-CH$_2$, adamantane), 1.83 (2 H, m; H$_A$-6, colch), 1.85 (6 H, s; 17-CH$_3$, colch), 2.01 (2 H, m; H$_B$-6, colch), 2.17 (2 H, m; H$_A$-5, colch), 2.52 (2 H, m; H$_B$-5, colch), 3.48 (6 H, s; 13-OCH$_3$, colch)*, 3.65 (2 H, br s; secondary amine N–H), 3.77 (6 H, s; 15-OCH$_3$, colch)*, 3.82 (6 H, s; 14-OCH$_3$, colch)*, 4.26 (br m; 8-CH$_2$, m-xylylene), 4.32–4.39 (2 H, br m; H-7, colch), 4.76 (s; 7-CH$_2$, m-xylylene), 6.73 (2 H, s; H-4, colch), 7.03 (2 H, br m; H-11, colch), 7.06 (2 H, s; H-8, colch), 7.12–7.72 (br m; H-4, H-6, H-5, H-2, m-xylylene), 7.17 (2 H, br m; H-12, colch), 8.54 (2 H, d; ^3J = 7.7 Hz;

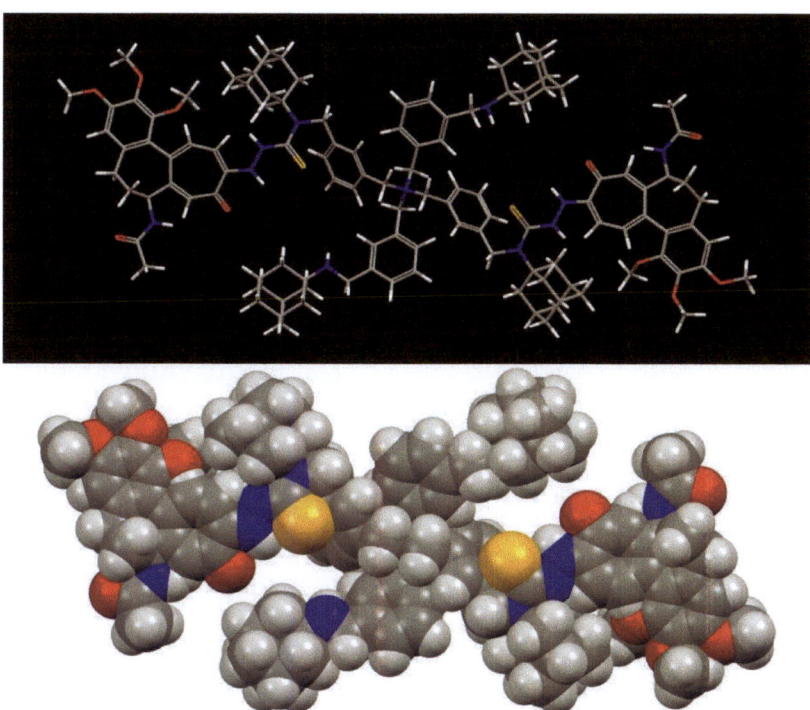

Fig. 26. Molecular modeling {ACD/Chem Sketch version 12.01 with integrated ACD/3D Viewer (Advanced Chemistry Development, Inc., Toronto, Ontario, Canada) and processed with Mercury 3.1 version 3.1.1 [The Cambridge Crystallographic Data Centre (CCDC), Cambridge, UK]} of compound **3** [**PT167 (NSC 799315)**] = $C_{116}H_{142}N_{11}O_{10}S_2^+ \times Cl^- \times 5$ $H_2O = C_{116}H_{152}ClN_{11}O_{15}S_2$ (M = 2040.10 g/mol) without the chloride counteranion (Cl^-) and the water of crystallization (pentahydrate). An intramolecular interaction between the β-methylene and γ-methine structural elements of the adamantanamine cages with H-11 of the 10-(thiosemicarbazide)-substituted tropone ring in compound **3** [**PT167 (NSC 799315)**] could be demonstrated.

N–H acetamide, colch), 9.59 (4 H, s; 1′-N–H, 2′-N–H, hydrazinecarbothioamide) [colch = the colchic(in)oid part of **PT167**; * these assignments are tentative and interchangeable (they could not be assigned unequivocally to the individual methoxy groups); the adamantane resonances δ 2.00 ppm (β-CH$_2$) and 2.14 ppm (γ-CH) were not detected due to paramagnetic compression].

The specimen of **PT167** (**NSC 799315**) which was synthesized by *Andreas J. Kesel* at Saturday, May 27th, 2017, was investigated by proton NMR (Fig. 27) at Wednesday, August 23rd, 2023, after over six years storage at +0−4 °C in the refrigerator. The specimen was newly dried over CaCl$_2$ *in vacuo* for 19 h. The proton resonances were measured as chemical shifts δ (ppm): δ 1.14 (1 H, s; hydroxytropyl radical O–H), 1.45–1.81 (24 H, br m; δ-CH$_2$, adamantane), 1.83 (2 H, m; H$_A$-6, colch), 1.85 (6 H, s; 17-CH$_3$, colch), 1.91 (2 H, m; H$_B$-6, colch), 2.02–2.14 (12 H, br m; γ-CH), 2.18 (2 H, br m; H$_A$-5, colch), 2.55 (2 H, br m; H$_B$-5, colch), 2.86–3.08 [7 H, br s; 7-CH$_2$, *m*-xylylene CH$_2$ including ammonium ylide R−(CH⁻)N⁺(CH$_2$R)$_3$], 3.49 (6 H, s; 13-OCH$_3$, colch)*, 3.67 (1 H, s; secondary amine N–H), 3.78 (6 H, s; 15-OCH$_3$, colch)*, 3.82 (6 H, s; 14-OCH$_3$, colch)*, 4.26–4.39 (8 H, br m; H-7, colch; 3 × 8-CH$_2$ *m*-xylylene), 4.76 (2 H, s; 1 × 8-CH$_2$, *m*-xylylene at 8-NH⁺• radical cation), 6.72 (2 H, s; H-4, colch), 6.99 (2 H, br s; H-11, colch), 7.06 (2 H, s; H-8, colch), 7.17 (2 H, br s; H-12, colch), 7.30–7.37 (12 H, br m; H-4, H-6, H-2, *m*-xylylene), 7.51 (4 H, br s; H-5, *m*-xylylene), 8.14 (1 H, s; 8-NH⁺• radical cation N–H), 8.48 (2 H, d; ^3J = 7.9 Hz; N–H acetamide, colch), 9.56 (4 H, br s; 1′-N–H, 2′-N–H, hydrazinecarbothioamide) [colch = the colchic(in)oid part of **PT167**; * these assignments are tentative and interchangeable

Fig. 27 (next page). The 499.86 MHz ^{1}H-NMR spectrum of newly dried (CaCl$_2$, *in vacuo*, 19 h) **PT167** (**NSC 799315**) in DMSO-d_6 after storing the substance over six years at +0−4 °C in the refrigerator. The spectrum was measured at ϑ = 35 °C on a Varian Unity INOVA 500 instrument. Yellow marked are the solvent DMSO-d_6 residual resonance [DMSO] and the water broad singlet resonance at δ 3.25 ppm [Water]. Only traces of the utilized synthesis solvent acetone (singlet, δ 2.08 ppm) are present.

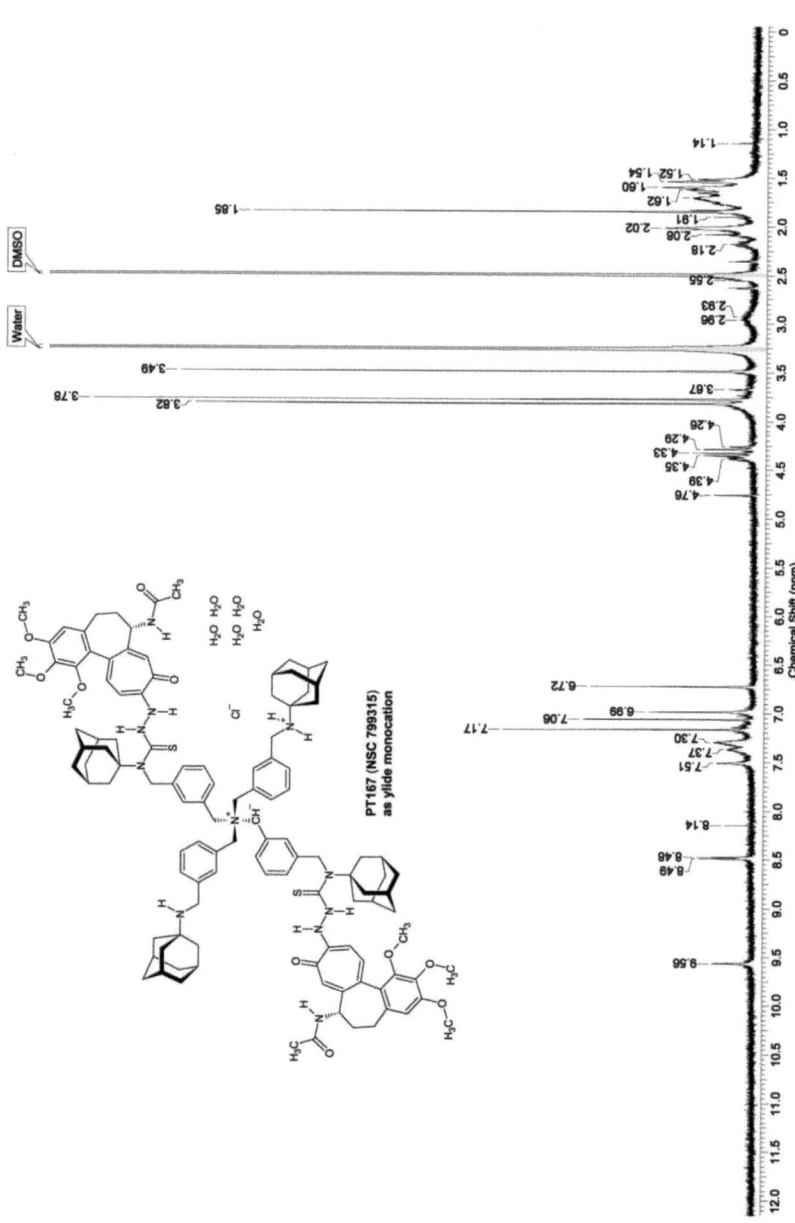

(they could not be assigned unequivocally to the individual methoxy groups); the adamantane β-CH$_2$ resonance δ 2.00 ppm was not detected due to paramagnetic compression].

The ^{1}H-NMR spectrum of newly dried (CaCl$_2$, *in vacuo*, 19 h) **PT167** (**NSC 799315**) in DMSO-d_6 after storing the substance over six years at +0–4 °C in the refrigerator (Fig. 27) convincingly proves that (i) the substance is very pure even after six years storage, (ii) exhibits the chemical structure given by me, and (iii) points to proton transfer during storage yielding the ylide monocation (ylide monohydrochloride) with discernible resonances (7 H) for the ylide R–(CH$^-$)N$^+$(CH$_2$R)$_3$.

This substance bears a peculiar magnetic property. During NMR spectrometer shim it was detected that newly dried (CaCl$_2$, *in vacuo*, 19 h) **PT167** (**NSC 799315**) is, in part, paramagnetic, because there were considerable difficulties in shimming the NMR spectrometer probe magnetic field (personal communication *Robbin Schnieders*). The operator told me that the DMSO-d_6 solution of newly dried (CaCl$_2$, *in vacuo*, 19 h) **PT167** (**NSC 799315**) had to be strongly diluted with DMSO-d_6, and that the spectrum acquisition time had to be elongated considerably. This pointed to inclusion of a paramagnetic partial structure in newly dried (CaCl$_2$, *in vacuo*, 19 h) **PT167** (**NSC 799315**). Indeed, the ^{1}H-NMR spectrum (Fig. 27) gives evidence for that interpretation which is depicted in **Fig. 28**. The colchic(in)oid part of the molecule picks up one electron from the ylide monocation (ylide monohydrochloride) (Fig. 28, in blue) yielding a resonance-stabilized   1-hydroxycyclohepta-2,4,6-trien-1-yl

Fig. 28 (next page). The electron transfer in **PT167** (**NSC 799315**) yielding a partially paramagnetic molecular species. The colchic(in)oid part of the molecule picks up one electron from the ylide monocation yielding a resonance-stabilized 1-hydroxycyclohepta-2,4,6-trien-1-yl radical (hydroxytropyl radical) producing the 8-NH$^{+\bullet}$ radical cation.

PT167 (NSC 799315) as ylide monocation

PT167 (NSC 799315) as ylide with one radical cation center and one hydroxytropyl radical

radical (hydroxytropyl radical) producing in consequence the $8\text{-NH}^{+\bullet}$ radical cation (Fig. 28, in red).

1.3. The liquid chromatographic (HPLC) investigation of **PT167** (**NSC 799315**)

The specimen of **PT167** (**NSC 799315**) which was synthesized by *Andreas J. Kesel* at Saturday, May 27th, 2017, was investigated at Friday, July 21st, 2023, after over six years storage at $+0-4$ °C in the refrigerator. The high-performance liquid chromatography (HPLC) (Fig. 29, Fig. S1) was performed with a reversed phase C_8 (RP8, *n*-octyl) column and gradient elution with eluent A = water/0.1% (*v/v*) formic acid (HCOOH) and eluent B = acetonitrile/0.1% (*v/v*) formic acid (HCOOH). The flowrate was 0.5 ml/min and the linear eluent gradient was t_{0min} = 95% eluent A/5% eluent B to t_{13min} = 5% eluent A/95% eluent B, t_{16min} = stop. A 5 µl volume of a 50 µM **PT167** (**NSC 799315**) solution in acetonitrile (N≡C–CH$_3$) was injected (0.25 nmol, 510.025 ng).

The total ion current (TIC) chromatogram is shown in **Fig. 29**, the chromatogram with UV detection at λ = 335 nm is depicted in **Fig. S1**. Multiple ionic species of **PT167** (**NSC 799315**) were separated (Table 2) due to the complicated ionization kinetics of **PT167** (**NSC 799315**) dissolved in acetonitrile (N≡C–CH$_3$) with presence of 0.1% (*v/v*) HCOOH. The quaternary ammonium compound **PT167** (**NSC 799315**) can be protonated once or twice, or being not protonated like the *in situ* substance (Table 2). Moreover, **PT167** (**NSC 799315**) can exist in equilibrium as a neutral nitrogen ylide [3–5] at the central quaternary ammonium cation. This nitrogen ylide can be protonated once or twice, or being not protonated (neutral nitrogen ylide) (Table 2). The substance **PT167** (**NSC 799315**) was quite pure as judged from the chromatogram with UV detection at λ = 335 nm (Fig. S1).

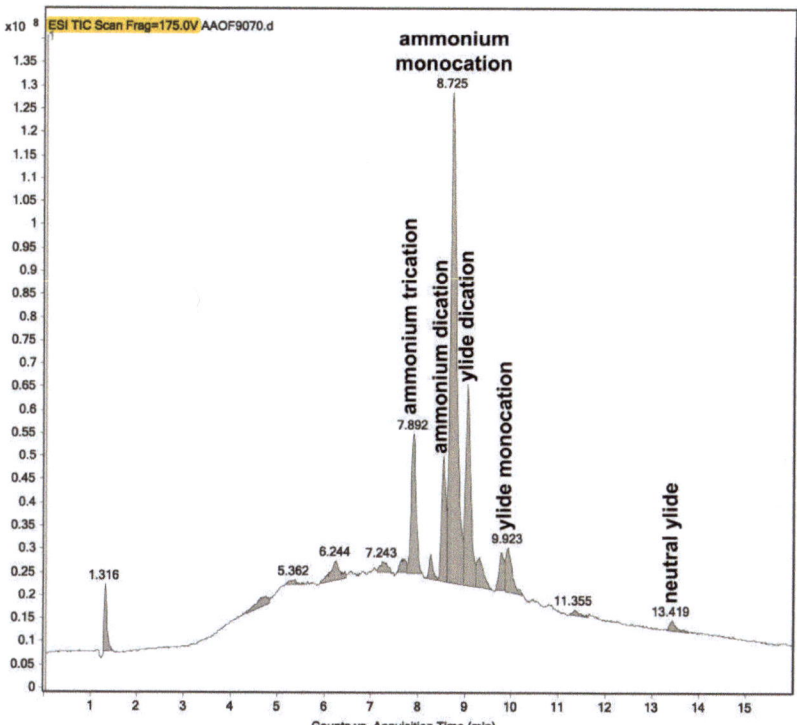

Fig. 29. The total ion current (TIC) chromatogram of the liquid chromatographic (HPLC)/electrospray ionization (ESI) time–of–flight (ToF) mass spectrometric investigation of **PT167** (**NSC 799315**) after storing the substance over six years at +0–4 °C in the refrigerator. The high-performance liquid chromatography (HPLC) of **PT167** (**NSC 799315**) was performed on a reversed phase C_8 (RP8, *n*-octyl) column with gradient elution [eluent A = water/0.1% (*v/v*) formic acid (HCOOH), eluent B = acetonitrile/0.1% (*v/v*) formic acid (HCOOH)]. The flowrate was 0.5 ml/min and the linear eluent gradient was t_{0min} = 95% eluent A/5% eluent B to t_{13min} = 5% eluent A/95% eluent B, t_{16min} = stop. Indicated are the presumed multiple ionic species of **PT167** (**NSC 799315**) (see Table 2) which were separated due to the complicated ionization kinetics of the macromolecular substance **PT167** (**NSC 799315**) dissolved in acetonitrile ($N≡C–CH_3$) with presence of 0.1% (*v/v*) HCOOH in the HPLC eluents.

Table 2. The liquid chromatographic (HPLC)/electrospray ionization (ESI) time–of–flight (ToF) mass spectrometric investigation of **PT167** (**NSC 799315**) after storing the substance over six years at +0–4 °C in the refrigerator. Given are the HPLC peak regions in the total ion current (TIC) chromatogram (Fig. 29) which were scanned in the ESI mass spectrometer with the observed fragmentation peaks (in parentheses: relative peak intensity of the 100% base peak), and the presumed ionization identities of the ionized species of **PT167** (**NSC 799315**) dissolved in acetonitrile (N≡C–CH$_3$) with presence of 0.1% (v/v) HCOOH in the HPLC eluents. The m/z 922.0098 is an internal control substance (reference cation) added to the analysis for auto-calibration of the mass spectrometer.

HPLC peak (min)	Peak identity	ESI–MS fragment peaks (m/z) (relative peak intensity of the 100% base peak)
7.842–7.925	ammonium trication	290.1670 (100%), 678.3662 (12.5%), 135.1157 (9.6%)
8.508–8.558	ammonium dication	712.3545 (100%), 123.0807 (16.5%), 356.6799 (2.1%), 483.2713 (1.3%)
8.608–8.658	ammonium monocation	712.3550 (100%), 543.3511 (27.9%), 356.6804 (18.1%), 123.0806 (14.2%), 653.3701 (5.4%), 483.2714 (2.5%), 409.2404 (1.7%)
8.691–8.741	ammonium monocation	712.3558 (100%), 356.6814 (19.1%), 578.2448 (6.3%), 135.1165 (5.8%)
9.024–9.074	ylide dication	483.2727 (100%), 965.5391 (80.9%), 712.3534 (19.5%), 123.0798 (14.1%), 356.6793 (5.0%), 831.4260 (4.3%), 577.2110 (3.4%), 213.1784 (2.3%)
9.740–9.973	ylide monocation	227.2000 (100%), 123.0804 (47.2%), 609.8644 (31.0%), 712.3522 (6.6%), 398.7700 (5.8%), 1218.7191 (5.0%), 796.5327 (4.0%), 483.2712 (2.5%)
13.386–13.453	neutral ylide	123.0805 (100%), 637.3055 (45.6%), 227.1988 (7.1%), 439.2038 (5.8%), 712.3521 (3.2%)

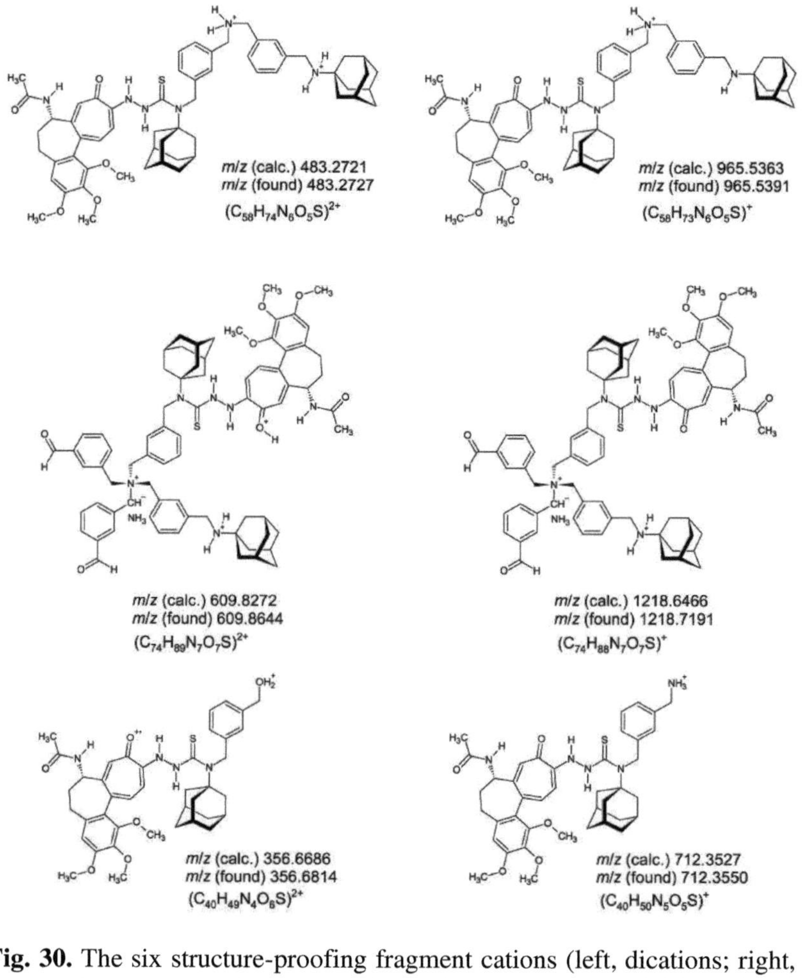

Fig. 30. The six structure-proofing fragment cations (left, dications; right, monocations) in the electrospray ionization (ESI) time−of−flight (ToF) mass spectrometric investigation of **PT167** (**NSC 799315**) after storing the substance over six years at +0−4 °C in the refrigerator. The m/z 483.2727 (100%) (generated from ylide dication), m/z 965.5391 (80.9%) (generated from ylide dication), m/z 609.8644 (31.0%) (generated from ylide monocation), m/z 1218.7191 (5.0%) (generated from ylide monocation), m/z 356.6814 (19.1%) (generated from ammonium monocation), and m/z 712.3550 (100%) (generated from ammonium monocation) are the major, structure-proofing fragments of **PT167** (**NSC 799315**) produced in the ESI−ToF mass spectrometer under the fragmentor voltage V_f = 175 V.

1.4. The electrospray ionization (ESI) mass spectrometric investigation of **PT167** (**NSC 799315**) after HPLC separation

The six structure-proofing fragment cations in the electrospray ionization (ESI) time–of–flight (ToF) mass spectrometric investigation of **PT167** (**NSC 799315**) following HPLC separation on a RP8 column (LC/MS coupling) are shown in **Fig. 30** (left, dications; right, monocations). The cations $(C_{58}H_{74}N_6O_5S)^{2+}$ m/z 483.2727 (100%) (generated from ylide dication), $(C_{58}H_{73}N_6O_5S)^+$ m/z 965.5391 (80.9%) (generated from ylide dication), $(C_{74}H_{89}N_7O_7S)^{2+}$ m/z 609.8644 (31.0%) (generated from ylide monocation), $(C_{74}H_{88}N_7O_7S)^+$ m/z 1218.7191 (5.0%) (generated from ylide monocation), $(C_{40}H_{49}N_4O_6S)^{2+}$ m/z 356.6814 (19.1%) (generated from ammonium monocation), and $(C_{40}H_{50}N_5O_5S)^+$ m/z 712.3550 (100%) (generated from ammonium monocation) are the major, structure-proofing fragments of **PT167** (**NSC 799315**) created in the ESI–ToF mass spectrometer under the fragmentor voltage V_f = 175 V. The molecule cation $(C_{116}H_{142}N_{11}O_{10}S_2)^+$ m/z 1913.0382 (or a higher protonated form) was not observed due to extensive molecule fragmentation.

The two peaks $(C_{74}H_{89}N_7O_7S)^{2+}$ m/z 609.8644 (31.0%) (generated from ylide monocation) and $(C_{74}H_{88}N_7O_7S)^+$ m/z 1218.7191 (5.0%) (generated from ylide monocation) (Fig. 30) are to be formulated as ammonia (NH_3) coordination-stabilized [3,4] nitrogen ylides [5] being in equilibrium with a mass spectrometric generated species exhibiting pentavalent nitrogen [6–8] according to **Fig. S12**.

The fragment cations $(C_{18}H_{21}NNaO)^+$ m/z 290.17 [(3-{[(adamantan-1-yl)imino-κN]methyl}benzaldehyde-κO) sodium(1+)], $(C_8H_7O_2)^+$ m/z 135.12 [protonated isophthal(di)aldehyde], $(C_8H_{11}O)^+$ m/z 123.08 [protonated m-xylyl alcohol (3-methylbenzyl alcohol)], and $(C_{16}H_{21}N)^{+\bullet}$ m/z 227.20 [N-phenyladamantan-1-amine radical cation], accompany the greater fragments pointing to extensive fragmentation force under the fragmentor voltage V_f = 175 V. The N-phenyladamantan-1-amine radical cation results from 1-{[(adamantan-1-yl)amino]methyliumyl}cyclopenta-2,4-dien-1-ide ($C_{16}H_{21}N$, a zwitterionic fulvene) created from the benzyl species N-{[3-(aminomethyl)phenyl]methyl} adamantan-1-amine ($C_{18}H_{26}N_2$) through loss of C_2H_5N and fulvene−to−benzene rearrangement [9,10].

In summary, the chemical structure **PT167** (**NSC 799315**) could be substantiated as derivative of colchiceine hydrazide (10-hydrazinyl-10-demethoxycolchicine) [11,12] bridged over a thiocarbonyl to the **PT162** (**NSC 796018**) core, being quite pure. None **PT166** (**NSC 750423**) and **PT162** (**NSC 796018**), the synthesis starting substances, or colchiceine hydrazide, a possible degradation product, could be detected in the **PT167** (**NSC 799315**) preparation by highly sensitive detection methods.

2. References

[1] A.J. Kesel, Broad-spectrum antiviral activity including human immunodeficiency and hepatitis C viruses mediated by a novel retinoid thiosemicarbazone derivative, *Eur. J. Med. Chem.* **46** (2011) 1656–1664.

[2] A.J. Kesel, et al., Retinazone inhibits certain blood-borne human viruses including Ebola virus Zaire, *Antivir. Chem. Chemother.* **23** (2014) 197–215.

[3] A.W. Johnson, Organic chemistry, Vol. 7, Ylid chemistry, 1st ed., Academic Press, New York, London, 1966, pp. 251–283, ISBN 978-0123864505.

[4] W.K. Musker, R.R. Stevens, Nitrogen ylides. V. Coordination chemistry of trimethylammonium methylide, *Inorg. Chem.* **8** (1969) 255–264.

[5]   G. Wittig, M.-H. Wetterling, Darstellung und Eigenschaften des Trimethyl-ammonium-methylids, *Justus Liebigs Ann. Chem.* **557** (1947) 193–201.

[6]   B.V. Nekrasov, Pentavalent nitrogen, *Bull. Acad. Sci. U. S. S. R., Div. Chem. Sci. (Russ. Chem. Bull.)* **28** (1979) 1789–1790, https://doi.org/10.1007/BF00952448.

[7]   D. Kurzydłowski, P. Zaleski-Ejgierd, Hexacoordinated nitrogen(V) stabilized by high pressure, *Sci. Rep.* **6** (2016), 36049, https://doi.org/10.1038/srep36049.

[8]   C. Yan, et al., Synthesis and properties of hypervalent electron-rich pentacoordinate nitrogen compounds, *Chem. Sci.* **11** (2020) 5082–5088, https://doi.org/10.1039/D0SC00002G.

[9]   E. Ikeda, R.S. Tranter, J.H. Kiefer, R.D. Kern, H.J. Singh, Q. Zhang, The pyrolysis of methylcyclopentadiene: Isomerization and formation of aromatics, *Proc. Combust. Inst.* **28** (2000) 1725–1732.

[10] B. Hanamirian, A. Della Libera, L. Pratali Maffei, C. Cavallotti, Investigation of methylcyclopentadiene reactivity: Abstraction reactions and methylcyclopentadienyl radical unimolecular decomposition, *J. Phys. Chem. A* **127** (2023) 1314–1328.

[11] T. Nozoe, T. Ikemi, S. Itô, Some derivatives from colchicine, *Proc. Japan Acad. (Nippon-gakushiin-kiyô, Tokyo)* **30** (1954) 609–613.

[12] T. Nozoe, T. Ikemi, S. Itô, Derivatives of colchicine, *Sci. Rep. Tôhoku Univ. Ser. 1 (Tôhoku-daigaku-rika-hôkoku, dai 1-shû, kagaku, Sendai)* **38** (1954) 117–129.

CHAPTER FOUR

ANTINEOPLASTIC ACTIVITIES OF
PT162, **PT166** AND **PT167**

1. NCI 60 Cell Five-Dose Screen with the Drugs PT162, PT166 and PT167

1.1. National Cancer Institute (NCI) Developmental Therapeutics Program (DTP) 60-cancer cell 5-dose testing

- **First page:** graphic allover presentation of second page with **All Cell Lines** in one graphic and molar concentrations expressed in logarithmic $\log_{10}$ unit. The earlier the colored curves aspire to the bottom, the more potent is the drug. The more the curves strive from $\pm 0\%$ to -100%, the more the tumor is actually killed by the drug.

- **Second page:** inhibition curves for tumor cell lines summarized in terms of tumor type. The **Sample Concentration**s are given at the x-axis in $\log_{10}$ units ($-9 = 1$ nM, $-8 = 10$ nM, $-7 = 100$ nM, $-6 = 1$ µM, $-5 = 10$ µM, $-4 = 100$ µM, $-3 = 1000$ µM $= 1$ mM). The **Percentage Growth** are given at the y-axis in %, and spans from $+100\%$ to -100%. **0% Growth** means that the tumor is still there but not growing anymore. **-100% Growth** means that the tumor cells are all dead and had died by apoptosis or necrosis, this is the ideal outcome. The smoother the curve, the more reliable is the tumor inhibition. Generally, it is not sufficient to reach only **0% Growth**, since the tumor is still there. Ideal is **-100% Growth**, since the tumor cells were completely killed by the drug, but only few antineoplastic drugs in clinical use reach this. Cytostatics in clinical use generally reach only **0% Growth**, this is called cytostasis (therefore the name cytostatics).

- **Third page:** the actual used concentrations in $\log_{10}$ unit are given for five doses (<u>Note</u>: mostly these are not smooth values, but technically created values). Then the Mean Optical Densities of the used vital stain sulforhodamine B (SRB) retained in the cells are given. The higher the SRB optical density, the more is the number of living tumor cells. Then the **Percent Growth** is given again. The **GI50 (Growth inhibition 50%), TGI (Total Growth Inhibition = 0% Growth),** and **LC50 (Lethal Concentration 50% = –50% Growth)** are given in linear concentration ($E-6 = 10^{-6}$ M = μM, $E-5 = 10^{-5}$ M...) units. A > 1.00E–X (for example: > 1.00E–4 = > 100 μM) means that the corresponding defined criterion is not reached by the drug = failure to reach the defind tumor inhibition criterion (**GI50, TGI,** or **LC50**). The **NSC number** of the test drug is given at the heading. The **NSC Number** is a standardized system of all anticancer compounds tested by NCI. The **NSC number** can be used for unequivocal identification and definition of all anticancer drugs, if registered and tested by NCI.

- **Fourth page:** this is the summary of the results expressed in $\log_{10}$ units. The defined tumor inhibition criterion (**GI50, TGI,** or **LC50**) is recalculated in $\log_{10}$ expression, and the the colored bars which indicate then the sensitivity of the individual tumor cell line to the agent are given in $\log_{10}$ units. **Bar to the left: less sensitive than mean, Bar to the right: more sensitive than mean.** The most important feature is at the bottom of the page: the **MID (Mean of Inhibition Data)** indicates the mean concentration for all tested cell lines required for the drug to reach the defined tumor inhibition criterion (**GI50, TGI,** or **LC50**). It is given in **Log₁₀GI50, Log₁₀TGI** and **Log₁₀LC50**. From that values the corresponding **MID** is calculated. The more negative the **MID**, the more potent is the drug. The **MID** can be transformed from logarithmic into linear concentrations by the formula: $c = 10^{MID}$. The Delta and Range of the MID correspond to these definitions, expressed in logarithmic $\log_{10}$ unit:

The **Delta** is defined as:

Delta = Mean — Growth Percent of the drug's most inhibited cell line

The **Range** is defined as:
Range = (Growth Percent of the drug's least inhibited cell line **— Mean) + Delta**

1.2. Overall NCI 60 cell five-dose screen results with the drugs **PT162, PT166** and **PT167**

Compound **1** (**PT162, NSC 796018**), compound **2** (**PT166, NSC 750423**) and compound **3** (**PT167, NSC 799315**) were screened in the NCI DTP 60-cancer cell 5-dose testing program. The results are summarized in the **Table 3**. Compound **1** (**PT162, NSC 796018**) and compound **3** (**PT167, NSC 799315**) generally started to inhibit cancer cell growth in the submicromolar range, whereby compound **3** (**PT167, NSC 799315**) was slightly more potent than compound **1** (**PT162, NSC 796018**). The responses of compound **1** (**PT162, NSC 796018**) and compound **3** (**PT167, NSC 799315**) regarding inhibition of cancer cell growth were remarkably smooth, regular and consistent. Nearly all cancer cell lines were inhibited by compound **1** (**PT162, NSC 796018**) and compound **3** (**PT167, NSC 799315**) in a very consistent fashion, including leukemia cell lines for compound **3** (**PT167**, **NSC 799315**). In contrast, the inhibiting effect of compound **2** (**PT166**, **NSC 750423**) on cancer cell growth was widely variable. Importantly, compound **1** (**PT162**, **NSC 796018**) and compound **3** (**PT167**, **NSC 799315**), including leukemia cell lines for compound **3** (**PT167**, **NSC 799315**), induced consistent cancer cell death in almost all cancer cell lines. In contrast, compound **2** (**PT166**, **NSC 750423**) failed to induce cancer cell death in nearly all cancer cell lines. The **GI50** for compound **1** (**PT162**, **NSC 796018**) was 1.288 µM, for compound **2** (**PT166**, **NSC 750423**) 0.933 µM, and for compound **3** (**PT167**, **NSC 799315**) 1.349 µM (Table 3). The **TGI** for compound **1** (**PT162**, **NSC 796018**) was 4.677 µM, for compound **2** (**PT166**, **NSC 750423**) 32.359 µM, and for compound **3** (**PT167**, **NSC 799315**) 4.571 µM (Table 3). The **LC50** for compound **1** (**PT162**, **NSC 796018**) was 16.596 µM, for compound **2** (**PT166**, **NSC 750423**) 95.499 µM, and for compound **3** (**PT167**, **NSC 799315**) 15.849 µM (Table 3).

As can be clearly seen from these data compound **2** [**PT166** (**NSC 750423**)] failed to induce cancer cell death and acts only cytostatic, whereas compound **1** (**PT162**, **NSC 796018**) and compound **3** (**PT167**, **NSC 799315**) successfully induced cancer cell death to nearly −100% cancer cell growth and can be classified as tumoricidal.

Compound **1** (**PT162**, **NSC 796018**) and compound **3** (**PT167**, **NSC 799315**) were consistently active versus wild-type p53-containing cancer cell lines and cancer cell lines with mutant or lost p53 protein (Table 3). The p53 status of the individual cancer cell lines in the NCI DTP 60-cancer cell 5-dose testing cell line panel was taken as published [1,2].

2. National Cancer Institute (NCI) Developmental Therapeutics Program (DTP) 60-Cancer Cell 5-Dose Testing Results with the Drugs PT162, PT166 and PT167

2.1. National Cancer Institute (NCI) Developmental Therapeutics Program (DTP) 60-cancer cell 5-dose testing results with compound **1** (**PT162, NSC 796018**)

The four pages of the National Cancer Institute (NCI) Developmental Therapeutics Program (DTP) 60-cancer cell 5-dose testing results for compound **1** (**PT162, NSC 796018**) are given in succession. **First page** (Fig. 31): graphic allover presentation of page two with **All Cell Lines** in one graphic. **Second page** (Fig. 32): inhibition curves for tumor cell lines arranged/ordered for general tumor type. **Third page** (Fig. 33): the Mean Optical Densities of the utilized vital stain sulforhodamine B (SRB) retained in the cells, the actual used concentrations in $\log_{10}$ unit for five doses, and the **Percent Growth** are given. The **GI50 (Growth inhibition 50%)**, **TGI (Total Growth Inhibition = 0% Growth)**, and **LC50 (Lethal Concentration 50% = –50% Growth)** are given in linear concentration units. **Fourth page** (Fig. 34): this is the summary of the results expressed in $\log_{10}$ units. The defined tumor inhibition criterion (**GI50, TGI, or LC50**) is recalculated in $\log_{10}$ expression, and the the colored bars which indicate then the sensitivity of the individual tumor cell line to the agent are given in $\log_{10}$ units.

Table 3. National Cancer Institute (NCI) Developmental Therapeutics Program (DTP) 60-cancer cell 5-dose testing of compound 1 (**PT162**), compound 2 (**PT166**), and compound 3 (**PT167**) (with cellular p53 status).

Cancer cell line	Compound	GI50 (μM)	TGI (μM)	LC50 (μM)
Leukemia (p53 status: *, termination; del, deletion; fs, frame shift; Lit., Literature)				
CCRF-CEM	1	1.46	> 50	> 50
mutant p53	2	0.422	> 100	> 100
R175H, R248Q	3	0.904	2.47	14.9
HL-60 (TB)	1	0.87	2.71	> 50
mutant p53	2	0.113	1.26	> 100
p.M1_*394del	3	0.168	1.03	6.85
K-562	1	1.46	36.2	> 50
mutant p53	2	0.362	> 100	> 100
p.Q136fs*13	3	—	—	—
MOLT-4	1	1.32	4.09	> 50
mutant p53	2	0.548	> 100	> 100
Lit. uncertain	3	0.562	1.93	13.3
RPMI-8226	1	1.32	3.99	> 50
mutant p53	2	0.349	8.65	> 100
E285K	3	0.757	1.76	> 33.3
SR	1	1.49	> 50	> 50
wild-type p53	2	0.279	> 100	> 100
	3	—	—	—
Non-small-cell lung cancer (p53 status: *, termination; del, deletion; fs, frame shift)				
A549	1	2.13	8.70	24.2
wild-type p53	2	3.23	> 100	> 100
	3	1.61	6.00	18.2
EKVX	1	—	—	—
mutant p53	2	—#	> 100	> 100
splicing defect	3	2.68	8.46	23.6
HOP-62	1	2.66	10.1	29.7
mutant p53	2	0.700	> 100	> 100
splicing defect	3	2.14	7.43	20.2
HOP-92	1	1.14	3.06	12.6
mutant p53	2	—	—	—
R175L	3	0.897	4.08	15.1
NCI-H226	1	2.76	10.8	31.2
Lit.	2	1.74	> 100	> 100
inconclusive	3	1.96	9.97	> 33.3
NCI-H23	1	1.53	6.36	28.2
mutant p53	2	0.438	> 100	> 100
M246I	3	1.38	5.33	16.4
NCI-H322M	1	1.26	5.10	16.0
mutant p53	2	0.619	> 100	> 100
R248L	3	2.57	7.03	16.3
NCI-H460	1	1.19	2.71	17.9
wild-type p53	2	0.429	> 100	> 100
	3	1.22	3.79	13.5

NCI-H522	1	0.731	1.55	3.30
mutant p53	2	0.550	> 100	> 100
p.P191fs*56	3	0.699	1.88	8.33
Colon cancer (p53 status: *, termination; del, deletion; fs, frame shift; Lit., Literature)				
COLO 205	1	1.09	3.13	24.8
mutant p53	2	0.280	0.622	9.13
Lit. uncertain	3	0.683	1.52	3.61
HCC-2998	1	1.22	5.31	22.6
mutant p53	2	0.272	0.674	> 100
R213X	3	0.635	1.47	3.55
HCT-116	1	0.728	2.01	6.47
wild-type p53	2	0.377	10.6	> 100
	3	0.896	3.07	11.0
HCT-15	1	1.10	3.91	18.4
mutant p53	2	4.03	> 100	> 100
Lit. uncertain	3	1.56	5.96	17.2
HT29	1	0.857	2.82	14.6
mutant p53	2	0.336	> 100	> 100
R273H	3	0.958	2.81	11.3
KM-12	1	1.65	6.75	20.6
mutant p53	2	0.255	0.801	> 100
Lit. uncertain	3	1.08	4.52	22.5
SW-620	1	1.25	3.95	17.2
mutant p53	2	0.369	> 100	> 100
R273H, P309S	3	0.814	2.06	8.74
CNS cancer (brain tumor) (p53 status: *, termination; del, deletion; fs, frame shift)				
SF-268	1	1.53	5.41	30.8
mutant p53	2	0.581	> 100	> 100
R273H	3	1.37	6.54	29.9
SF-295	1	3.05	10.4	28.2
mutant p53	2	0.549	> 100	> 100
R248Q	3	1.53	5.92	15.4
SF-539	1	1.01	2.48	7.59
mutant p53	2	0.418	20.5	> 100
Lit. uncertain	3	1.14	4.30	13.8
SNB-19	1	1.92	7.27	19.9
mutant p53	2	0.686	> 100	> 100
R273H	3	1.65	6.20	19.5
SNB-75	1	2.34	9.73	27.9
mutant p53	2	0.441	> 100	> 100
E258K	3	1.40	6.68	20.1
U251	1	1.12	2.69	8.79
mutant p53	2	0.479	> 100	> 100
R273H	3	—	—	—
Melanoma (p53 status: *, termination; del, deletion; fs, frame shift; Lit., Literature)				
LOX IMVI	1	0.505	1.27	3.18
wild-type p53	2	0.710	> 100	> 100
	3	0.873	2.86	14.3

MALME-3M	**1**	0.839	1.86	4.12
wild-type p53	**2**	0.394	> 100	> 100
	3	0.830	3.04	14.4
M14	**1**	0.803	2.08	6.82
mutant p53	**2**	0.284	0.735	> 100
G266E	**3**	0.822	2.26	9.06
MDA-MB-435	**1**	0.825	2.11	6.50
mutant p53	**2**	0.233	0.838	> 100
G266E	**3**	0.779	3.50	12.4
SK-MEL-2	**1**	1.06	3.20	15.6
mutant p53	**2**	> 100	> 100	> 100
G245S	**3**	0.861	2.76	12.4
SK-MEL-28	**1**	1.66	7.91	21.9
mutant p53	**2**	—	> 100	> 100
L145R	**3**	1.02	4.07	13.6
SK-MEL-5	**1**	1.52	6.28	18.6
wild-type p53	**2**	0.373	4.71	> 100
	3	0.810	2.25	8.65
UACC-257	**1**	3.08	10.8	29.4
wild-type p53	**2**	0.646	> 100	> 100
	3	4.51	10.3	23.6
UACC-62	**1**	1.16	3.68	14.2
wild-type p53	**2**	0.625	> 100	> 100
	3	1.61	6.38	18.0
Ovarian cancer (p53 status: *, termination; del, deletion; fs, frame shift; Lit., Literature)				
IGROV1	**1**	0.886	2.34	8.65
mutant p53	**2**	1.18	> 100	> 100
Lit. uncertain	**3**	1.45	5.95	20.9
OVCAR-3	**1**	1.04	2.82	9.97
mutant p53	**2**	0.217	0.459	—
R248Q	**3**	1.66	6.53	18.5
OVCAR-4	**1**	1.16	5.45	18.4
mutant p53	**2**	0.507	> 100	> 100
Lit. uncertain	**3**	2.17	8.94	30.0
OVCAR-5	**1**	0.977	2.76	10.8
Lit.	**2**	9.67	> 100	> 100
inconclusive	**3**	1.17	5.03	14.2
OVCAR-8	**1**	2.07	8.48	35.3
mutant p53	**2**	0.970	> 100	> 100
splicing defect	**3**	2.03	7.49	24.3
NCI/ADR-RES	**1**	1.44	4.55	> 50
mutant p53	**2**	25.3	> 100	> 100
splicing defect	**3**	5.43	12.5	28.6
SK-OV-3	**1**	5.11	11.4	25.5
no p53 protein	**2**	1.39	> 100	> 100
expressed	**3**	3.00	7.51	17.6

Renal cancer (p53 status: *, termination; del, deletion; fs, frame shift; Lit., Literature)				
786-0	1	0.848	1.85	4.05
mutant p53	2	0.818	> 100	> 100
Lit. uncertain	3	1.30	5.28	17.6
A498	1	1.19	7.05	21.2
wild-type p53	2	2.09	> 100	> 100
	3	1.07	3.28	12.4
ACHN	1	0.874	2.14	5.55
wild-type p53	2	8.50	> 100	> 100
	3	3.68	7.99	17.3
CAKI-1	1	1.28	4.70	15.4
wild-type p53	2	7.12	> 100	> 100
	3	3.20	7.37	16.5
RXF 393	1	0.811	1.56	3.02
mutant p53	2	0.298	0.747	> 100
R175H	3	1.70	6.65	20.9
SN12C	1	1.41	4.43	15.8
mutant p53	2	0.828	> 100	> 100
E336X	3	2.23	6.90	17.4
TK-10	1	1.85	7.17	21.5
mutant p53	2	6.77	> 100	> 100
L264R	3	3.66	8.35	19.0
UO-31	1	0.817	1.96	4.73
wild-type p53	2	> 100	> 100	> 100
	3	2.16	7.20	18.3
Prostate cancer (p53 status: *, termination; del, deletion; fs, frame shift; ⁻, null p53 protein)				
PC-3	1	1.40	5.17	21.4
mutant p53⁻	2	0.255	> 100	> 100
p.K139fs*31	3	1.45	5.64	17.1
DU-145	1	1.47	4.61	15.2
mutant p53	2	0.341	1.44	> 100
P223L, V274F	3	2.46	7.10	17.3
Breast cancer (p53 status: *, termination; del, deletion; fs, frame shift)				
MCF7	1	1.07	6.19	45.8
wild-type p53	2	0.415	> 100	> 100
	3	0.862	3.44	> 33.3
MDA-MB-231	1	2.09	7.41	22.7
mutant p53	2	0.359	1.88	> 100
R280K	3	0.994	2.99	12.4
HS 578T	1	1.92	11.8	> 50
mutant p53	2	> 100	> 100	> 100
V157F	3	1.22	6.76	> 33.3
BT-549	1	1.02	2.77	10.2
mutant p53	2	0.294	0.924	> 100
R249S	3	1.55	5.89	16.5
T-47D	1	1.34	6.72	38.0
mutant p53	2	> 100	> 100	> 100
L194F	3	1.83	9.40	> 33.3

MDA-MB-468	1	0.797	1.68	3.55
mutant p53	2	0.158	0.464	> 100
R273H	3	0.657	1.75	10.7
Mean of Inhibition Data (MID)		**GI50** (μM)	**TGI** (μM)	**LC50** (μM)
10^{-MID}	**1**	1.288	4.677	16.596
10^{-MID}	**2**	0.933	32.359	95.499
10^{-MID}	**3**	1.349	4.571	15.849

[#], The **GI50** value could not being calculated due to positive growth.

——, Not tested, because cancer cell line not available at NCI test facility.

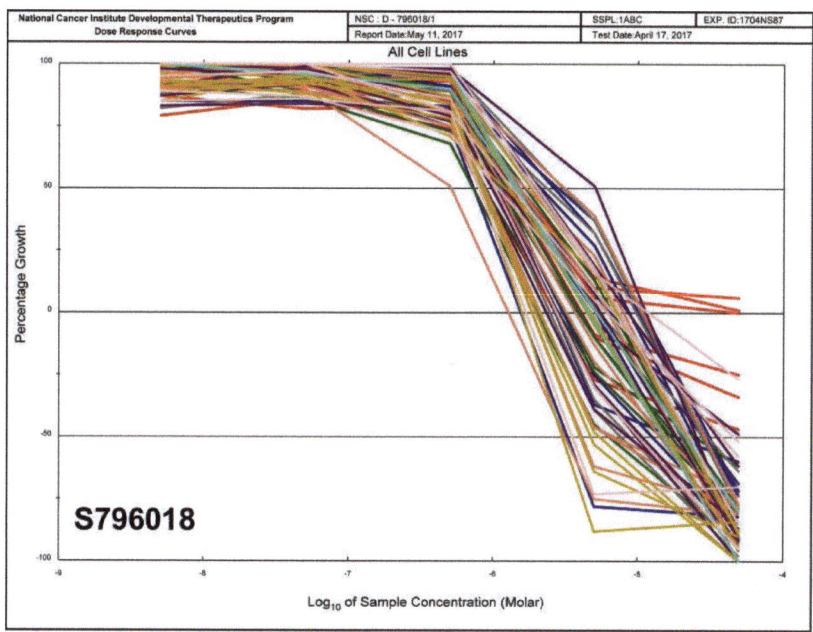

Fig. 31. Graphic allover presentation of the antineoplastic activity in the National Cancer Institute (NCI) Developmental Therapeutics Program (DTP) 60-cancer cell 5-dose testing exhibited by the pure drug compound **1** (**PT162**, **NSC 796018**) with **All Cell Lines** in one graphic.

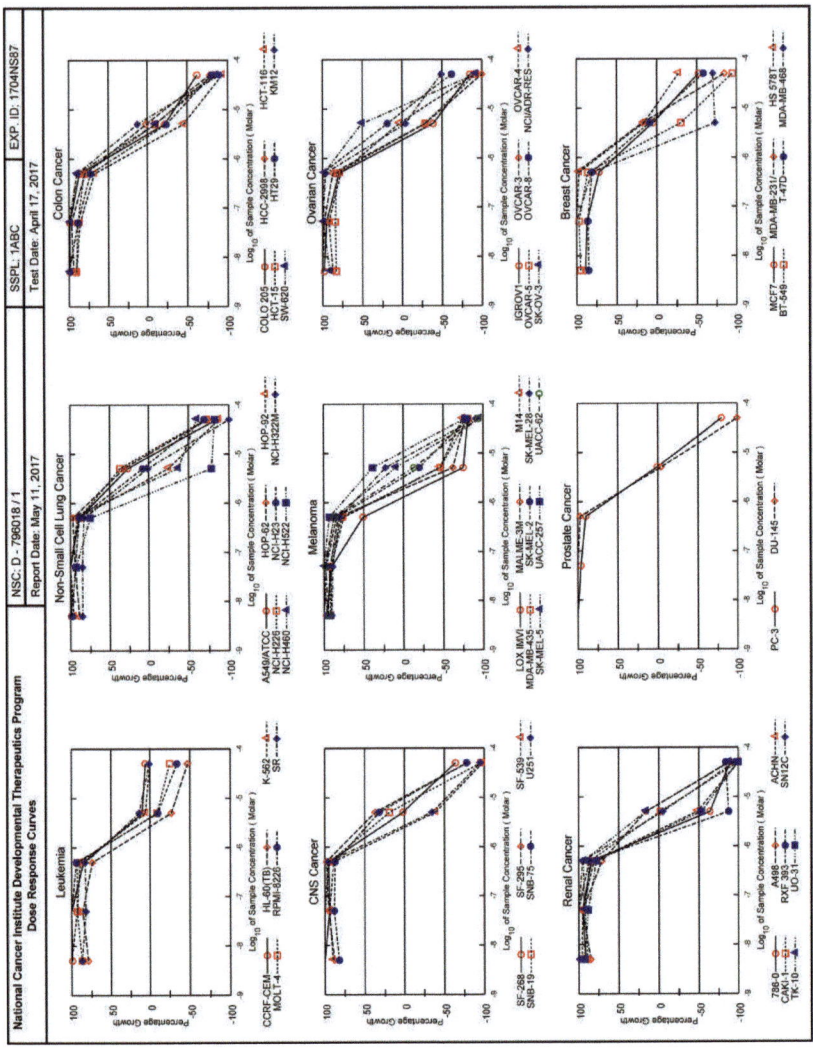

Fig. 32. Graphic presentation of the antineoplastic activity exhibited by the pure drug compound **1** (**PT162**, **NSC 796018**) in the National Cancer Institute (NCI) Developmental Therapeutics Program (DTP) 60-cancer cell 5-dose testing with the inhibition curves for sixty tumor cell lines arranged/ordered in terms of general tumor type.

National Cancer Institute Developmental Therapeutics Program In-Vitro Testing Results				
NSC : D - 796018 / 1	Experiment ID : 1704NS87	Test Type : 08	Units : Molar	
Report Date : May 11, 2017	Test Date : April 17, 2017	QNS :	MC :	
COMI : PT162	Stain Reagent : SRB Dual-Pass Related	SSPL : 1ABC		

Panel/Cell Line	Time Zero	Ctrl	Mean Optical Densities (Log10 Concentration)					Percent Growth					GI50	TGI	LC50
			-8.3	-7.3	-6.3	-5.3	-4.3	-8.3	-7.3	-6.3	-5.3	-4.3			
Leukemia															
CCRF-CEM	0.434	1.625	1.618	1.661	1.441	0.557	0.503	99	103	85	10	6	1.46E-6	> 5.00E-5	> 5.00E-5
HL-60(TB)	0.750	2.047	1.769	1.864	1.715	0.548	0.396	79	86	74	-27	-47	8.70E-7	2.71E-6	> 5.00E-5
K-562	0.269	1.764	1.761	1.653	1.593	0.354	0.267	100	93	89	6		1.46E-6	3.62E-5	> 5.00E-5
MOLT-4	0.735	2.452	2.235	2.332	2.332	0.670	0.553	87	93	93	-9	-25	1.32E-6	4.09E-6	> 5.00E-5
RPMI-8226	0.587	2.220	2.252	2.299	2.117	0.526	0.386	102	105	94	-10	-34	1.32E-6	3.99E-6	> 5.00E-5
SR	0.441	1.725	1.564	1.491	1.504	0.615	0.457	87	82	83	14	1	1.49E-6	> 5.00E-5	> 5.00E-5
Non-Small Cell Lung Cancer															
A549/ATCC	0.361	1.704	1.693	1.730	1.557	0.724	0.083	99	102	89	27	-85	2.13E-6	8.70E-6	2.42E-5
HOP-62	0.745	2.044	1.904	1.969	2.004	1.165	0.193	89	94	97	32	-74	2.66E-6	1.01E-5	2.97E-5
HOP-92	1.114	1.649	1.626	1.647	1.603	0.837	0.142	96	100	91	-25	-87	1.14E-6	3.06E-6	1.26E-5
NCI-H226	0.841	1.823	1.875	1.867	1.711	1.200	0.233	105	105	89	37	-72	2.76E-6	1.08E-5	3.12E-5
NCI-H23	0.511	1.825	1.804	1.748	1.686	0.616	0.157	98	94	89	8	-69	1.53E-6	6.36E-6	2.82E-5
NCI-H322M	0.874	2.125	1.936	1.933	1.909	0.885	-0.004	95	85	83	1	-100	1.26E-6	5.10E-6	1.60E-5
NCI-H460	0.221	2.164	2.313	2.308	2.213	0.139	0.088	108	107	103	-37	-60	1.19E-6	2.71E-6	1.79E-5
NCI-H522	0.892	2.118	2.215	2.030	1.815	0.200	0.162	108	93	75	-78	-82	7.31E-7	1.55E-6	3.30E-6
Colon Cancer															
COLO 205	0.508	1.801	1.785	1.795	1.634	0.396	0.192	99	99	87	-22	-62	1.09E-6	3.13E-6	2.48E-5
HCC-2998	0.694	2.339	2.238	2.288	2.016	0.729	0.156	94	97	80	-2	-78	1.22E-6	5.31E-6	2.26E-5
HCT-116	0.195	1.586	1.457	1.393	1.147	0.108	0.014	91	86	68	-45	-93	7.28E-7	2.01E-6	6.47E-6
HCT-15	0.192	1.407	1.294	1.276	1.176	0.174	0.037	91	89	81	-10	-81	1.10E-6	3.91E-6	1.84E-5
HT29	0.230	1.418	1.436	1.288	1.093	0.175	0.047	102	89	73	-24	-80	8.57E-7	2.82E-6	1.46E-5
KM12	0.508	2.477	2.465	2.492	2.271	0.774	0.052	99	101	90	13	-90	1.65E-6	6.75E-6	2.06E-5
SW-620	0.265	1.779	1.766	1.710	1.625	0.238	0.041	99	90	90	-10	-85	1.25E-6	3.95E-6	1.72E-5
CNS Cancer															
SF-268	0.537	1.916	1.923	1.840	1.847	0.568	0.194	101	94	95	2	-64	1.53E-6	5.41E-6	3.08E-5
SF-295	0.604	2.260	2.086	2.200	2.241	1.223	0.129	88	95	98	37	-79	3.05E-6	1.04E-5	2.82E-5
SF-539	1.012	2.658	2.490	2.556	2.486	0.614	0.018	90	94	89	-39	-98	1.01E-6	2.48E-6	7.99E-6
SNB-19	0.445	1.952	1.950	1.949	1.867	0.726	0.019	100	100	94	19	-96	1.92E-6	7.27E-6	1.99E-5
SNB-75	0.886	1.781	1.618	1.671	1.668	1.169	0.198	82	88	87	32	-78	2.34E-6	9.73E-6	2.79E-5
U251	0.334	1.564	1.609	1.612	1.515	0.216	0.016	104	104	96	-35	-95	1.12E-6	2.69E-6	8.79E-6
Melanoma															
LOX IMVI	0.333	2.352	2.284	2.153	1.354	0.085	0.063	97	90	51	-75	-81	5.05E-7	1.27E-6	3.18E-6
MALME-3M	0.572	1.296	1.261	1.241	1.169	0.217	0.126	95	92	82	-62	-78	8.39E-7	1.86E-6	4.12E-6
M14	0.420	1.538	1.434	1.433	1.258	0.226	0.108	91	91	75	-46	-74	8.03E-7	2.08E-6	6.82E-6
MDA-MB-435	0.592	2.489	2.328	2.357	2.047	0.320	0.114	92	93	77	-46	-81	8.25E-7	2.11E-6	6.50E-6
SK-MEL-2	1.031	2.002	2.045	1.977	1.848	0.822	0.202	104	97	84	-20	-80	1.06E-6	3.20E-6	1.56E-5
SK-MEL-28	0.753	2.281	2.125	2.119	1.976	1.098	0.071	90	89	80	23	-91	1.66E-6	7.91E-6	2.19E-5
SK-MEL-5	0.632	2.957	2.993	2.933	2.653	0.876	0.030	102	99	87	10	-95	1.52E-6	6.28E-6	1.96E-5
UACC-257	1.062	2.071	2.030	2.114	1.997	1.452	0.250	96	104	93	39	-77	3.08E-6	1.08E-5	2.94E-5
UACC-62	0.631	2.480	2.374	2.437	2.232	0.548	0.037	94	98	87	-13	-94	1.16E-6	3.68E-6	1.42E-5
Ovarian Cancer															
IGROV1	0.375	1.786	1.742	1.690	1.480	0.229	0.055	98	95	79	-39	-85	8.86E-7	2.34E-6	8.65E-6
OVCAR-3	0.417	1.444	1.440	1.423	1.309	0.298	0.001	100	98	87	-29	-100	1.04E-6	2.82E-6	9.97E-6
OVCAR-4	0.826	1.689	1.578	1.616	1.489	0.857	0.073	87	92	77	4	-91	1.16E-6	5.45E-6	1.84E-5
OVCAR-5	0.581	1.404	1.263	1.273	1.259	0.414	0.045	83	84	82	-29	-92	9.77E-7	2.76E-6	1.08E-5
OVCAR-8	0.581	2.276	2.357	2.368	2.279	0.894	0.220	105	106	101	19	-62	2.07E-6	8.46E-6	3.53E-5
NCI/ADR-RES	0.487	1.643	1.650	1.641	1.596	0.467	0.251	101	100	96	-4	-49	1.44E-6	4.55E-6	> 5.00E-5
SK-OV-3	0.894	1.876	1.787	1.867	1.854	1.399	0.071	91	99	98	51	-92	5.11E-6	1.14E-5	2.55E-5
Renal Cancer															
786-0	0.403	1.759	1.632	1.687	1.540	0.147	0.041	91	95	84	-64	-90	8.48E-7	1.85E-6	4.05E-6
A498	1.422	2.245	2.125	2.205	2.005	1.551	0.159	85	95	71	16	-89	1.19E-6	7.05E-6	2.12E-5
ACHN	0.379	1.642	1.589	1.581	1.405	0.199	-0.002	96	95	81	-48	-100	8.74E-7	2.14E-6	5.55E-6
CAKI-1	0.767	2.753	2.532	2.597	2.481	0.749	0.004	89	92	86	-2	-100	1.28E-6	4.70E-6	1.54E-5
RXF 393	0.685	1.323	1.358	1.334	1.239	0.080	0.112	105	102	87	-88	-84	8.11E-7	1.56E-6	3.02E-6
SN12C	0.391	1.784	1.773	1.781	1.719	0.371	0.020	99	100	95	-5	-95	1.41E-6	4.43E-6	1.58E-5
TK-10	0.865	1.676	1.618	1.621	1.630	0.998	0.100	93	93	94	16	-88	1.85E-6	7.17E-6	2.15E-5
UO-31	0.608	2.142	2.029	1.962	1.804	0.285	-0.007	93	88	78	-53	-100	8.17E-7	1.96E-6	4.73E-6
Prostate Cancer															
PC-3	0.440	1.517	1.515	1.477	1.406	0.453	0.089	100	96	90	1	-80	1.40E-6	5.17E-6	2.14E-5
DU-145	0.338	1.467	1.493	1.480	1.437	0.326	-0.002	102	101	97	-4	-100	1.47E-6	4.61E-6	1.52E-5
Breast Cancer															
MCF7	0.346	2.158	1.966	1.929	1.650	0.443	0.166	89	87	72	5	-52	1.07E-6	6.19E-6	4.58E-5
MDA-MB-231/ATCC	0.547	1.458	1.511	1.536	1.487	0.707	0.081	106	108	103	18	-85	2.09E-6	7.41E-6	2.27E-5
HS 578T	0.815	1.655	1.671	1.681	1.631	0.952	0.593	102	103	97	16	-27	1.92E-6	1.16E-5	> 5.00E-5
BT-549	1.139	2.003	1.962	1.978	1.880	0.603	0.053	95	97	86	-30	-95	1.02E-6	2.77E-6	1.02E-5
T-47D	0.703	1.599	1.461	1.471	1.429	0.780	0.296	85	86	81	9	-58	1.34E-6	6.72E-6	3.80E-5
MDA-MB-468	0.640	1.327	1.331	1.332	1.198	0.174	0.190	101	101	81	-73	-70	7.97E-7	1.68E-6	3.55E-6

Fig. 33. Tabular list of the antineoplastic activity exhibited by the pure drug compound **1** (**PT162, NSC 796018**) in the National Cancer Institute (NCI) Developmental Therapeutics Program (DTP) 60-cancer cell 5-dose testing with the Mean Optical Densities of the used vital stain sulforhodamine B (SRB) retained in the cells given. **Percent Growth, GI50 (Growth inhibition 50%)**, **TGI (Total Growth Inhibition = 0% Growth)**, and **LC50 (Lethal Concentration 50% = –50% Growth)** are given in linear concentration units.

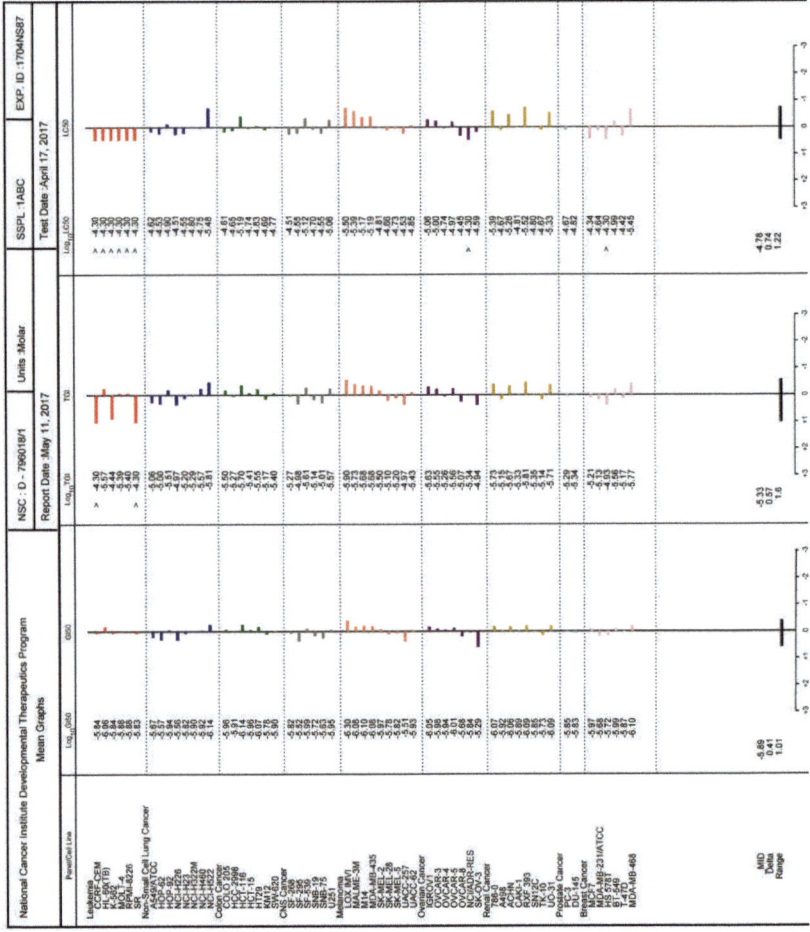

Fig. 34. Graphic table presentation of the antineoplastic activity exhibited by the pure drug compound **1** (**PT162, NSC 796018**) in the National Cancer Institute (NCI) Developmental Therapeutics Program (DTP) 60-cancer cell 5-dose testing with the **Percent Growth, GI50 (Growth inhibition 50%), TGI (Total Growth Inhibition = 0% Growth)**, and **LC50 (Lethal Concentration 50% = –50% Growth)** given in linear concentration units. This is the summary of the results expressed in $\log_{10}$ units. The defined tumor inhibition criterion (**GI50, TGI**, or **LC50**) is recalculated in $\log_{10}$ expression, and the colored bars which indicate then the sensitivity of the individual tumor cell line to the agent are given, but

in $\log_{10}$ units. **Bar to the left: less sensitive than mean, Bar to the right: more sensitive than mean.** The most important feature is at the bottom of the page: the **MID** (**Mean of Inhibition Data**) indicates the mean concentration for all tested cell lines required for the drug to reach the defined tumor inhibition criterion (**GI50, TGI**, or **LC50**). It is given in **Log$_{10}$GI50, Log$_{10}$TGI** and **Log$_{10}$LC50**. From that values the corresponding **MID** is calculated. The more negative the **MID**, the more potent is the drug. The **MID** can be transformed from logarithmic into linear concentrations by the formula: $c = 10^{MID}$.

2.2. National Cancer Institute (NCI) Developmental Therapeutics Program (DTP) 60-cancer cell 5-dose testing results with compound 2 (PT166, NSC 750423)

The four pages of the National Cancer Institute (NCI) Developmental Therapeutics Program (DTP) 60-cancer cell 5-dose testing results for compound **2** (**PT166, NSC 750423**) are given in succession. **First page** (Fig. 35): graphic allover presentation of page two with **All Cell Lines** in one graphic. **Second page** (Fig. 36): inhibition curves for tumor cell lines arranged/ordered for general tumor type. **Third page** (Fig. 37): the Mean Optical Densities of the utilized vital stain sulforhodamine B (SRB) retained in the cells, the actual used concentrations in $\log_{10}$ unit for five doses, and the **Percent Growth** are given. The **GI50 (Growth inhibition 50%)**, **TGI (Total Growth Inhibition = 0% Growth)**, and **LC50 (Lethal Concentration 50% = –50% Growth)** are given in linear concentration units. **Fourth page** (Fig. 38): this is the summary of the results expressed in $\log_{10}$ units. The defined tumor inhibition criterion (**GI50, TGI**, or **LC50**) is recalculated in $\log_{10}$ expression, and the the colored bars which indicate then the sensitivity of the individual tumor cell line to the agent are given in $\log_{10}$ units.

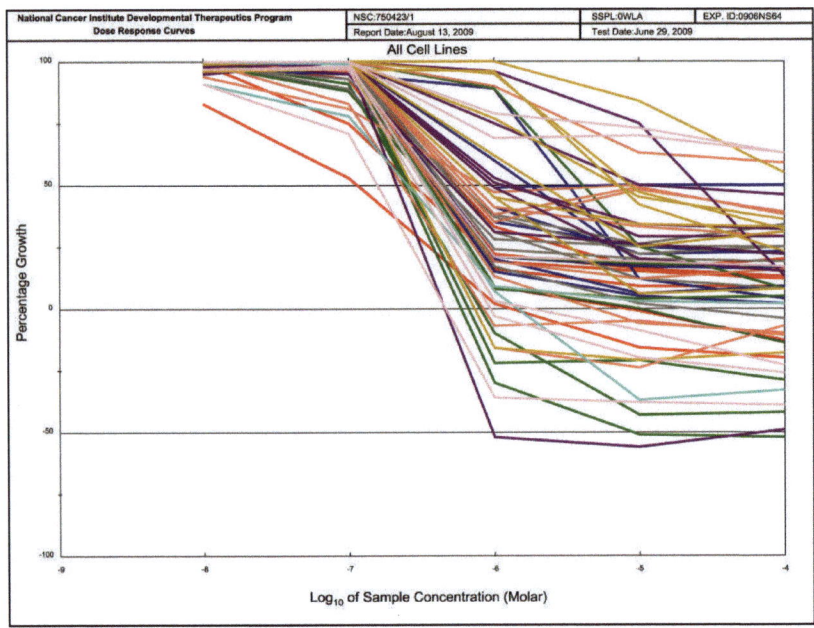

Fig. 35. Graphic allover presentation of the antineoplastic activity in the National Cancer Institute (NCI) Developmental Therapeutics Program (DTP) 60-cancer cell 5-dose testing exhibited by the drug compound **2** (**PT166, NSC 750423**) with **All Cell Lines** in one graphic.

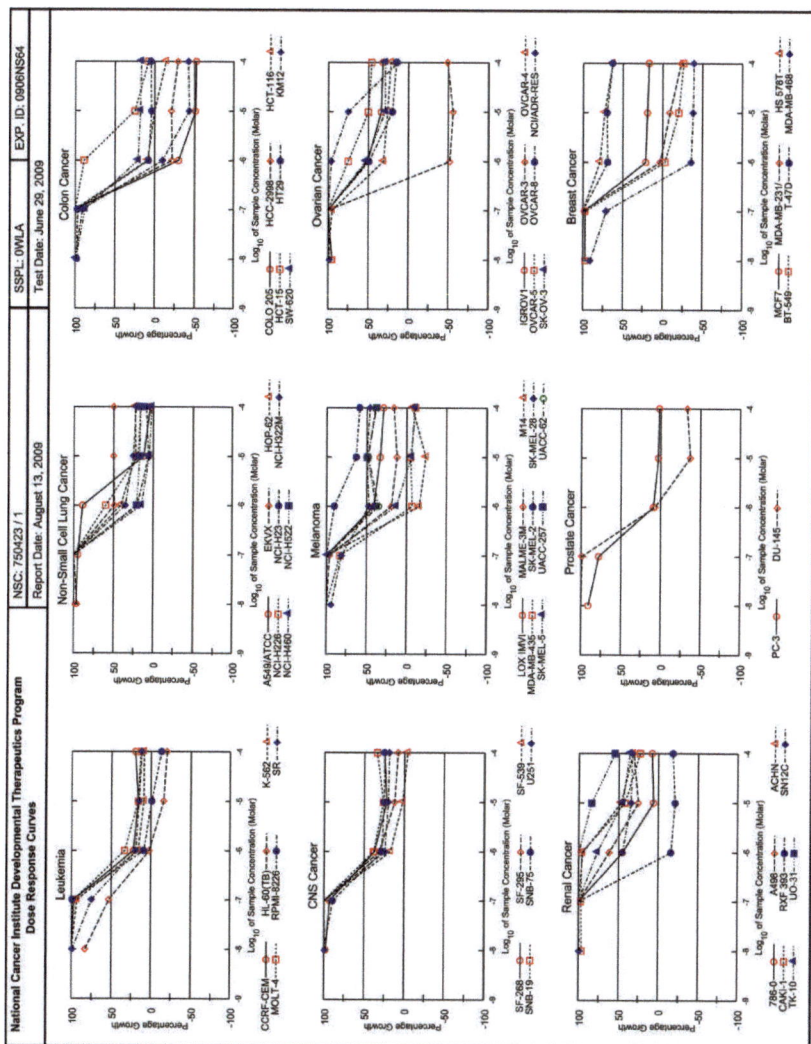

Fig. 36. Graphic presentation of the antineoplastic activity exhibited by the drug compound **2** (**PT166**, **NSC 750423**) in the National Cancer Institute (NCI) Developmental Therapeutics Program (DTP) 60-cancer cell 5-dose testing with the inhibition curves for sixty tumor cell lines arranged/ordered in terms of general tumor type.

National Cancer Institute Developmental Therapeutics Program
In-Vitro Testing Results

NSC : 750423 / 1	Experiment ID : 0906NS64	Test Type : 08	Units : Molar
Report Date : August 13, 2009	Test Date : June 29, 2009	QNS :	MC :
COMI : colch-TSC (84886)	Stain Reagent : SRB Dual-Pass Related	SSPL : 0WLA	

Panel/Cell Line	Time Zero	Ctrl	Mean Optical Densities					Percent Growth					GI50	TGI	LC50
			-8.0	-7.0	-6.0	-5.0	-4.0	-8.0	-7.0	-6.0	-5.0	-4.0			
Leukemia															
CCRF-CEM	0.356	1.223	1.293	1.199	0.545	0.496	0.531	108	97	22	16	20	4.22E-7	> 1.00E-4	> 1.00E-4
HL-60(TB)	0.825	2.422	2.153	1.668	0.854	0.694	0.664	83	53	2	-16	-20	1.13E-7	1.26E-6	> 1.00E-4
K-562	0.287	1.715	1.711	1.622	0.510	0.417	0.422	100	93	16	9	9	3.62E-7	> 1.00E-4	> 1.00E-4
MOLT-4	0.609	1.986	2.143	1.948	1.068	0.825	0.792	111	97	33	16	13	5.46E-7	> 1.00E-4	> 1.00E-4
RPMI-8226	0.864	1.665	1.739	1.658	0.933	0.859	0.751	109	99	9	-1	-13	3.49E-7	8.85E-6	> 1.00E-4
SR	0.312	1.029	1.020	0.850	0.449	0.417	0.400	99	75	19	15	12	2.79E-7	> 1.00E-4	> 1.00E-4
Non-Small Cell Lung Cancer															
A549/ATCC	0.337	1.197	1.167	1.154	1.102	0.444	0.375	97	95	89	12	4	3.23E-6	> 1.00E-4	> 1.00E-4
EKVX	0.663	1.690	1.653	1.702	1.171	1.172	1.182	96	101	49	50	50		> 1.00E-4	> 1.00E-4
HOP-82	0.341	1.030	1.041	1.039	0.621	0.495	0.496	102	101	41	22	23	7.00E-7	> 1.00E-4	> 1.00E-4
NCI-H226	0.619	1.115	1.148	1.182	0.915	0.716	0.699	107	113	60	19	16	1.74E-6	> 1.00E-4	> 1.00E-4
NCI-H23	0.352	0.990	1.015	1.018	0.477	0.391	0.412	104	104	20	6	9	4.38E-7	> 1.00E-4	> 1.00E-4
NCI-H322M	0.533	1.061	1.061	1.090	0.720	0.665	0.649	100	106	35	25	22	6.16E-7	> 1.00E-4	> 1.00E-4
NCI-H460	0.117	1.142	1.287	1.240	0.275	0.165	0.138	114	110	15	5	2	4.29E-7	> 1.00E-4	> 1.00E-4
NCI-H522	0.482	1.412	1.668	1.706	0.682	0.639	0.633	127	132	21	17	16	5.50E-7	> 1.00E-4	> 1.00E-4
Colon Cancer															
COLO 205	0.180	0.657	0.737	0.727	0.127	0.089	0.087	117	115	-30	-51	-52	2.80E-7	6.22E-7	9.13E-6
HCC-2998	0.536	1.610	1.614	1.667	0.420	0.424	0.382	100	105	-22	-29	-29	2.72E-7	6.74E-7	> 1.00E-4
HCT-116	0.147	1.082	1.131	1.140	0.229	0.151	0.127	105	106	9		-14	3.77E-7	1.08E-5	> 1.00E-4
HCT-15	0.264	1.537	1.587	1.568	1.394	0.595	0.380	104	102	89	25	8	4.03E-6	> 1.00E-4	> 1.00E-4
HT29	0.209	1.360	1.338	1.328	0.298	0.259	0.262	98	97	8	4	5	3.36E-7	> 1.00E-4	> 1.00E-4
KM12	0.237	1.196	1.231	1.110	0.214	0.135	0.138	104	91	-10	-43	-42	2.55E-7	8.01E-7	> 1.00E-4
SW-620	0.180	1.104	1.096	0.995	0.355	0.328	0.321	99	88	21	18	17	3.69E-7	> 1.00E-4	> 1.00E-4
CNS Cancer															
SF-268	0.444	1.433	1.412	1.360	0.809	0.660	0.693	98	93	37	22	25	5.81E-7	> 1.00E-4	> 1.00E-4
SF-295	0.687	2.195	2.253	2.266	1.151	0.869	0.812	104	104	31	12	8	5.49E-7	> 1.00E-4	> 1.00E-4
SF-539	0.373	1.398	1.401	1.442	0.546	0.393	0.357	100	104	17	2	-4	4.18E-7	2.05E-5	> 1.00E-4
SNB-19	0.607	1.561	1.625	1.665	0.971	0.852	0.928	107	111	38	26	34	6.86E-7	> 1.00E-4	> 1.00E-4
SNB-75	0.502	0.959	0.968	0.908	0.632	0.617	0.617	102	89	28	25	25	4.41E-7	> 1.00E-4	> 1.00E-4
U251	0.207	1.094	1.088	1.141	0.421	0.388	0.380	99	105	24	20	19	4.79E-7	> 1.00E-4	> 1.00E-4
Melanoma															
LOX IMVI	0.261	1.596	1.631	1.653	0.802	0.706	0.650	103	104	41	33	29	7.10E-7	> 1.00E-4	> 1.00E-4
MALME-3M	0.417	0.566	0.574	0.560	0.445	0.436	0.442	106	96	19	12	16	3.94E-7	> 1.00E-4	> 1.00E-4
M14	0.317	1.044	1.086	1.080	0.266	0.240	0.294	106	105	-16	-24	-7	2.84E-7	7.35E-7	> 1.00E-4
MDA-MB-435	0.370	1.324	1.361	1.163	0.345	0.351	0.329	104	83	-7	-5	-11	2.33E-7	8.38E-7	> 1.00E-4
SK-MEL-2	0.484	0.922	0.992	1.029	0.879	0.758	0.740	116	125	90	63	59	> 1.00E-4	> 1.00E-4	> 1.00E-4
SK-MEL-28	0.262	0.870	0.832	0.754	0.546	0.569	0.543	94	81	47	50	46		> 1.00E-4	> 1.00E-4
SK-MEL-5	0.571	2.052	2.059	2.045	0.764	0.535	0.514	100	99	13	-6	-10	3.73E-7	4.71E-6	> 1.00E-4
UACC-257	0.448	0.815	0.816	0.818	0.588	0.629	0.589	100	101	38	49	38	6.46E-7	> 1.00E-4	> 1.00E-4
UACC-62	0.821	2.155	2.248	2.246	1.294	1.457	1.338	107	107	35	48	39	6.25E-7	> 1.00E-4	> 1.00E-4
Ovarian Cancer															
IGROV1	0.360	1.694	1.624	1.727	1.043	0.815	0.784	95	102	51	34	32	1.18E-6	> 1.00E-4	> 1.00E-4
OVCAR-3	0.320	0.943	0.965	0.952	0.154	0.140	0.165	104	101	-52	-56	-49	2.17E-7	4.59E-7	
OVCAR-4	0.463	1.261	1.315	1.219	0.713	0.672	0.635	107	95	31	26	22	5.07E-7	> 1.00E-4	> 1.00E-4
OVCAR-5	0.348	0.719	0.699	0.722	0.626	0.532	0.518	95	100	75	50	46	9.87E-6	> 1.00E-4	> 1.00E-4
OVCAR-8	0.507	1.475	1.514	1.642	0.984	0.702	0.650	104	107	49	20	15	9.70E-7	> 1.00E-4	> 1.00E-4
NCI/ADR-RES	0.222	0.710	0.702	0.714	0.690	0.589	0.284	98	101	96	75	13	2.53E-5	> 1.00E-4	> 1.00E-4
SK-OV-3	0.510	1.213	1.385	1.453	0.886	0.715	0.712	124	134	53	29	29	1.39E-6	> 1.00E-4	> 1.00E-4
Renal Cancer															
786-0	0.371	1.447	1.471	1.491	0.854	0.440	0.461	102	104	45	6	8	8.18E-7	> 1.00E-4	> 1.00E-4
A498	0.688	1.527	1.621	1.608	1.207	0.897	0.949	111	110	62	25	31	2.09E-6	> 1.00E-4	> 1.00E-4
ACHN	0.320	1.117	1.222	1.221	1.076	0.692	0.574	113	113	95	47	32	8.50E-6	> 1.00E-4	> 1.00E-4
CAKI-1	0.659	1.875	1.821	1.835	1.822	1.171	0.942	96	97	96	42	23	7.12E-6	> 1.00E-4	> 1.00E-4
RXF 393	0.650	0.840	0.858	0.858	0.547	0.514	0.535	110	109	-16	-21	-18	2.98E-7	7.47E-7	> 1.00E-4
SN12C	0.370	1.309	1.301	1.362	0.793	0.691	0.678	99	106	45	34	33	8.28E-7	> 1.00E-4	> 1.00E-4
TK-10	0.504	0.957	1.011	1.036	0.852	0.706	0.669	112	117	77	45	36	6.77E-6	> 1.00E-4	> 1.00E-4
UO-31	0.645	1.192	1.278	1.279	1.251	1.105	0.944	116	116	111	84	55	> 1.00E-4	> 1.00E-4	> 1.00E-4
Prostate Cancer															
PC-3	1.013	2.121	2.023	1.875	1.118	1.048	1.039	91	78	9	3	2	2.55E-7	> 1.00E-4	> 1.00E-4
DU-145	0.296	1.074	1.079	1.068	0.350	0.187	0.199	101	99	7	-37	-33	3.41E-7	1.44E-6	> 1.00E-4
Breast Cancer															
MCF7	0.241	1.345	1.312	1.320	0.468	0.447	0.434	97	98	21	19	17	4.15E-7	> 1.00E-4	> 1.00E-4
MDA-MB-231/ATCC	0.446	0.922	0.990	0.962	0.462	0.408	0.342	114	108	3	-9	-23	3.59E-7	1.88E-6	> 1.00E-4
HS 578T	0.568	1.728	1.974	1.959	1.484	1.418	1.299	121	120	79	73	63	> 1.00E-4	> 1.00E-4	> 1.00E-4
BT-549	0.938	1.523	1.506	1.506	0.906	0.749	0.698	97	97	-3	-20	-26	2.94E-7	9.24E-7	> 1.00E-4
T-47D	0.646	1.231	1.240	1.234	1.047	1.054	1.012	102	101	69	70	63	> 1.00E-4	> 1.00E-4	> 1.00E-4
MDA-MB-468	0.476	1.315	1.241	1.074	0.306	0.295	0.289	91	71	-36	-38	-39	1.58E-7	4.64E-7	> 1.00E-4

Fig. 37. Tabular list of the antineoplastic activity exhibited by the drug compound **2** (**PT166, NSC 750423**) in the National Cancer Institute (NCI) Developmental Therapeutics Program (DTP) 60-cancer cell 5-dose testing with the Mean Optical Densities of the used vital stain sulforhodamine B (SRB) retained in the cells given. **Percent Growth, GI50 (Growth inhibition 50%), TGI (Total Growth Inhibition = 0% Growth)**, and **LC50 (Lethal Concentration 50% = –50% Growth)** are given in linear concentration units.

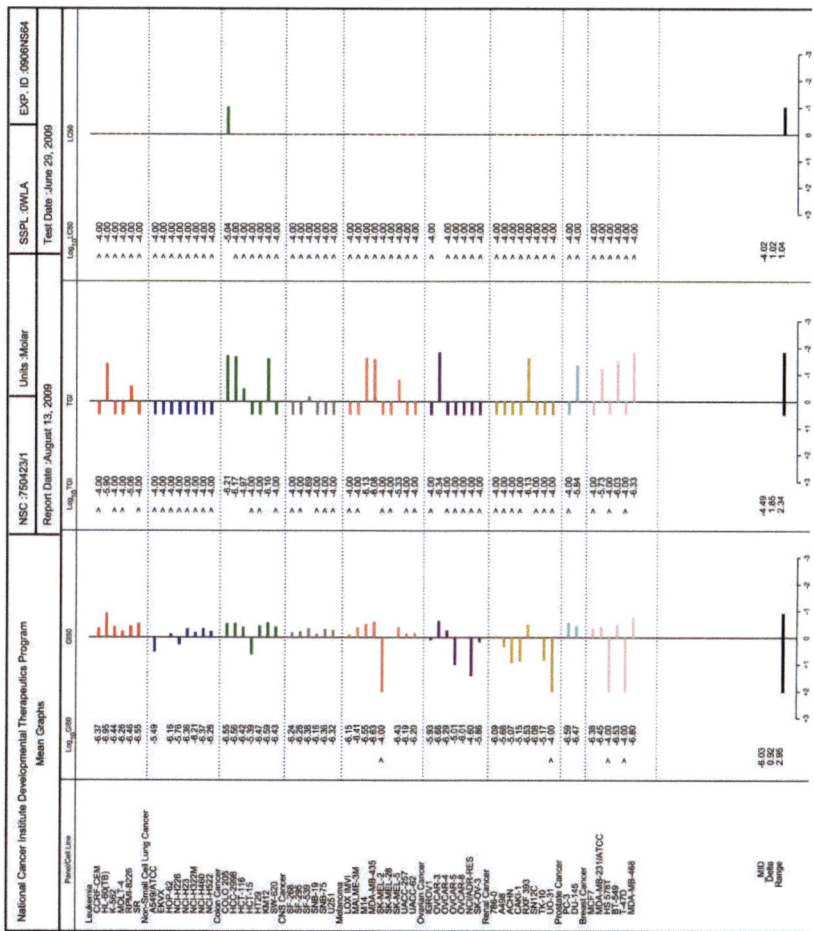

Fig. 38. Graphic table presentation of the antineoplastic activity exhibited by the drug compound **2** (**PT166, NSC 750423**) in the National Cancer Institute (NCI) Developmental Therapeutics Program (DTP) 60-cancer cell 5-dose testing with the **Percent Growth, GI50 (Growth inhibition 50%), TGI (Total Growth Inhibition = 0% Growth)**, and **LC50 (Lethal Concentration 50% = –50% Growth)** given in linear concentration units. This is the summary of the results expressed in $\log_{10}$ units. The defined tumor inhibition criterion (**GI50, TGI, or LC50**) is recalculated in $\log_{10}$ expression, and the colored bars which indicate then the sensitivity of the individual tumor cell line to the agent are given, but

in $\log_{10}$ units. **Bar to the left: less sensitive than mean, Bar to the right: more sensitive than mean.** The most important feature is at the bottom of the page: the **MID (Mean of Inhibition Data)** indicates the mean concentration for all tested cell lines required for the drug to reach the defined tumor inhibition criterion (**GI50, TGI,** or **LC50**). It is given in **Log₁₀GI50, Log₁₀TGI** and **Log₁₀LC50**. From that values the corresponding **MID** is calculated. The more negative the **MID**, the more potent is the drug. The **MID** can be transformed from logarithmic into linear concentrations by the formula: $c = 10^{MID}$.

2.3. National Cancer Institute (NCI) Developmental Therapeutics Program (DTP) 60-cancer cell 5-dose testing results with compound **3** (**PT167, NSC 799315**)

The four pages of the National Cancer Institute (NCI) Developmental Therapeutics Program (DTP) 60-cancer cell 5-dose testing results for compound **3** (**PT167, NSC 799315**) are given in succession. **First page** (Fig. 39): graphic allover presentation of page two with **All Cell Lines** in one graphic. **Second page** (Fig. 40): inhibition curves for tumor cell lines arranged/ordered for general tumor type. **Third page** (Fig. 41): the Mean Optical Densities of the utilized vital stain sulforhodamine B (SRB) retained in the cells, the actual used concentrations in $\log_{10}$ unit for five doses, and the **Percent Growth** are given. The **GI50 (Growth inhibition 50%), TGI (Total Growth Inhibition = 0% Growth),** and **LC50 (Lethal Concentration 50% = –50% Growth)** are given in linear concentration units. **Fourth page** (Fig. 42): this is the summary of the results expressed in $\log_{10}$ units. The defined tumor inhibition criterion (**GI50, TGI,** or **LC50**) is recalculated in $\log_{10}$ expression, and the the colored bars which indicate then the sensitivity of the individual tumor cell line to the agent are given in $\log_{10}$ units.

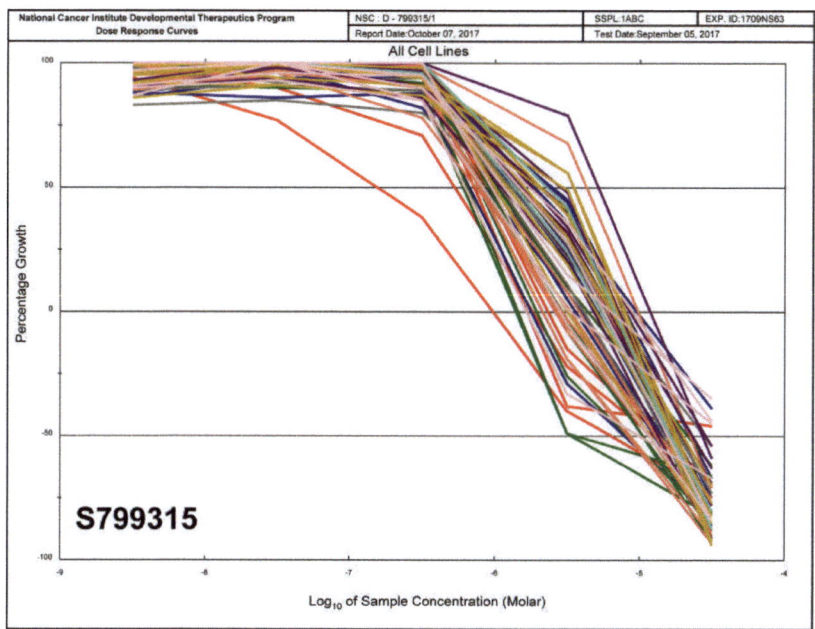

Fig. 39. Graphic allover presentation of the antineoplastic activity in the National Cancer Institute (NCI) Developmental Therapeutics Program (DTP) 60-cancer cell 5-dose testing exhibited by the drug compound **3** (**PT167, NSC 799315**) with **All Cell Lines** in one graphic.

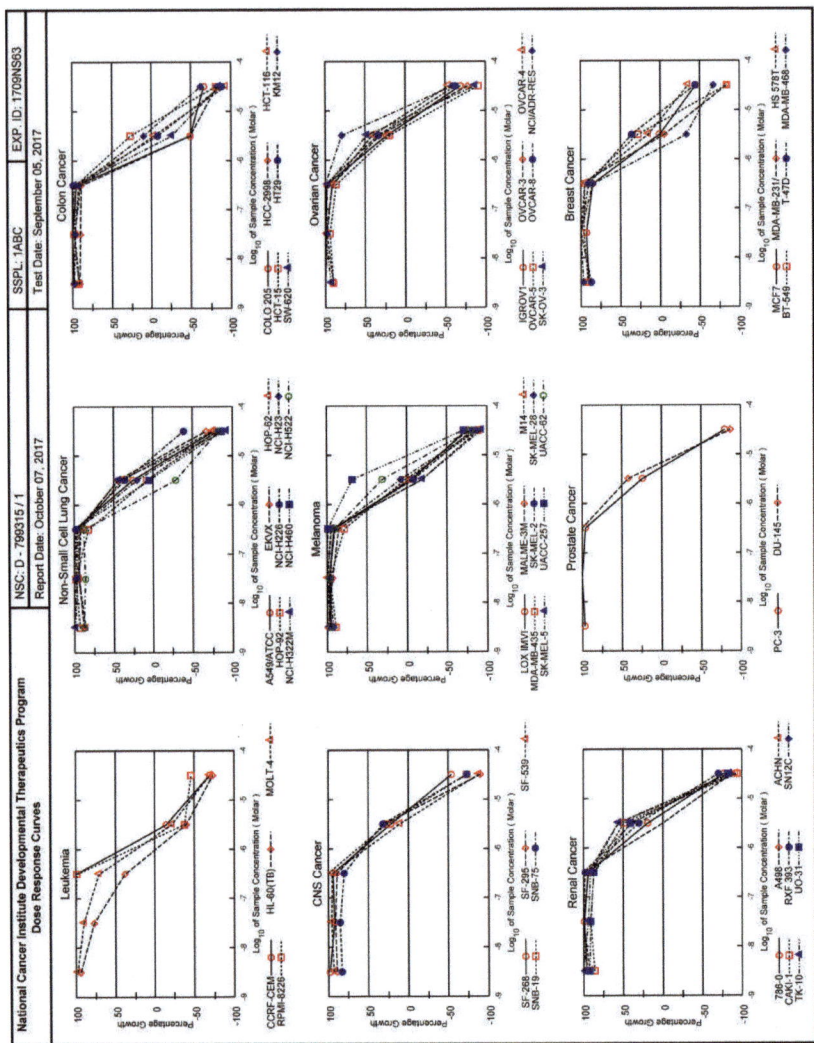

Fig. 40. Graphic presentation of the antineoplastic activity exhibited by the drug compound **3** (**PT167**, **NSC 799315**) in the National Cancer Institute (NCI) Developmental Therapeutics Program (DTP) 60-cancer cell 5-dose testing with the inhibition curves for sixty tumor cell lines arranged/ordered in terms of general tumor type.

National Cancer Institute Developmental Therapeutics Program In-Vitro Testing Results				
NSC : D - 799315 / 1	Experiment ID : 1709NS63		Test Type : 08	Units : Molar
Report Date : October 07, 2017	Test Date : September 05, 2017		QNS :	MC :
COMI : PT167	Stain Reagent : SRB Dual-Pass Related		SSPL : 1ABC	

Panel/Cell Line	Time Zero	Ctrl	Mean Optical Densities −8.5	−7.5	−6.5	−5.5	−4.5	Percent Growth −8.5	−7.5	−6.5	−5.5	−4.5	GI50	TGI	LC50
Leukemia															
CCRF-CEM	0.461	2.449	2.482	2.556	2.443	0.393	0.144	102	105	100	−15	−69	9.04E-7	2.47E-6	1.49E-5
HL-60(TB)	0.857	3.020	2.897	2.528	1.689	0.517	0.236	94	77	38	−40	−73	1.68E-7	1.03E-6	6.85E-6
MOLT-4	0.638	2.703	2.656	2.504	2.108	0.498	0.201	98	90	71	−22	−69	5.62E-7	1.93E-6	1.33E-5
RPMI-8226	0.451	1.817	1.889	1.916	1.799	0.281	0.242	105	107	99	−38	−46	7.57E-7	1.76E-6	> 3.33E-5
Non-Small Cell Lung Cancer															
A549/ATCC	0.341	1.522	1.533	1.524	1.532	0.654	0.078	101	100	101	26	−77	1.61E-6	6.00E-6	1.82E-5
EKVX	0.693	2.180	2.008	2.089	2.090	1.368	0.231	88	94	94	45	−67	2.68E-6	8.46E-6	2.36E-5
HOP-62	0.633	1.719	1.565	1.652	1.632	1.068	0.159	86	94	92	40	−75	2.14E-6	7.43E-6	2.02E-5
HOP-92	1.136	1.750	1.704	1.738	1.639	1.184	0.223	93	98	82	8	−80	8.97E-7	4.08E-6	1.51E-5
NCI-H226	0.603	1.414	1.429	1.431	1.398	0.893	0.366	102	102	98	36	−39	1.95E-6	9.97E-6	> 3.33E-5
NCI-H23	0.495	1.655	1.654	1.628	1.620	0.739	0.091	100	98	97	21	−82	1.38E-6	5.33E-6	1.64E-5
NCI-H322M	0.700	1.763	1.748	1.716	1.717	1.170	0.055	99	96	96	44	−92	2.57E-6	7.03E-6	1.63E-5
NCI-H460	0.246	1.834	1.927	1.994	1.961	0.327	0.036	106	110	108	5	−86	1.22E-6	3.76E-6	1.35E-5
NCI-H522	0.948	2.248	2.098	2.062	2.086	0.673	0.174	88	86	88	−29	−82	6.99E-7	1.88E-6	8.33E-6
Colon Cancer															
COLO 205	0.433	1.448	1.425	1.472	1.398	0.219	0.147	98	102	95	−49	−66	6.83E-7	1.52E-6	3.61E-6
HCC-2998	0.479	1.564	1.468	1.450	1.440	0.244	0.085	91	90	89	−49	−82	6.35E-7	1.47E-6	3.55E-6
HCT-116	0.152	1.300	1.211	1.263	1.187	0.147	0.010	92	97	90	−3	−93	8.96E-7	3.07E-6	1.10E-5
HCT-15	0.218	1.575	1.470	1.543	1.523	0.590	0.042	92	98	96	27	−81	1.56E-6	5.96E-6	1.72E-5
HT29	0.184	0.975	0.982	0.980	0.968	0.170	0.023	101	101	99	−8	−88	9.58E-7	2.81E-6	1.13E-5
KM12	0.366	1.900	1.874	1.856	1.782	0.513	0.138	98	97	92	10	−82	1.06E-6	4.52E-6	2.25E-5
SW-620	0.245	1.570	1.638	1.631	1.544	0.182	0.040	105	105	98	−26	−84	8.14E-7	2.06E-6	8.74E-6
CNS Cancer															
SF-268	0.648	2.073	2.041	1.963	1.990	0.965	0.301	98	92	94	22	−54	1.37E-6	6.54E-6	2.99E-5
SF-295	0.787	2.563	2.370	2.402	2.368	1.323	0.075	89	91	89	30	−90	1.53E-6	5.92E-6	1.54E-5
SF-539	0.784	2.356	2.243	2.299	2.275	0.956	0.097	93	96	95	11	−88	1.14E-6	4.30E-6	1.38E-5
SNB-19	0.422	1.532	1.536	1.626	1.553	0.723	0.113	100	108	102	27	−73	1.65E-6	6.20E-6	1.95E-5
SNB-75	0.874	1.816	1.657	1.677	1.631	1.172	0.237	83	85	80	32	−73	1.40E-6	6.68E-6	2.01E-5
Melanoma															
LOX IMVI	0.360	2.108	2.017	2.054	1.943	0.337	0.089	95	97	91	−6	−75	8.73E-7	2.86E-6	1.43E-5
MALME-3M	0.535	1.269	1.265	1.218	1.160	0.517	0.125	99	93	85	−3	−77	8.30E-7	3.04E-6	1.44E-5
M14	0.339	1.194	1.148	1.183	1.148	0.275	0.033	95	99	95	−19	−90	8.22E-7	2.26E-6	9.06E-6
MDA-MB-435	0.461	2.023	1.847	1.965	1.680	0.493	0.051	89	96	78	2	−89	7.79E-7	3.50E-6	1.24E-5
SK-MEL-2	0.961	2.171	2.118	2.127	2.059	0.884	0.177	96	96	91	−8	−82	8.61E-7	2.70E-6	1.24E-5
SK-MEL-28	0.593	1.761	1.665	1.727	1.641	0.690	0.177	92	97	90	8	−87	1.02E-6	4.07E-6	1.36E-5
SK-MEL-5	0.640	2.822	2.761	2.828	2.681	0.517	0.043	97	100	94	−19	−93	8.10E-7	2.25E-6	8.65E-6
UACC-257	1.116	2.133	2.086	2.182	2.119	1.811	0.327	95	105	99	68	−71	4.51E-6	1.03E-5	2.36E-5
UACC-62	0.845	2.428	2.362	2.385	2.274	1.342	0.171	98	97	90	31	−80	1.61E-6	6.38E-6	1.80E-5
Ovarian Cancer															
IGROV1	0.536	1.959	2.009	1.995	1.925	0.865	0.169	103	103	98	23	−69	1.45E-6	5.95E-6	2.09E-5
OVCAR-3	0.498	1.651	1.697	1.643	1.547	0.870	0.110	104	99	91	32	−78	1.66E-6	6.53E-6	1.85E-5
OVCAR-4	0.624	1.245	1.185	1.232	1.188	0.877	0.286	90	98	91	41	−54	2.17E-6	8.94E-6	3.00E-5
OVCAR-5	0.527	1.467	1.371	1.411	1.338	0.715	0.046	90	94	86	20	−91	1.17E-6	5.03E-6	1.42E-5
OVCAR-8	0.403	1.457	1.515	1.528	1.336	0.765	0.148	105	107	107	34	−63	2.03E-6	7.49E-6	2.43E-5
NCI/ADR-RES	0.428	1.273	1.280	1.252	1.278	1.069	0.175	101	98	101	79	−59	5.43E-6	1.25E-5	2.86E-5
SK-OV-3	0.689	1.473	1.417	1.479	1.449	1.064	0.087	93	101	97	48	−87	3.00E-6	7.51E-6	1.76E-5
Renal Cancer															
786-0	0.443	1.813	1.755	1.803	1.737	0.706	0.104	96	99	94	19	−77	1.30E-6	5.28E-6	1.76E-5
A498	1.401	1.875	1.938	1.910	1.883	1.393	0.178	113	107	102		−87	1.07E-6	3.28E-6	1.24E-5
ACHN	0.423	1.617	1.516	1.612	1.544	1.098	0.033	92	100	94	56	−92	3.68E-6	7.99E-6	1.73E-5
CAKI-1	0.470	2.123	1.894	1.967	1.908	1.286	0.030	86	91	87	49	−94	3.20E-6	7.37E-6	1.65E-5
RXF 393	0.723	1.364	1.317	1.374	1.336	0.912	0.214	95	104	98	30	−70	1.70E-6	6.65E-6	2.09E-5
SN12C	0.570	1.726	1.713	1.791	1.741	1.024	0.087	99	106	101	39	−85	2.23E-6	6.90E-6	1.74E-5
TK-10	0.681	1.672	1.687	1.610	1.581	1.233	0.110	101	94	91	56	−84	3.66E-6	8.35E-6	1.90E-5
UO-31	0.517	1.694	1.601	1.592	1.542	1.005	0.092	92	91	87	41	−82	2.16E-6	7.20E-6	1.83E-5
Prostate Cancer															
PC-3	0.366	1.536	1.498	1.536	1.494	0.644	0.074	97	100	96	24	−80	1.45E-6	5.64E-6	1.71E-5
DU-145	0.330	1.311	1.319	1.359	1.314	0.746	0.045	101	105	100	42	−87	2.46E-6	7.10E-6	1.73E-5
Breast Cancer															
MCF7	0.402	2.309	2.117	2.178	2.018	0.414	0.223	90	93	85	1	−45	8.62E-7	3.44E-6	> 3.33E-5
MDA-MB-231/ATCC	0.623	1.590	1.619	1.624	1.587	0.593	0.101	103	104	100	−5	−84	9.94E-7	2.99E-6	1.24E-5
HS 578T	0.856	1.542	1.544	1.584	1.508	0.970	0.567	100	106	95	15	−35	1.22E-6	6.76E-6	> 3.33E-5
BT-549	0.768	1.785	1.696	1.740	1.730	1.065	0.124	91	96	95	28	−84	1.55E-6	5.89E-6	1.65E-5
T-47D	0.691	1.313	1.232	1.332	1.248	0.915	0.388	87	103	90	44	−44	1.83E-6	9.40E-6	> 3.33E-5
MDA-MB-468	0.748	1.767	1.734	1.778	1.611	0.502	0.250	97	101	85	−33	−67	6.57E-7	1.75E-6	1.07E-5

Fig. 41. Tabular list of the antineoplastic activity exhibited by the drug compound **3** (**PT167, NSC 799315**) in the National Cancer Institute (NCI) Developmental Therapeutics Program (DTP) 60-cancer cell 5-dose testing with the Mean Optical Densities of the used vital stain sulforhodamine B (SRB) retained in the cells given. **Percent Growth, GI50 (Growth inhibition 50%), TGI (Total Growth Inhibition = 0% Growth)**, and **LC50 (Lethal Concentration 50% = –50% Growth)** are given in linear concentration units.

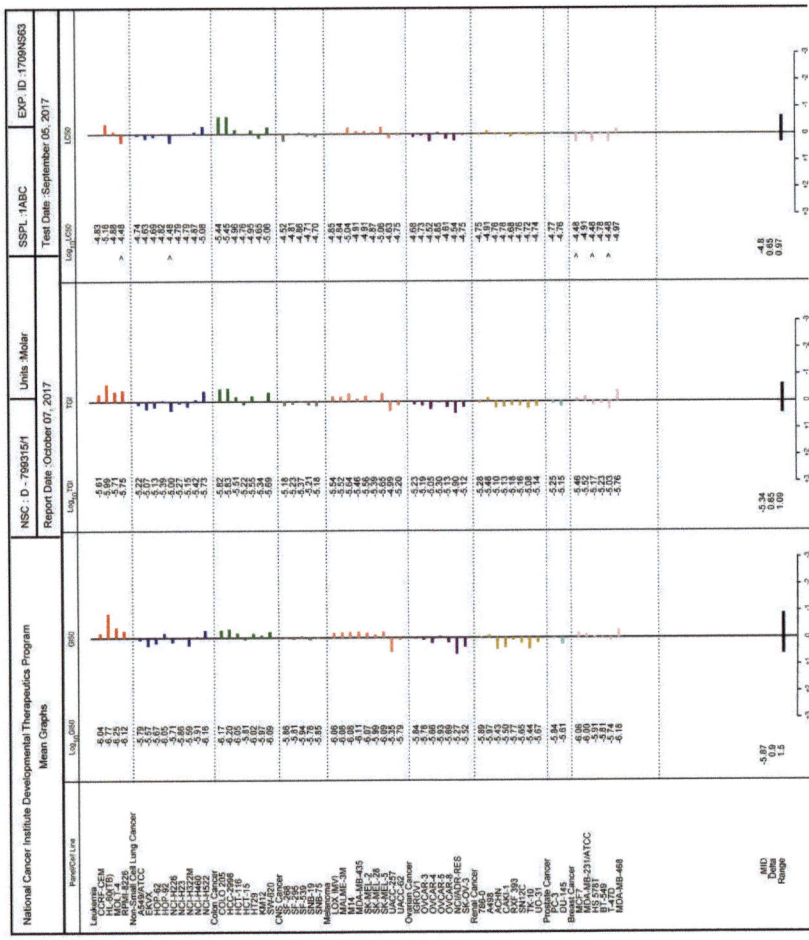

Fig. 42. Graphic table presentation of the antineoplastic activity exhibited by the drug compound **3** (**PT167, NSC 799315**) in the National Cancer Institute (NCI) Developmental Therapeutics Program (DTP) 60-cancer cell 5-dose testing with the **Percent Growth, GI50 (Growth inhibition 50%), TGI (Total Growth Inhibition = 0% Growth)**, and **LC50 (Lethal Concentration 50% = –50% Growth)** given in linear concentration units. This is the summary of the results expressed in log$_{10}$ units. The defined tumor inhibition criterion (**GI50, TGI, or LC50**) is recalculated in log$_{10}$ expression, and the colored bars which indicate then the sensitivity of the individual tumor cell line to the agent are given, but

in $\log_{10}$ units. **Bar to the left: less sensitive than mean, Bar to the right: more sensitive than mean.** The most important feature is at the bottom of the page: the **MID** (**Mean of Inhibition Data**) indicates the mean concentration for all tested cell lines required for the drug to reach the defined tumor inhibition criterion (**GI50, TGI,** or **LC50**). It is given in **Log₁₀GI50, Log₁₀TGI** and **Log₁₀LC50**. From that values the corresponding **MID** is calculated. The more negative the **MID**, the more potent is the drug. The **MID** can be transformed from logarithmic into linear concentrations by the formula: $c = 10^{\mathrm{MID}}$.

3. Cytochrome *c* Assay (Mitochondrial and Cytosolic) with the Drugs PT162, PT166 and PT167 in the Human Prostate Cancer Cell Lines PC-3 and DU-145

To assess the nature of the cancer cell death-inducing effect of the drugs compound **1** (**PT162, NSC 796018**), compound **2** (**PT166, NSC 750423**), and compound **3** (**PT167, NSC 799315**), and to verify the failure to induce cancer cell death of compound **2** (**PT166, NSC 750423**), the cellular compartment of cytochrome *c* in the prostate cancer cell lines PC-3 and DU-145 under the action of compound **1** (**PT162, NSC 796018**), compound **2** (**PT166, NSC 750423**), and compound **3** (**PT167, NSC 799315**) was investigated (Fig. 43). Compound **1** (**PT162, NSC 796018**) readily induced cytochrome *c* translocation from mitochondria into the cytosol at 25.0 µM concentration in PC-3 cells (Fig. 43A) and 5.0 µM concentration in DU-145 cells (Fig. 43B). Compound **2** (**PT166, NSC 750423**) failed to induce a significant difference in the cytochrome *c*-residing cellular compartment in PC-3 cells (Fig. 43C) and, less significant, in DU-145 cells (Fig. 43D). Compound **3** (**PT167, NSC 799315**) readily induced cytochrome *c* translocation from mitochondria into the cytosol at 5.0 µM concentration in PC-3 cells (Fig. 43E) and 25.0 µM concentration in DU-145 cells (Fig. 43F). At 25.0 µM concentration compound **1** (**PT162, NSC 796018**) in DU-145 cells (Fig. 43B) and compound **3**

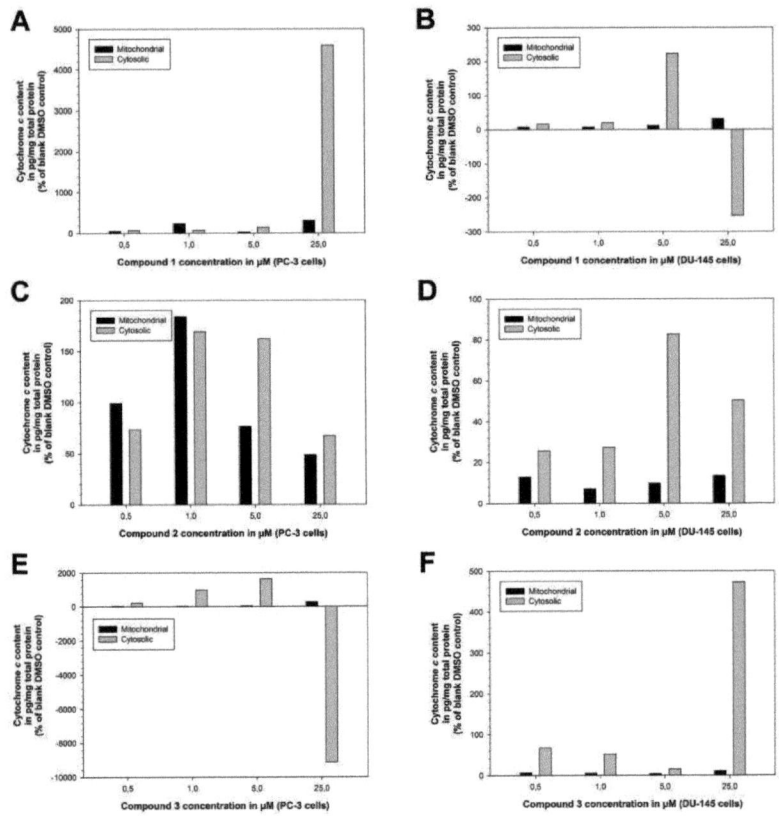

Fig. 43. Compound **1** (**PT162**, **NSC 796018**) and compound **3** (**PT167**, **NSC 799315**) induce cytochrome *c* translocation from mitochondria into the cytosol, a hallmark of the intrinsic pathway of apoptosis, whereas compound **2** (**PT166**, **NSC 750423**) fails to induce apoptotic cytochrome *c* translocation. The cytochrome *c* assays (mitochondrial and cytosolic) were performed with compound **1**, **2** and **3** in the human prostate cancer cell lines PC-3 and DU-145. The protein content for each cellular fraction was calculated to determine the mass content of cytochrome *c* in each fraction (pg cytochrome *c*/mg total protein). The mass content of cytochrome *c* (pg cytochrome *c*/mg total protein) was normalized towards the corresponding blank DMSO control and is given in percent (%) of blank DMSO control. Each experiment was representative for the effects of compound **1** (**PT162**, **NSC 796018**), compound **2** (**PT166**, **NSC 750423**), and compound **3** (**PT167**, **NSC 799315**) in the human prostate cancer cell lines

PC-3 and DU-145. Legend: **A,** experiment compound **1** (**PT162, NSC 796018**) in PC-3 cells. **B,** experiment compound **1** (**PT162, NSC 796018**) in DU-145 cells. **C,** experiment compound **2** (**PT166, NSC 750423**) in PC-3 cells. **D,** experiment compound **2** (**PT166, NSC 750423**) in DU-145 cells. **E,** experiment compound **3** (**PT167, NSC 799315**) in PC-3 cells. **F,** experiment compound **3** (**PT167, NSC 799315**) in DU-145 cells.

(**PT167, NSC 799315**) in PC-3 cells (Fig. 43E) both induced complete cell death which resulted in massive depletion of cytochrome c in the cytosol, very probably by apoptotic degradation of cytochrome c protein by effector caspases.

4. HIV-1$_{LAI}$ Replication Reverse Transcriptase Assay with the Drug PT162 in Primary PBL Cells

Compound **1** (**PT162, NSC 796018**) is inhibitory towards human immunodeficieny virus type 1 (HIV-1) strain LAI (HIV-1$_{LAI}$) (= HIV-1$_{BRU}$ = LAV-1) replication in freshly explanted, primary human peripheral blood lymphocytes (PBL cells) (see Appendix, Table S1). The effective inhibitory concentration 50% (EC$_{50}$) in PBL cells was 0.56 µM, the effective inhibitory concentration 90% (EC$_{90}$) in PBL cells was 4.3 µM. The cyctotoxic concentration 50% (CC$_{50}$) for the PBL cells was 2.2 µM, this yields a selectivity index 50% (SI$_{50}$) = CC$_{50}$/EC$_{50}$ of 3.9. The r^2 coefficient of determination (r^2 measure of goodness–of–fit) on EC$_{50}$ and EC$_{90}$ was 0.93. As a positive control served AZT (zidovudine, 3'-azido-3'-deoxythymidine). The given effective inhibitory concentrations (µM ± s.d.) for the positive control AZT were averaged and treated statistically from four (n = 4) independent determinations (see Appendix, Table S1). Furthermore, the cytotoxicity of compound **1** (**PT162, NSC 796018**) towards CCRF−CEM cells (ATCC CCL-119™, acute lymphoblastic leukemia cells, tumorigenic CD4$^+$ T lymphoblasts) [3] and Vero cells [African green monkey (grivet) *Chlorocebus aethiops* (SYN. *Cercopithecus aethiops*) kidney epithelial cells] was determined (see Appendix, Table S1). The cyctotoxic concentration 50% (CC_{50}) for the CCRF−CEM cells was < 1 µM with 60.0% growth inhibition of CCRF−CEM cells at 1 µM. The cytotoxic concentration 50% (CC_{50}) for the Vero cells was 1.8 µM.

The inhibitory action of p53 on HIV-1 replication is well established [4−6]. Compound **1** (**PT162, NSC 796018**) clearly inhibits HIV-1$_{LAI}$ replication by inducing p53 and its associated cyclin-dependent kinase inhibitor p21^{Waf1}/p21^{Cip1} [7]. The latter factor p21^{Waf1}/p21^{Cip1} is induced by p53 activation [8] and inhibits HIV-1 replication [9,10]. In addition, tumor suppressor protein p53 interacts with HIV-1 *trans*-activator protein Tat (*trans*-activator of transcription) [11−13], HIV-1 Nef (negative regulatory factor) accessory protein [14], and HIV-1 Vpr (viral protein R, viral protein rapid) accessory protein [10,15]. The marked cytotoxic action of compound **1** (**PT162, NSC 796018**) on CCRF−CEM acute lymphoblastic leukemia cells clearly stems from its strong antileukemic/antineoplastic activity.

5. References

[1]   H. Berglind, Y. Pawitan, S. Kato, C. Ishioka, T. Soussi, Analysis of p53 mutation status in human cancer cell lines. A paradigm for cell line cross-contamination, *Cancer Biol. Ther.* **7** (2008) 699–708, https://doi.org/10.4161/cbt.7.5.5712.

[2]   P.A.J. Muller, K.H. Vousden, Mutant p53 in cancer: New functions and therapeutic opportunities, *Cancer Cell* **25** (2014) 304–317, https://doi.org/10.1016/j.ccr.2014.01.021.

[3]   G.E. Foley, H. Lazarus, S. Farber, B.G. Uzman, B.A. Boone, R.E. McCarthy, Continuous culture of human

lymphoblasts from peripheral blood of a child with acute leukemia, *Cancer* **18** (1965) 522–529.

[4]   M.A. Subler, D.W. Martin, S. Deb, Inhibition of viral and cellular promoters by human wild-type p53, *J. Virol.* **66** (1992) 4757–4762.

[5]   M.A. Subler, D.W. Martin, S. Deb, Activation of the human immunodeficiency virus type 1 long terminal repeat by transforming mutants of human p53, *J. Virol.* **68** (1994) 103–110.

[6]   L. Duan, I. Ozaki, J.W. Oakes, J.P. Taylor, K. Khalili, R.J. Pomerantz, The tumor suppressor protein p53 strongly alters human immunodeficiency virus type 1 replication, *J. Virol.* **68** (1994) 4302–4313.

[7]   R. Altschul, N. Theise, PopTest Oncology LLC/Palisades Therapeutics (Cliffside Park, NJ, USA), Palisades Therapeutics announces new anti-cancer drug-PT162, a p53-reactivating cell cycle checkpoint inhibitor, EINPresswire.com (January 3rd, 2023), https://www.einpresswire.com/article/609163965/palisa des-therapeutics-announces-new-anti-cancer-drug-pt162-a-p53-reactivating-cell-cycle-checkpoint-inhibitor.

[8]   W.S. el-Deiry, et al., *WAF1*, a potential mediator of p53 tumor suppression, *Cell* **75** (1993) 817–825.

[9]   B. Shi, et al., Inhibition of HIV early replication by the p53 and its downstream gene p21, *Virol. J.* **15** (2018), 53, https://doi.org/10.1186/s12985-018-0959-x.

[10] I.H. Chowdhury, et al., HIV-1 Vpr activates cell cycle inhibitor p21/Waf1/Cip1: A potential mechanism of G2/M cell cycle arrest, *Virology* **305** (2003) 371–377.

[11] C.J. Li, C. Wang, D.J. Friedman, A.B. Pardee, Reciprocal modulations between p53 and Tat of human immunodeficiency virus type 1, *Proc. Natl. Acad. Sci. U. S. A.* **92** (1995) 5461–5464.

[12] F. Longo, M.A. Marchetti, L. Castagnoli, P.A. Battaglia, F. Gigliani, A novel approach to protein–protein interaction: Complex formation between the p53 tumor suppressor and the HIV Tat proteins, *Biochem. Biophys. Res. Commun.* **206** (1995) 326–334.

[13] Y. Ariumi, A. Kaida, M. Hatanaka, K. Shimotohno, Functional cross-talk of HIV-1 Tat with p53 through its C-terminal domain, *Biochem. Biophys. Res. Commun.* **287** (2001) 556–561.

[14] A.L. Greenway, et al., Human immunodeficiency virus type 1 Nef binds to tumor suppressor p53 and protects cells against p53-mediated apoptosis, *J. Virol.* **76** (2002) 2692–2702.

[15] B.E. Sawaya, K. Khalili, W.E. Mercer, L. Denisova, S. Amini, Cooperative actions of HIV-1 Vpr and p53 modulate viral gene transcription, *J. Biol. Chem.* **273** (1998) 20052–20057.

MATERIALS AND METHODS, CHEMICAL SYNTHESIS, EXPERIMENTAL INSTRUCTIONS AND SUPPLEMENTARY DATA

1. Materials and Methods

1.1. Materials

1-Adamantanammonium chloride (INN: amantadine hydrochloride) (1-aminoadamantane hydrochloride) [Lot: S4247215; w (m/m) = 100.0% (argentometric titration), mp > 360 °C (dec.)] and absolute ethanol *pro analysi* EMPLURA® [Lot: K48011060; w (n/n) = 99.9% (gas chromatography, area%), ρ_4^{20} = 0.789–0.790 g/ml, w (H_2O) (m/m) = 0.06%, non-volatile matter < 0.0001%] were purchased from Merck KGaA–EMD Millipore Corp. (Darmstadt, Germany). Sodium hydroxide (NaOH) pearls pure (Ph.Eur., BP, Food Grade) [Lot: 2J002792; w (m/m) = 99.31% (titration), sodium carbonate < 0.5%, SiO_2 < 0.001%, NaCl < 0.008%, Na_2SO_4 < 0.0025%, As < 0.00001 %, heavy metals (Cu, Fe, Mn, Ni, Pb, Hg) < 0.001%], 10.27 M [32% (m/m)] aqueous hydrochloric acid *pro analysi* [Lot: 3A001639; w (m/m) = 33.09% (titration), bromide < 0.005%, phosphate < 0.00005%, sulfate < 0.0001%, As < 0.000001 %, Fe < 0.00002%, heavy metals (Ni, Pb, Zn) < 0.000005%], sodium hydrogen carbonate (sodium bicarbonate) *pro analysi* $NaHCO_3$ [Lot: 4W000829; w (m/m) = 100.42% (titration), pH (5% in H_2O) 8.04 (20 °C), chloride ≤ 0.001%, sulfate ≤ 0.005%, phosphate ≤ 0.005%, cations (K, Mg, Ca) ≤ 0.005%, As ≤ 0.0001%, heavy metals

(Cu, Fe, Pb) $\leq$ 0.0005%], and (–)-colchicine sesquihydrate ($\times$ 1½ H_2O) = colchicine *BioChemica* [w (m/m) $\geq$ 98% (HPLC), $[\alpha]_D^{20}$ = –240° to –250° (c = 1 in EtOH), w (H_2O) (m/m) $\leq$ 3% (Karl Fischer titration)] were purchased from AppliChem (Darmstadt, Germany). Acetone (USP, BP, Ph.Eur.) Pharma Quality [Lot: 0000869897; w (n/n) = 99.9% (gas chromatography, area%), ρ_{20}^{20} = 0.791 g/ml, ρ_{25}^{25} < 0.789 g/ml, w (H_2O) (m/m) = 0.3%, non-volatile matter 0.0002%, methanol < 0.05%, propan-2-ol < 0.05%, benzene < 0.0002%, ethanol < 500 ppm, heavy metals (Fe, Zn) < 1,300 ppm, heavy metals (Cu, Mn) < 250 ppm], ethyl acetate *pro analysi* [Lot: 0000518022; w (n/n) = 99.9% (gas chromatography, area%), w (H_2O) (m/m) = 0.01% (Karl Fischer titration), ethanol < 0.1%, methanol < 0.02%, methyl acetate < 0.02%, trace elements (Cr, Fe, Ni, Pb, Zn, P, S, K, Mg) < 0.00001%, Si < 0.00002%, Na < 0.0002%, non-volatile matter < 0.001%, acidity/alkalinity < 0.0005 meq/g] were purchased from PanReac AppliChem GmbH (Darmstadt, Germany). 1,3-Bis(chloromethyl)benzene (α,α'-dichloro-*m*-xylene) *purum* $\geq$ 98% (GC) [Lot: 385191/1; w (m/m) = 100.6% (argentometric titration after oxygen combustion), w (n/n) = 99.9% (gas chromatography, area %), mp 33.2–34.0 °C] was purchased from Fluka Chemie AG (Buchs, Switzerland). Thiosemicarbazide *puriss. p.a.* [Lot: 1167177V (Fluka); w (m/m) = 100.1% (iodometric titration), mp 181 °C (dec.), residue on ignition < 0.05%, metal trace analysis (inductively coupled plasma mass spectrometry) $\leq$ 50–5 mg/kg] was purchased from Sigma-Aldrich Corp. (St. Louis, MO, USA).

1.2. Methods

The *Fourier*-transform infrared (FT–IR) spectra were recorded with neat substance on JASCO FT/IR–4100 type A and FT/IR–6100 type A spectrometers (JASCO International

Co. Ltd., Tokyo, Japan). Given FT–IR absorbance bands, expressed in wavenumbers $\tilde{v}$ (cm^{-1}), are characterized in intensity as strong (str), middle (m), weak (w), and broad (br). The proton nuclear magnetic resonance (^{1}H-NMR), carbon-13 nuclear magnetic resonance (^{13}C-NMR) and ^{13}C-Distortionless Enhancement by Polarization Transfer Including Detection of Quaternary Nuclei (DEPTQ ^{13}C-NMR) [1,2] NMR spectroscopy experiments were recorded at a temperature of 25 °C using a Bruker Avance 700 III HD nuclear magnetic resonance spectrometer (Bruker BioSpin GmbH, Rheinstetten, Germany) [^{1}H-NMR (700.43 MHz), ^{13}C-NMR (176.12 MHz)]. The spectra were referenced to the center of the NMR solvent signal [^{1}H-NMR: δ 2.51 (DMSO-d_6); ^{13}C-NMR: δ 39.41 (DMSO-d_6)]. Additional ^{1}H-NMR, ^{13}C-NMR, DEPTQ ^{13}C-NMR, gradient-selected Correlation Spectroscopy (gs-COSY) [2], gradient-selected Heteronuclear Multiple Quantum Coherence (gs-HMQC) [2] and gradient-selected Heteronuclear Multiple Bond Correlation (gs-HMBC) [2] spectra were recorded using a Bruker Avance III HD 400 nuclear magnetic resonance spectrometer (Bruker BioSpin GmbH, Rheinstetten, Germany) [^{1}H-NMR (400.13 MHz), ^{13}C-NMR (100.62 MHz)] at a temperature of 300.0 K. The spectra were referenced to the center of the NMR solvent signal [^{1}H-NMR: δ 2.50 (DMSO-d_6); ^{13}C-NMR: δ 39.52 (DMSO-d_6)]. Given chemical shifts δ [from tetramethylsilane (TMS): δ = 0] are specified as singlet (s), broad singlet (br s), doublet (d), triplet (t), quartet (q), multiplet (m), and broad multiplet (br m). Electrospray ionization time–of–flight mass spectrometry (ESI–ToF–MS) of **PT167** was conducted in positive ion mode on an Agilent LC–ESI–ToF instrument using an Agilent 1260 Infinity II liquid chromatography (LC) stack with an Agilent ZORBAX 300SB–C8 (4.6 mm ID × 50 mm) column (pore size 300 Å, particle size 5 μm) coupled to an Agilent 6230B time–of–flight LC/MS (LC/ToF) system

(Agilent Technologies, Inc., Santa Clara, CA, USA). Source settings were ϑ (dry gas) = 350 °C, gas flow 10 l/min, nebulizer pressure p_n = 35 psi (2.4132 bar). Capillary voltage was set to V_c = 3,500 V and fragmentor voltage was set to V_f = 175 V. The scan range was m/z 105−3000. Elemental analyses (C, H, N, S, O) were conducted on the EURO EA3000 CHNS–O elemental analyser (EuroVector SpA, Milan, Italy) by HEKAtech GmbH (Wegberg, Germany).

1.3. Software

Crystal data visualization and molecular modeling was performed with ACD/Chem Sketch version 2022.1.0 with integrated ACD/3D Viewer (Advanced Chemistry Development, Inc., Toronto, Ontario, Canada) and processed with Mercury 2022.3.0 [The Cambridge Crystallographic Data Centre (CCDC), Cambridge, UK]. Additional molecular modeling was performed with ACD/Chem Sketch version 12.01 with integrated ACD/3D Viewer (Advanced Chemistry Development, Inc., Toronto, Ontario, Canada) and processed with Mercury 3.1 version 3.1.1 [The Cambridge Crystallographic Data Centre (CCDC), Cambridge, UK]. The mass spectrometric m/z values were calculated with the Scripps Research Core Service Molar Mass Calculator (The Scripps Research Institute, Center for Metabolomics and Mass Spectrometry, San Diego, CA, USA).

2. Chemical Synthesis

2.1. Salt-containing tetrakis{3-[(tricyclo[3.3.1.1^{3,7}]decan-1-ammonio)methyl]benzyl}ammonium pentachloride (compound **1** × 1.5 NaCl, **PT162** × 1.5 NaCl)

2.50 g 1-Aminoadamantane hydrochloride (13.32 mmol) and 3.50 g 1,3-bis(chloromethyl)benzene (α,α′-

dichloro-*m*-xylene) (19.99 mmol) were dissolved in 30 ml of 90% (*v/v*) aqueous ethanol. A solution of 1.60 g sodium hydroxide (40.00 mmol) in 40 ml of water was added, and the mixture was refluxed for 3 h. After 20 min and 40 min reflux, 20 ml of acetone, each, were added through the reflux condensor. After 60 min, 80 min, and 100 min reflux, 40 ml of acetone, each, were added through the reflux condensor. After 120 min reflux, additional 20 ml of acetone were added through the reflux condensor. Then, after 10 min pre-cooling at +0–2 °C, the colorless solution with few suspended impurities was warm filtrated. The filtrate (pH 9) was mixed with 100 ml of water, and was evaporated *in vacuo* from the acetone to a volume of ca. 170 ml. Afterwards, 2 ml of 10.27 M [32% (*m/v*)] hydrochloric acid (20.54 mmol) were added, and the colorless solution (pH 2–3) was evaporated further *in vacuo* to a volume of ca. 120 ml.

Then the turbid suspension was mixed with 20 ml of water and was extracted with 100 ml of ethyl acetate (EtOAc) to remove unreacted 1,3-bis(chloromethyl)benzene (α,α'-dichloro-*m*-xylene). The aqueous phase was isolated and further evaporated *in vacuo* to a volume of ca. 50 ml. The aqueous phase was then frozen at −25 °C for 1½ h. The evolved white precipitate of crude compound **1** × 1.5 NaCl (**PT162** × 1.5 NaCl) was filtered and dried over $CaCl_2$ *in vacuo* (from the filtrate additional substance could be obtained which was treated as before). From the separated EtOAc phase by cooling at +0–2 °C for 3 h additional crude compound **1** × 1.5 NaCl (**PT162** × 1.5 NaCl) could be obtained which was treated as before.

The combined crude product (730 mg) was dissolved in 50 ml of 80% (*v/v*) aqueous acetone by short (5 min) refluxing, and was hot filtrated to remove few impurities. The filtrate was transferred and mixed with 40 ml of 50% (*v/v*) aqueous acetone. Afterwards, the filtrate was evaporated *in vacuo* from the acetone. The resulting solution (pH 5) was acidified to pH 0–1 by addition of 0.6 ml of 10.27 M [32% (*m/v*)] hydrochloric acid (6.16 mmol). Instantly, a white precipitate formed. The suspension was supplemented with 10 ml of 50% (*v/v*) aqueous acetone and was frozen at –25 °C for 2½ h. The evolved white precipitate of compound **1** × 1.5 NaCl (**PT162** × 1.5 NaCl) was filtered and dried over $CaCl_2$ *in vacuo*.

Compound:	Compound **1** × 1.5 NaCl (**PT162** × 1.5 NaCl)	
Molecular formula:	$C_{72}H_{100}N_5Cl_5$ × 1.5 NaCl	
Molecular weight:	1,300.54 g/mol	
Yield:	13%	
Elemental analysis:	calculated:	C 66.49% H 7.75% N 5.38% O 0.00%
	found:	C 66.47% H 7.54% N 4.25% O 0.82%
		C 66.51% H 7.53% N 4.24% O 0.80%
FT–IR (cm⁻¹):	2925, 2850, 2760, 2710, 2436, 1610, 1585, 1494, 1459, 1269, 1108, 1074, 1011, 973, 794, 777, 762, 731, 693	
¹H-NMR: (DMSO-d_6, ppm)	1.62 (3 H, d; $^2J_{gem}$ = –12.1 Hz; δ-CH$_{axial}$), 1.69 (3 H, d; $^2J_{gem}$ = –12.4 Hz; δ-CH$_{equatorial}$), 2.02 (6 H, s; β-CH$_2$), 2.15 (3 H, s; γ-CH), 4.10 (2 H, t; $^3J_{vicinal}$ = 6.3 Hz; 8-CH$_2$), 4.78 (2 H, s; 7-CH$_2$), 7.42–7.49 (2 H, m; H-4, H-6), 7.65 (1 H, d; $^3J_{ortho}$ = 7.1 Hz; H-5), 7.69 (1 H, s; H-2), 9.24 (2 H, br s; 8-NH$_2^+$)	
¹³C-NMR: (DMSO-d_6, ppm)	28.50 (γ-CH), 35.25 (δ-CH$_2$), 37.35 (β-CH$_2$), 42.31 (8-CH$_2$), 45.84 (7-CH$_2$), 57.06 (α-C), 128.87 (C-4)*, 129.14 (C-6)*, 130.36 (C-2)*, 130.62 (C-5)*, 133.22 (C-3), 137.84 (C-1)	

* these assignments are tentative and interchangeable (they could not be assigned unequivocally to the individual carbons)

2.2. Pure (salt-free) tetrakis{3-[(tricyclo[3.3.1.1³,⁷]decan-1-ammonio)methyl]benzyl}ammonium pentachloride (**PT162, NSC 796018**)

1-Aminoadamantane hydrochloride (M = 187.71 g/mol, 10.075 g, 53.6732 mmol) was dissolved in water (100 ml). A solution of sodium hydroxide NaOH (2.160 g, 54.0000 mmol) in water (20 ml) was added. Residues were transferred with water (20 ml). A heavy precipitate of the free base 1-aminoadamantane formed instantly. The suspension was frozen at –25 °C for 1 h. The evolved white precipitate of the yield of 1-aminoadamantane (free base) was filtered and vacuum-sucked dry (ca. 1 h).

The still wet 1-aminoadamantane (free base) and 1,3-bis(chloromethyl)benzene (α,α′-dichloro-m-xylene) (M = 175.06 g/mol, 7.498 g, 42.8310 mmol) were suspended in absolute ethanol (200 ml). The suspension was refluxed for 3 h. After 40 min reflux a clear colorless solution formed. After 5 min pre-cooling at +0–2 °C, the colorless solution with few suspended impurities was hot filtrated through one layer of filter paper. Residues were transferred and rinsed with absolute ethanol (10 ml) and acetone (30 ml). The filtrate was mixed with acetone (300 ml), 10.27 M [32% (m/v)] hydrochloric acid (3,200 µl, 32.8640 mmol), and ethyl acetate (EtOAc) (200 ml), and was frozen at –25 °C for 2.5 h. Afterwards, water (200 ml) and EtOAc (1,000 ml) were added, the mixture was shaken vigorously for 1 min, and was frozen at –25 °C for 2.5 h. Then 10.27 M [32% (m/v)] hydrochloric acid (3,000 µl, 30.8100 mmol) was added, the mixture was shaken vigorously for 1 min, and it was frozen at –25 °C for 30 min. The upper phase was then decanted and the lower aqueous phase was isolated. The isolated upper EtOAc phase was re-extracted with water (90 ml), the aqueous phase was isolated after phase separation, and was combined with the first aqueous phase. Finally, the isolated upper EtOAc phase was re-extracted with acidified {3,000 µl 10.27 M [32% (m/v)] hydrochloric acid, 30.8100 mmol} water (100 ml), the aqueous phase was isolated after phase separation, and was combined with the two prior aqueous phases. The combined aqueous phases ($V = 500$ ml) were then evaporated *in vacuo* at the lowest possible temperature to a volume of 200 ml until heavy crystallization started. The crystallizing suspension was then cooled at +0–2 °C for 6 h, and frozen at –25 °C for 20 min, to complete crystallization. The evolved first yield (1.543 g) of white crystals were filtered and dried over $CaCl_2$ *in vacuo*. The filtrate was cooled at +0–2 °C for 50 h. The evolved second yield (62 mg) of white crystals was filtered and dried over $CaCl_2$ *in vacuo*. Both yields were combined.

Compound:	Compound **1** (**PT162, NSC 796018**)	
Molecular formula:	$C_{72}H_{100}Cl_5N_5$	
Molecular weight:	1,212.86 g/mol	
Yield:	1.605 g (12.4%)	
Elemental analysis:	calculated:	C 71.30% H 8.31% N 5.77% O 0.000%
	found:	C 65.67% H 7.76% N 4.29% O 0.669%
		C 65.66% H 7.74% N 4.27% O 0.691%
FT–IR (cm^{-1}):	2925, 2850, 2760, 2710, 2436, 1610, 1585, 1494, 1459, 1269, 1108, 1074, 1011, 973, 794, 777, 762, 731, 693	
^{1}H-NMR: (DMSO-d_6, ppm)	1.61 (3 H, d; $^2J_{gem} = -11.7$ Hz; δ-CH$_{axial}$), 1.68 (3 H, d; $^2J_{gem} = -11.7$ Hz; δ-CH$_{equatorial}$), 2.00 (6 H, s; β-CH$_2$), 2.14 (3 H, s; γ-CH), 4.09 (2 H, t; $^3J_{vicinal} = 6.4$ Hz; 8-CH$_2$), 4.77 (2 H, s; 7-CH$_2$), 7.43–7.48 (2 H, m; H-4, H-6), 7.64 (1 H, d; $^3J_{ortho} = 7.1$ Hz; H-5), 7.68 (1 H, s; H-2), 9.24 (2 H, br s; 8-NH$_2^+$ ammonium)	
^{13}C-NMR: (DMSO-d_6, ppm)	28.50 (γ-CH), 35.25 (δ-CH$_2$), 37.35 (β-CH$_2$), 42.31 (8-CH$_2$), 45.84 (7-CH$_2$), 57.06 (α-C), 128.87 (C-4)*, 129.14 (C-6)*, 130.36 (C-2)*, 130.62 (C-5)*, 133.22 (C-3), 137.84 (C-1)	

* these assignments are tentative and interchangeable (they could not be assigned unequivocally to the individual carbons)

2.3.   (*M*)-10-(2-Carbamothioylhydrazinyl)-10-demethoxy-colchicine monohydrate × ⅔ (ethyl acetate) = *N*-[(a*S*,7*S*)-10-

(2-carbamothioylhydrazinyl)-1,2,3-trimethoxy-9-oxo-5,6,7,9-tetrahydrobenzo[*a*]heptalen-7-yl]acetamide monohydrate × ⅔ (ethyl acetate) (**PT166, NSC 750423**)

5.00 g (–)-Colchicine sesquihydrate (× 1½ H_2O) (M = 426.46 g/mol, 11.72 mmol) and 1.08 g thiosemicarbazide (M = 91.13 g/mol, 11.85 mmol) were dissolved in 25 ml of 90% (*v/v*) aqueous ethanol by refluxing for 5 min. After adding a solution of 0.48 g sodium hydroxide (12.00 mmol) in 2 ml of water, the deep orange-red solution was refluxed for 5 min. The cold deep orange-red solution solution, after pre-cooling at –25 °C for 20 min, was titrated by dropwise addition of 1.1 ml of 10.27 M [32% (*m/v*)] hydrochloric acid (11.30 mmol) which was diluted with 2 ml of water. Afterwards, the volume of the solution was reduced *in vacuo* approximately by one half. The reddish-brown solution was then mixed with 100 ml of water, and was titrated with 1.1 ml of 10.27 M [32% (*m/v*)] hydrochloric acid (11.30 mmol) which was diluted with 2 ml of water. The oily emulsion was extracted with 50 ml of ethyl acetate (EtOAc). The separated aqueous layer (pH 2) was additionally extracted with 40 ml of EtOAc. After neutralization of this aqueous phase with sodium hydrogen carbonate $NaHCO_3$, the aqueous phase (pH 7–8) was extracted twice with 40 ml of EtOAc each. The EtOAc phases were combined and washed twice with 100 ml of water each. The washed EtOAc phase, which already precipitated, was mixed with 50 ml of acetone and was frozen at –25 °C for 10 h. If precipitation did not start spontaneously, the volume of the solution was reduced *in vacuo* until coagulation started. The evolved yellow precipitate of **PT166** was filtered (1.01 g) and dried over $CaCl_2$ *in vacuo*. From the combined aqueous phases by cooling two days at +0–2 °C a second crop of **PT166** could be obtained (1.75 g). It was treated as before and combined with the main yield.

Compound:	Compound **2** (**PT166, NSC 750423**)	
Molecular formula:	$C_{22}H_{26}N_4O_5S \times H_2O \times \frac{2}{3}(C_4H_8O_2)$	
Molecular weight:	535.28 g/mol	
Yield:	2.76 g (44%)	
Elemental analysis:	calculated:	C 55.35% H 6.28% N 10.47% S 5.99%
	found:	C 55.34% H 6.29% N 10.35% S 6.00%
		C 55.38% H 6.14% N 10.34% S 6.00%
FT–IR (cm^{-1}):	3421, 3249, 2934, 1727, 1703, 1660, 1601, 1543, 1488, 1449, 1432, 1402, 1375, 1350, 1322, 1282, 1241, 1193, 1142, 1091, 1042, 917, 899, 863, 781	
^{1}H-NMR: (DMSO-d_6, ppm)	1.18 (1.5 H, t; ^3J = 7.1 Hz; O–CH$_2$–CH$_3$ ethyl acetate), 1.85 (1 H, m; H$_A$-6), 1.86 (3 H, s; 17-CH$_3$), 1.99 (1.5 H, s; ROOC–CH$_3$ ethyl acetate), 2.05 (1 H, m; H$_B$-6), 2.19 (1 H, m; H$_A$-5), 2.57 (1 H, m; H$_B$-5), 3.51 (3 H, s; 13-OCH$_3$)*, 3.79 (3 H, s; 15-OCH$_3$)*, 3.83 (3 H, s; 14-OCH$_3$)*, 4.03 (1 H, q; ^3J = 7.1 Hz; O–CH$_2$–CH$_3$ ethyl acetate), 4.37 (1 H, m; H-7), 6.60 (1 H, d; ^3J = 11.1 Hz; H-11), 6.76 (1 H, s; H-4), 7.14 (1 H, s; H-8), 7.20 (1 H, d; ^3J = 10.9 Hz; H-12), 7.56 (1 H, br s; H$_2$N–C=S amino, 4'-H$_A$), 7.96 (1 H, br s; H$_2$N–C=S amino, 4'-H$_B$), 8.56 (1 H, d; ^3J = 7.6 Hz; N–H acetamide), 9.06 (1 H, s; 1'-N–H), 9.59 (1 H, s; 2'-N–H)	
^{13}C-NMR: (DMSO-d_6, ppm)	14.05 (O–CH$_2$–CH$_3$ ethyl acetate), 20.72 (ROOC–CH$_3$ ethyl acetate), 22.49 (C-17, CH$_3$ acetamide), 29.33 (C-5), 36.34 (C-6), 51.38 (C-7), 55.84 (14-OCH$_3$)**, 59.72 (O–CH$_2$–CH$_3$ ethyl acetate), 60.62 (13-OCH$_3$, 15-OCH$_3$)**, 107.61 (C-4), 108.27 (C-11), 126.23 (C-8), 131.57 (C-1a), 134.26 (C-4a), 137.21 (C-12), 140.71 (C-3)***, 150.34 (C-1)***, 150.40 (C-10), 150.46 (C-12a), 152.61 (C-2)***, 152.73 (C-7a), 168.39 (C-16, HN–C=O amide), 170.30 (C=O ester carbonyl, ethyl acetate), 174.81 (C-9, C=O carbonyl), 181.86 (C-3', C=S thiocarbonyl)	

*, **, *** these assignments are tentative and interchangeable (they could not be assigned unequivocally to the individual protons or carbons, respectively)

2.4. [(Bis{3-[(tricyclo[3.3.1.1^{3,7}]decan-1-ylamino)methyl]benzyl}ammonio)bis(methanediylbenzene-3,1-diylmethane-diyl)]di-2-[(aS,7S)-7-(acetylamino)-1,2,3-trimethoxy-9-oxo-5,6,7,9-tetrahydrobenzo[a]heptalen-10-yl]-N-(tricyclo[3.3.1.1^{3,7}]decan-1-yl)hydrazinecarbothioamide chloride pentahydrate (PT167, NSC 799315) (synthesized by *Andreas J. Kesel* at Saturday, May 27th, 2017)

Materials:
- **(PT162, NSC 796018)** = tetrakis{3-[(tricyclo[3.3.1.1^{3,7}]decan-1-ammonio)methyl]benzyl}ammonium pentachloride ($C_{72}H_{100}Cl_5N_5$) (M = 1,212.86 g/mol) [w (n/n) ≥ 99% (^{1}H-NMR and elemental analysis)], synthesized by *A.J. Kesel* at Friday, December 30th, 2016.
- **(PT166, NSC 750423)** = N-[(7S)-10-(2-carbamothioylhydrazinyl)-1,2,3-trimethoxy-9-oxo-5,6,7,9-tetrahydrobenzo[a]heptalen-7-yl]acetamide monohydrate × ⅔ (ethyl acetate) [$C_{22}H_{26}N_4O_5S$ × H_2O × ⅔ ($C_4H_8O_2$)] (M = 535.28 g/mol) [w (n/n) ≥ 98% (^{1}H-NMR and elemental analysis)], synthesized by *A.J. Kesel* at Thursday, January 29th, 2009.

PT162 (NSC 796018) (M = 1,212.86 g/mol, 300 mg, 247.3492 µmol) and **PT166 (NSC 750423)** (M = 535.28 g/mol, 300 mg, 560.4543 µmol) were suspended in absolute ethanol (20 ml), and the yellow suspension was heated to 40–50 °C for 4 min (heatgun). Then water (1,000 µl) was added under stirring and all material dissolved to give a bright yellow solution. Afterwards, a solution of sodium hydroxide (37 mg, 925.0000 µmol) in water (2,000 µl) was added under stirring. The color of the solution changed to orange-yellow. After cooling at +0–2 °C for 12 min, the mixture was frozen at –25 °C for 10 min. After adding water (10 ml), the precipitating emulsion was frozen at –25 °C for 2 h. The evolved first yield (212 mg) of the bright yellow, amorphous substance **PT167** was filtered, carefully dried by vacuum suction for 30 min on the sintered glass filter filter, and dried over $CaCl_2$ *in vacuo*. The filtrate was transferred with water (20 ml), and was frozen at –25 °C for 30 min. After cooling at

+0–2 °C for 1 h, the evolved second yield (17 mg) of the bright yellow, amorphous substance **PT167** was filtered [the initial turbid filtrate was transferred with water (10 ml), and was re-filtered on the same sintered glass filter used before], carefully dried by vacuum suction for 30 min on the sintered glass filter filter, and dried over $CaCl_2$ *in vacuo*. Both yields were combined.

Compound:	Compound 3 (**PT167, NSC 799315**)	
Molecular formula:	$C_{116}H_{142}ClN_{11}O_{10}S_2 \times 5\ H_2O$	
Molecular weight:	2,040.10 g/mol	
Yield:	229 mg (45%)	
Elemental analysis:	calculated:	C 68.29% H 7.51% N 7.55% S 3.14% O 11.76%
	found:	C 60.31% H 6.68% N 8.01% S 3.34% O 11.84%
		C 60.24% H 6.45% N 7.98% S 3.38% O 11.64%
¹H-NMR: (DMSO-d_6, ppm)	1.48–1.68 (24 H, br m; δ-CH_2, adamantane), 1.83 (2 H, m; H_A-6, colch), 1.85 (6 H, s; 17-CH_3, colch), 2.01 (2 H, m; H_B-6, colch), 2.17 (2 H, m; H_A-5, colch), 2.52 (2 H, m; H_B-5, colch), 3.48 (6 H, s; 13-OCH_3, colch)*, 3.65 (2 H, br s; secondary amine N–H), 3.77 (6 H, s; 15-OCH_3, colch)*, 3.82 (6 H, s; 14-OCH_3, colch)*, 4.26 (br m; 8-CH_2, *m*-xylylene), 4.32–4.39 (2 H, br m; H-7, colch), 4.76 (s; 7-CH_2, *m*-xylylene), 6.73 (2 H, s; H-4, colch), 7.03 (2 H, br m; H-11, colch), 7.06 (2 H, s; H-8, colch), 7.12–7.72 (br m; H-4, H-6, H-5, H-2, *m*-xylylene), 7.17 (2 H, br m; H-12, colch), 8.54 (2 H, d; ^3J = 7.7 Hz; N–H acetamide, colch), 9.59 (4 H, s; 1'-N–H, 2'-N–H, hydrazinecarbo-thioamide)	

colch = the colchic(in)oid part of **PT167**; * these assignments are tentative and interchangeable (they could not be assigned unequivocally to the individual methoxy groups); the adamantane resonances at δ 2.00 ppm (24 H; β-CH_2) and δ 2.14 ppm (12 H; γ-CH) could not being detected due to paramagnetic compression

3. X-Ray Crystallographic Determination of the Crystal and Molecular Structure of (*M*)-10-(2-Carbamothioyl-hydrazinyl)-10-demethoxycolchicine Sesquihydrate × ½ (Ethyl Acetate) = *N*-[(a*S*,7*S*)-10-(2-Carbamothioyl-hydrazinyl)-1,2,3-trimethoxy-9-oxo-5,6,7,9-tetrahydro-benzo[*a*]heptalen-7-yl]acetamide Sesquihydrate × ½ (Ethyl Acetate) (Crystalline PT166)

3.1. Crystallization of **PT166** single crystals

PT166 was crystallized by atmospheric evaporation from ethyl acetate (EtOAc) overnight (time ~10 h) in an open *Petri* dish at room temperature (RT, ϑ = 14.0 °C). A suitable single crystal was selected and isolated under polarized light microscopic examination.

3.2. Crystal data of **PT166** single crystals

The crystal data of **PT166** were collected on a Bruker X8 *APEX*-II diffractometer with a CCD area detector and multi-layer mirror monochromated Mo$_{K\alpha}$ radiation. The structure was solved using direct methods, refined with the *SHELX* software package (G. Sheldrick, *Acta Cryst.*, **2008**, *A64*, 112–122) [3] and expanded using *Fourier* techniques. All non-hydrogen atoms were refined anisotropically. Hydrogen atoms were assigned to idealized positions and were included in structure factor calculations. The *Flack* parameter x_{Flack} (H.D. Flack, *Acta Cryst.*, **1983**, *A39*, 876–881) [4] was near zero indicating that the right absolute configuration was solved.

3.3. Crystallographic information file (cif-file) of **PT166**

The cif-file of **PT166** (cu144, colch-TSC) is documented at the following twenty-five pages:

data_cu144

1. Submission Details

_publ_contact_author_name   'Prof. Dr. Holger Braunschweig'
_publ_contact_author_address
;
Institut fuer Anorganische Chemie
Universitaet Wuerzburg
Am Hubland
97074 Wuerzburg, Germany
;
_publ_contact_author_email   'H.Braunschweig@mail.uni-wuerzburg.de'
_publ_contact_author_fax   +49-931-8884623
_publ_contact_author_phone   +49-931-8885260

_publ_requested_journal   ?
_publ_requested_category   ?
_publ_requested_coeditor_name   ?

_publ_contact_letter
;
?
;

_publ_section_title
;
?
;

_publ_section_abstract
;
?
;

loop_
_publ_author_name
_publ_author_address
    'Braunschweig, Holger'
;   Institut fuer Anorganische Chemie
    Universitaet Wuerzburg

Am Hubland
D-97074 Wuerzburg, Germany
;

'Kesel, Andreas'
;   Institut fuer Anorganische Chemie
Universitaet Wuerzburg
Am Hubland
D-97074 Wuerzburg, Germany
;

'Kupfer, Thomas'
;   Institut fuer Anorganische Chemie
Universitaet Wuerzburg
Am Hubland
D-97074 Wuerzburg, Germany
;

_audit_creation_method   SHELXL-97
_chemical_name_systematic
;
N-[10-(2-carbamothioylhydrazinyl)-1,2,3-trimethoxy-9-oxo-5,6,7,9-
tetrahydrobenzo[a]heptalen-7-yl]acetamide ethyl acetate solvate hydrate
;
_chemical_name_common
;
10-(2-carbamothioylhydrazinyl)-10-demethoxycolchicine ethyl acetate
solvate hydrate
;
_chemical_melting_point   ?
_chemical_formula_moiety
'2(C22 H26 N4 O5 S), C4 H8 O2, 3(H2 O)'
_chemical_formula_sum
'C48 H66 N8 O15 S2'
_chemical_absolute_configuration
'(aS,7S)'
_chemical_formula_weight   1059.23

loop_
 _atom_type_symbol
 _atom_type_description
 _atom_type_scat_dispersion_real
 _atom_type_scat_dispersion_imag

_atom_type_scat_source
'C' 'C' 0.0033 0.0016
'International Tables Vol C Tables 4.2.6.8 and 6.1.1.4'
'H' 'H' 0.0000 0.0000
'International Tables Vol C Tables 4.2.6.8 and 6.1.1.4'
'N' 'N' 0.0061 0.0033
'International Tables Vol C Tables 4.2.6.8 and 6.1.1.4'
'O' 'O' 0.0106 0.0060
'International Tables Vol C Tables 4.2.6.8 and 6.1.1.4'
'S' 'S' 0.1246 0.1234
'International Tables Vol C Tables 4.2.6.8 and 6.1.1.4'

_symmetry_cell_setting 'monoclinic'
_symmetry_space_group_name_H-M 'P2(1)'
_symmetry_space_group_name_Hall 'P 2yb'

loop_
 _symmetry_equiv_pos_as_xyz
'x, y, z'
'-x, y+1/2, -z'

_cell_length_a 9.1886(5)
_cell_length_b 20.9047(10)
_cell_length_c 13.9841(7)
_cell_angle_alpha 90.00
_cell_angle_beta 106.153(2)
_cell_angle_gamma 90.00
_cell_volume 2580.1(2)
_cell_formula_units_Z 2
_cell_measurement_temperature 100(2)
_cell_measurement_reflns_used 9271
_cell_measurement_theta_min 2.47
_cell_measurement_theta_max 25.90

_exptl_crystal_description 'plate'
_exptl_crystal_colour 'colourless'
_exptl_crystal_size_max 0.48
_exptl_crystal_size_mid 0.31
_exptl_crystal_size_min 0.04
_exptl_crystal_density_meas ?
_exptl_crystal_density_diffrn 1.363

```
_exptl_crystal_density_method   'not measured'
_exptl_crystal_F_000   1124
_exptl_absorpt_coefficient_mu   0.178
_exptl_absorpt_correction_type   'multi-scan'
_exptl_absorpt_correction_T_min   0.9193
_exptl_absorpt_correction_T_max   0.9929
_exptl_absorpt_process_details   'Sadabs 2008/1 (Sheldrick, 2008)'

_exptl_special_details
;
?
;

_diffrn_ambient_temperature   100(2)
_diffrn_radiation_wavelength   0.71073
_diffrn_radiation_type   MoK\a
_diffrn_radiation_source   'rotating anode'
_diffrn_radiation_monochromator   'multi-layer mirror'
_diffrn_measurement_device_type   'Bruker APEX-II CCD'
_diffrn_measurement_method   '\f and \w scans'
_diffrn_detector_area_resol_mean   ?
_diffrn_reflns_number   49598
_diffrn_reflns_av_R_equivalents   0.0423
_diffrn_reflns_av_sigmaI/netI   0.0368
_diffrn_reflns_limit_h_min   -11
_diffrn_reflns_limit_h_max   11
_diffrn_reflns_limit_k_min   -25
_diffrn_reflns_limit_k_max   25
_diffrn_reflns_limit_l_min   -14
_diffrn_reflns_limit_l_max   17
_diffrn_reflns_theta_min   1.80
_diffrn_reflns_theta_max   26.05
_reflns_number_total   9686
_reflns_number_gt   8639
_reflns_threshold_expression   >2sigma(I)

_computing_data_collection   'APEX2 ver. 2008.3 (Bruker AXS, 2008)'
_computing_cell_refinement   'Saint+ ver. 7.53A (Bruker AXS, 2008)'
_computing_data_reduction   'Saint+ ver. 7.53A (Bruker AXS, 2008)'
_computing_structure_solution   'SHELXS-97 (Sheldrick, 2008)'
_computing_structure_refinement   'SHELXL-97 (Sheldrick, 2008)'
```

_computing_molecular_graphics   'XP ver. 5.1 (Bruker AXS, 1998)'
_computing_publication_material   'SHELXL-97 (Sheldrick, 2008)'

_refine_special_details
;
Refinement of F^2^ against ALL reflections. The weighted R-factor wR
and goodness of fit S are based on F^2^, conventional R-factors R are
based on F, with F set to zero for negative F^2^. The threshold expression
of F^2^ > 2sigma(F^2^) is used only for calculating R-factors(gt) etc. and
is not relevant to the choice of reflections for refinement. R-factors based
on F^2^ are statistically about twice as large as those based on F, and R-
factors based on ALL data will be even larger.
;

_refine_ls_structure_factor_coef   Fsqd
_refine_ls_matrix_type   full
_refine_ls_weighting_scheme   calc
_refine_ls_weighting_details
'calc w=1/[\s^2^(Fo^2^)+(0.0657P)^2^+2.5438P] where
P=(Fo^2^+2Fc^2^)/3'
_atom_sites_solution_primary   direct
_atom_sites_solution_secondary   difmap
_atom_sites_solution_hydrogens   geom
_refine_ls_hydrogen_treatment   mixed
_refine_ls_extinction_method   none
_refine_ls_extinction_coef   ?
_refine_ls_abs_structure_details
'Flack H D (1983), Acta Cryst. A39, 876-881'
_refine_ls_abs_structure_Flack   0.09(6)
_refine_ls_number_reflns   9686
_refine_ls_number_parameters   693
_refine_ls_number_restraints   5
_refine_ls_R_factor_all   0.0594
_refine_ls_R_factor_gt   0.0506
_refine_ls_wR_factor_ref   0.1325
_refine_ls_wR_factor_gt   0.1269
_refine_ls_goodness_of_fit_ref   1.021
_refine_ls_restrained_S_all   1.021
_refine_ls_shift/su_max   0.000
_refine_ls_shift/su_mean   0.000

loop_
_atom_site_label
_atom_site_type_symbol
_atom_site_fract_x
_atom_site_fract_y
_atom_site_fract_z
_atom_site_U_iso_or_equiv
_atom_site_adp_type
_atom_site_occupancy
_atom_site_symmetry_multiplicity
_atom_site_calc_flag
_atom_site_refinement_flags
_atom_site_disorder_assembly
_atom_site_disorder_group
C1 C 0.0127(2) 0.19304(10) 0.49224(15) 0.0216(5) Uani 1 1 d . . .
C2 C -0.0838(2) 0.24185(10) 0.50354(16) 0.0240(5) Uani 1 1 d . . .
H2 H -0.0472 0.2750 0.5505 0.029 Uiso 1 1 calc R . .
C3 C -0.2336(2) 0.24210(11) 0.44628(18) 0.0278(5) Uani 1 1 d . . .
C4 C -0.2921(2) 0.19144(11) 0.38269(17) 0.0261(5) Uani 1 1 d . . .
C5 C -0.1936(2) 0.14258(10) 0.37113(16) 0.0225(5) Uani 1 1 d . . .
C6 C -0.0398(2) 0.14461(10) 0.42268(15) 0.0190(5) Uani 1 1 d . . .
C7 C 0.1761(2) 0.19181(10) 0.55548(16) 0.0221(5) Uani 1 1 d . . .
H7A H 0.1997 0.2325 0.5928 0.027 Uiso 1 1 calc R . .
H7B H 0.2437 0.1883 0.5116 0.027 Uiso 1 1 calc R . .
C8 C 0.2068(2) 0.13548(10) 0.62947(15) 0.0226(5) Uani 1 1 d . . .
H8A H 0.3176 0.1299 0.6570 0.027 Uiso 1 1 calc R . .
H8B H 0.1643 0.1457 0.6854 0.027 Uiso 1 1 calc R . .
C9 C 0.1379(2) 0.07307(10) 0.58118(14) 0.0196(5) Uani 1 1 d . . .
H9 H 0.0256 0.0764 0.5689 0.024 Uiso 1 1 calc R . .
C10 C 0.1691(2) 0.06321(9) 0.47960(14) 0.0175(5) Uani 1 1 d . . .
C11 C 0.0713(2) 0.09830(9) 0.39941(15) 0.0172(4) Uani 1 1 d . . .
C12 C 0.0736(2) 0.09670(10) 0.30182(16) 0.0217(5) Uani 1 1 d . . .
H12 H 0.0001 0.1233 0.2587 0.026 Uiso 1 1 calc R . .
C13 C 0.1661(2) 0.06244(11) 0.25398(16) 0.0238(5) Uani 1 1 d . . .
H13 H 0.1429 0.0687 0.1841 0.029 Uiso 1 1 calc R . .
C14 C 0.2850(2) 0.02128(10) 0.29328(14) 0.0188(4) Uani 1 1 d . . .
C15 C 0.3476(2) 0.00316(9) 0.39760(15) 0.0199(5) Uani 1 1 d . . .
C16 C 0.2851(2) 0.02313(10) 0.47594(14) 0.0189(4) Uani 1 1 d . . .
H16 H 0.3348 0.0046 0.5386 0.023 Uiso 1 1 calc R . .
O1 O -0.33270(17) 0.29117(8) 0.44853(14) 0.0367(5) Uani 1 1 d . . .
C17 C -0.2702(3) 0.34688(12) 0.5037(2) 0.0377(6) Uani 1 1 d . . .

H17A H -0.2427 0.3372 0.5751 0.056 Uiso 1 1 calc R . .
H17B H -0.3454 0.3814 0.4890 0.056 Uiso 1 1 calc R . .
H17C H -0.1797 0.3603 0.4850 0.056 Uiso 1 1 calc R . .
O2 O -0.43976(17) 0.18990(8) 0.32414(13) 0.0340(4) Uani 1 1 d . . .
C18 C -0.5506(2) 0.18340(12) 0.3778(2) 0.0351(6) Uani 1 1 d . . .
H18A H -0.5368 0.1423 0.4128 0.053 Uiso 1 1 calc R . .
H18B H -0.6522 0.1852 0.3311 0.053 Uiso 1 1 calc R . .
H18C H -0.5387 0.2183 0.4262 0.053 Uiso 1 1 calc R . .
O3 O -0.25331(17) 0.09411(7) 0.30492(11) 0.0258(4) Uani 1 1 d . . .
C19 C -0.2461(2) 0.03176(11) 0.34992(16) 0.0264(5) Uani 1 1 d . . .
H19A H -0.1415 0.0226 0.3882 0.040 Uiso 1 1 calc R . .
H19B H -0.2801 -0.0006 0.2978 0.040 Uiso 1 1 calc R . .
H19C H -0.3119 0.0308 0.3944 0.040 Uiso 1 1 calc R . .
N1 N 0.18995(18) 0.02095(9) 0.65092(12) 0.0208(4) Uani 1 1 d . . .
H1 H 0.2721 0.0261 0.7008 0.025 Uiso 1 1 calc R . .
C20 C 0.1156(2) -0.03495(11) 0.64099(15) 0.0251(5) Uani 1 1 d . . .
C21 C 0.1818(3) -0.08466(12) 0.71874(19) 0.0374(7) Uani 1 1 d . . .
H21A H 0.1399 -0.0792 0.7755 0.056 Uiso 1 1 calc R . .
H21B H 0.2922 -0.0797 0.7412 0.056 Uiso 1 1 calc R . .
H21C H 0.1565 -0.1274 0.6902 0.056 Uiso 1 1 calc R . .
O4 O 0.00034(19) -0.04440(8) 0.57249(13) 0.0357(5) Uani 1 1 d . . .
O5 O 0.46057(16) -0.03400(7) 0.41738(11) 0.0258(4) Uani 1 1 d . . .
N2 N 0.3648(2) -0.00586(9) 0.23420(13) 0.0249(4) Uani 1 1 d . . .
H2A H 0.4516 -0.0251 0.2615 0.030 Uiso 1 1 calc R . .
N3 N 0.3087(2) -0.00295(10) 0.13085(13) 0.0283(5) Uani 1 1 d . . .
H3 H 0.2241 -0.0232 0.1016 0.034 Uiso 1 1 calc R . .
C22 C 0.3798(2) 0.02977(11) 0.07489(16) 0.0261(5) Uani 1 1 d . . .
S1 S 0.31565(6) 0.02436(3) -0.05146(4) 0.03298(14) Uani 1 1 d . . .
N4 N 0.4967(2) 0.06619(10) 0.11966(14) 0.0290(5) Uani 1 1 d D . .
H1NA H 0.551(2) 0.0873(11) 0.0838(14) 0.035 Uiso 1 1 d D . .
H1NB H 0.539(3) 0.0691(13) 0.1862(10) 0.035 Uiso 1 1 d D . .
C31 C 0.9015(2) 0.68843(11) 0.94575(15) 0.0248(5) Uani 1 1 d . . .
C32 C 0.9722(2) 0.63768(11) 1.00646(16) 0.0248(5) Uani 1 1 d . . .
H32 H 0.9150 0.6108 1.0372 0.030 Uiso 1 1 calc R . .
C33 C 1.1256(3) 0.62666(11) 1.02164(16) 0.0270(5) Uani 1 1 d . . .
C34 C 1.2114(3) 0.66616(12) 0.97854(17) 0.0297(6) Uani 1 1 d . . .
C35 C 1.1411(3) 0.71663(12) 0.91750(19) 0.0354(6) Uani 1 1 d . . .
C36 C 0.9841(3) 0.72738(11) 0.89925(16) 0.0272(5) Uani 1 1 d . . .
C37 C 0.7390(2) 0.70320(11) 0.93665(16) 0.0270(5) Uani 1 1 d . . .
H37A H 0.6927 0.6670 0.9632 0.032 Uiso 1 1 calc R . .
H37B H 0.6834 0.7087 0.8655 0.032 Uiso 1 1 calc R . .

C38 C 0.7246(3) 0.76447(11) 0.99415(17) 0.0273(5) Uani 1 1 d . . .
H38A H 0.7509 0.7546 1.0662 0.033 Uiso 1 1 calc R . .
H38B H 0.6181 0.7793 0.9732 0.033 Uiso 1 1 calc R . .
C39 C 0.8281(3) 0.81854(10) 0.97674(16) 0.0251(5) Uani 1 1 d . . .
H39 H 0.9349 0.8065 1.0120 0.030 Uiso 1 1 calc R . .
C40 C 0.8165(2) 0.82423(11) 0.86543(16) 0.0231(5) Uani 1 1 d . . .
C41 C 0.9044(2) 0.77878(10) 0.82966(17) 0.0255(5) Uani 1 1 d . . .
C42 C 0.9162(2) 0.77728(11) 0.73338(17) 0.0249(5) Uani 1 1 d . . .
H42 H 0.9835 0.7455 0.7222 0.030 Uiso 1 1 calc R . .
C43 C 0.8474(2) 0.81387(10) 0.64950(16) 0.0237(5) Uani 1 1 d . . .
H43 H 0.8805 0.8045 0.5924 0.028 Uiso 1 1 calc R . .
C44 C 0.7399(2) 0.86113(10) 0.63580(15) 0.0217(5) Uani 1 1 d . . .
C45 C 0.6699(2) 0.88719(10) 0.71000(16) 0.0234(5) Uani 1 1 d . . .
C46 C 0.7167(2) 0.86898(10) 0.81176(16) 0.0236(5) Uani 1 1 d . . .
H46 H 0.6684 0.8930 0.8518 0.028 Uiso 1 1 calc R . .
O31 O 1.20395(18) 0.57788(7) 1.07975(12) 0.0317(4) Uani 1 1 d . . .
C47 C 1.1185(3) 0.53722(11) 1.12644(18) 0.0330(6) Uani 1 1 d . . .
H47A H 1.0739 0.5629 1.1697 0.049 Uiso 1 1 calc R . .
H47B H 1.1855 0.5047 1.1663 0.049 Uiso 1 1 calc R . .
H47C H 1.0376 0.5162 1.0753 0.049 Uiso 1 1 calc R . .
O32 O 1.36479(18) 0.65571(9) 0.99539(13) 0.0380(4) Uani 1 1 d . . .
C48 C 1.4543(3) 0.67569(14) 1.09199(19) 0.0394(7) Uani 1 1 d . . .
H48A H 1.4469 0.7222 1.0979 0.059 Uiso 1 1 calc R . .
H48B H 1.5603 0.6637 1.1008 0.059 Uiso 1 1 calc R . .
H48C H 1.4168 0.6548 1.1433 0.059 Uiso 1 1 calc R . .
O33 O 1.2282(2) 0.76127(14) 0.88218(19) 0.1019(8) Uani 1 1 d . . .
C49 C 1.3190(4) 0.7474(2) 0.8313(3) 0.0819(13) Uani 1 1 d . . .
H49A H 1.3855 0.7123 0.8638 0.123 Uiso 1 1 calc R . .
H49B H 1.3805 0.7850 0.8267 0.123 Uiso 1 1 calc R . .
H49C H 1.2611 0.7341 0.7643 0.123 Uiso 1 1 calc R . .
N31 N 0.7928(2) 0.87662(9) 1.02238(13) 0.0283(5) Uani 1 1 d . . .
H31 H 0.6981 0.8839 1.0215 0.034 Uiso 1 1 calc R . .
C50 C 0.8995(3) 0.91988(11) 1.06617(17) 0.0340(6) Uani 1 1 d . . .
C51 C 0.8431(4) 0.97466(13) 1.11655(19) 0.0462(7) Uani 1 1 d . . .
H51A H 0.8948 0.9740 1.1880 0.069 Uiso 1 1 calc R . .
H51B H 0.7336 0.9703 1.1064 0.069 Uiso 1 1 calc R . .
H51C H 0.8643 1.0152 1.0880 0.069 Uiso 1 1 calc R . .
O34 O 1.0326(2) 0.91480(9) 1.06539(14) 0.0427(5) Uani 1 1 d . . .
O35 O 0.56844(17) 0.92891(8) 0.68098(11) 0.0289(4) Uani 1 1 d . . .
N32 N 0.68153(19) 0.88906(9) 0.54488(13) 0.0228(4) Uani 1 1 d . . .
H32A H 0.5966 0.9110 0.5330 0.027 Uiso 1 1 calc R . .

N33 N 0.7549(2) 0.88316(9) 0.47111(13) 0.0253(5) Uani 1 1 d . . .
H33 H 0.8457 0.8999 0.4808 0.030 Uiso 1 1 calc R . .
C52 C 0.6918(3) 0.85303(12) 0.38629(17) 0.0342(6) Uani 1 1 d . . .
S2 S 0.78074(10) 0.85155(4) 0.29517(5) 0.0540(2) Uani 1 1 d . . .
N34 N 0.5622(3) 0.82332(12) 0.37968(18) 0.0488(7) Uani 1 1 d D . .
H2NA H 0.504(2) 0.8370(14) 0.4176(15) 0.059 Uiso 1 1 d D . .
H2NB H 0.513(3) 0.8005(11) 0.3266(15) 0.059 Uiso 1 1 d D . .
C61 C 0.0489(4) 0.74943(16) 0.2160(2) 0.0613(10) Uani 1 1 d . . .
H61A H 0.0613 0.7954 0.2073 0.092 Uiso 1 1 calc R . .
H61B H -0.0193 0.7426 0.2579 0.092 Uiso 1 1 calc R . .
H61C H 0.0059 0.7295 0.1508 0.092 Uiso 1 1 calc R . .
C62 C 0.1996(3) 0.72021(14) 0.2647(2) 0.0454(7) Uani 1 1 d . . .
O61 O 0.3163(3) 0.74448(12) 0.2671(2) 0.0767(8) Uani 1 1 d . . .
O62 O 0.1873(2) 0.66330(9) 0.29871(13) 0.0406(5) Uani 1 1 d . . .
C63 C 0.3291(3) 0.62983(15) 0.3469(2) 0.0445(7) Uani 1 1 d . . .
H63A H 0.3990 0.6587 0.3944 0.053 Uiso 1 1 calc R . .
H63B H 0.3793 0.6157 0.2964 0.053 Uiso 1 1 calc R . .
C64 C 0.2908(3) 0.57393(16) 0.4000(2) 0.0501(8) Uani 1 1 d . . .
H64A H 0.2434 0.5886 0.4508 0.075 Uiso 1 1 calc R . .
H64B H 0.3834 0.5501 0.4319 0.075 Uiso 1 1 calc R . .
H64C H 0.2203 0.5461 0.3525 0.075 Uiso 1 1 calc R . .
O71 O 0.48970(16) 0.03129(8) 0.77440(12) 0.0311(4) Uani 1 1 d . . .
H1OA H 0.522(3) -0.0044(14) 0.754(2) 0.037 Uiso 1 1 d . . .
H1OB H 0.503(3) 0.0252(15) 0.836(2) 0.037 Uiso 1 1 d . . .
O72 O 0.4729(4) 0.88488(17) 1.0018(3) 0.1364(11) Uani 1 1 d G . .
H2OA H 0.4119 0.9209 0.9833 0.164 Uiso 1 1 d G . .
H2OB H 0.4953 0.8854 1.0672 0.164 Uiso 1 1 d G . .
O73 O 0.3109(6) 0.8477(3) 1.1349(5) 0.200(2) Uani 1 1 d G . .
H3OA H 0.2622 0.8870 1.1321 0.240 Uiso 1 1 d G . .
H3OB H 0.2674 0.8242 1.1714 0.240 Uiso 1 1 d G . .

loop_
 _atom_site_aniso_label
 _atom_site_aniso_U_11
 _atom_site_aniso_U_22
 _atom_site_aniso_U_33
 _atom_site_aniso_U_23
 _atom_site_aniso_U_13
 _atom_site_aniso_U_12
C1 0.0214(9) 0.0207(10) 0.0254(9) 0.0059(8) 0.0111(7) -0.0010(8)
C2 0.0255(9) 0.0171(10) 0.0328(10) -0.0010(9) 0.0137(8) -0.0002(8)

C3 0.0235(9) 0.0181(11) 0.0463(12) 0.0039(9) 0.0172(9) 0.0043(9)
C4 0.0171(9) 0.0217(11) 0.0394(12) 0.0047(9) 0.0077(8) 0.0019(8)
C5 0.0232(9) 0.0169(10) 0.0274(10) 0.0021(8) 0.0072(8) 0.0005(8)
C6 0.0203(9) 0.0151(10) 0.0231(9) 0.0034(8) 0.0084(7) -0.0007(8)
C7 0.0202(9) 0.0185(10) 0.0290(10) -0.0038(9) 0.0092(8) 0.0007(8)
C8 0.0240(9) 0.0199(10) 0.0238(10) -0.0031(8) 0.0063(8) -0.0004(8)
C9 0.0171(8) 0.0208(10) 0.0213(9) 0.0013(8) 0.0059(7) -0.0004(8)
C10 0.0164(8) 0.0146(9) 0.0213(9) -0.0023(8) 0.0047(7) -0.0046(8)
C11 0.0170(8) 0.0132(9) 0.0212(9) -0.0004(8) 0.0052(7) 0.0006(7)
C12 0.0178(9) 0.0205(10) 0.0260(10) 0.0038(9) 0.0046(8) 0.0030(8)
C13 0.0262(10) 0.0242(11) 0.0201(9) -0.0002(9) 0.0049(8) -0.0009(9)
C14 0.0161(8) 0.0169(9) 0.0245(9) -0.0037(8) 0.0076(7) -0.0031(8)
C15 0.0199(9) 0.0145(10) 0.0258(9) 0.0035(8) 0.0073(8) -0.0034(8)
C16 0.0180(8) 0.0148(9) 0.0221(9) 0.0038(8) 0.0025(7) -0.0003(8)
O1 0.0225(7) 0.0193(8) 0.0701(11) -0.0004(8) 0.0160(7) 0.0051(6)
C17 0.0342(11) 0.0209(12) 0.0617(15) -0.0047(11) 0.0196(11) 0.0068(10)
O2 0.0173(7) 0.0364(9) 0.0461(9) 0.0078(8) 0.0052(6) 0.0025(7)
C18 0.0194(10) 0.0338(13) 0.0513(14) -0.0023(11) 0.0084(10)
-0.0005(10)
O3 0.0241(7) 0.0217(8) 0.0280(7) 0.0022(6) 0.0015(6) 0.0014(6)
C19 0.0307(10) 0.0189(11) 0.0283(10) -0.0030(9) 0.0058(8) -0.0070(9)
N1 0.0211(7) 0.0210(8) 0.0196(7) 0.0028(7) 0.0043(6) -0.0009(7)
C20 0.0280(10) 0.0261(11) 0.0201(9) 0.0009(9) 0.0049(8) -0.0029(9)
C21 0.0429(13) 0.0298(13) 0.0354(12) 0.0086(11) 0.0040(11) -0.0054(11)
O4 0.0325(8) 0.0294(9) 0.0383(9) 0.0029(7) -0.0019(7) -0.0076(7)
O5 0.0256(7) 0.0222(8) 0.0332(7) 0.0071(6) 0.0144(6) 0.0075(6)
N2 0.0231(8) 0.0266(9) 0.0254(8) -0.0048(8) 0.0075(7) 0.0026(8)
N3 0.0295(9) 0.0361(11) 0.0212(8) -0.0078(8) 0.0100(7) -0.0054(8)
C22 0.0258(9) 0.0234(11) 0.0297(10) -0.0057(9) 0.0089(8) -0.0011(9)
S1 0.0316(3) 0.0439(3) 0.0239(2) -0.0066(3) 0.0085(2) -0.0031(3)
N4 0.0273(9) 0.0318(10) 0.0259(9) 0.0008(8) 0.0043(7) -0.0022(8)
C31 0.0312(10) 0.0220(11) 0.0198(9) -0.0017(9) 0.0049(8) 0.0039(9)
C32 0.0305(10) 0.0195(10) 0.0229(10) -0.0008(9) 0.0047(8) -0.0017(9)
C33 0.0367(11) 0.0206(11) 0.0204(10) -0.0011(9) 0.0025(9) 0.0084(10)
C34 0.0312(10) 0.0293(12) 0.0315(11) 0.0022(10) 0.0132(9) 0.0109(10)
C35 0.0346(11) 0.0329(13) 0.0425(12) 0.0125(11) 0.0174(10) 0.0150(10)
C36 0.0347(11) 0.0206(11) 0.0272(10) 0.0009(9) 0.0100(9) 0.0086(9)
C37 0.0291(10) 0.0247(11) 0.0262(10) 0.0031(9) 0.0060(9) 0.0047(9)
C38 0.0310(10) 0.0241(11) 0.0278(11) 0.0039(9) 0.0098(9) 0.0039(9)
C39 0.0307(10) 0.0199(11) 0.0246(10) -0.0004(9) 0.0073(9) 0.0040(9)
C40 0.0225(9) 0.0207(10) 0.0266(10) 0.0017(9) 0.0077(8) 0.0018(9)

C41 0.0266(10) 0.0185(11) 0.0320(11) 0.0040(9) 0.0094(8) 0.0069(9)
C42 0.0252(9) 0.0204(11) 0.0320(11) 0.0004(9) 0.0132(8) 0.0072(9)
C43 0.0257(10) 0.0196(11) 0.0268(10) -0.0026(9) 0.0092(8) 0.0030(9)
C44 0.0199(9) 0.0195(10) 0.0256(10) 0.0000(9) 0.0062(8) -0.0018(8)
C45 0.0207(9) 0.0186(10) 0.0325(11) -0.0025(9) 0.0099(8) 0.0041(8)
C46 0.0257(9) 0.0189(11) 0.0277(10) -0.0032(8) 0.0098(8) 0.0044(9)
O31 0.0316(8) 0.0217(8) 0.0368(9) 0.0058(7) 0.0014(7) 0.0074(7)
C47 0.0358(11) 0.0227(12) 0.0362(12) 0.0080(10) 0.0029(10) 0.0045(10)
O32 0.0334(8) 0.0447(10) 0.0396(8) 0.0099(8) 0.0164(7) 0.0194(8)
C48 0.0280(11) 0.0483(16) 0.0431(13) 0.0173(12) 0.0120(10) 0.0055(11)
O33 0.0591(10) 0.1474(19) 0.1240(14) 0.1071(13) 0.0667(10) 0.0700(12)
C49 0.061(2) 0.097(3) 0.092(3) 0.018(2) 0.0284(19) 0.004(2)
N31 0.0375(10) 0.0237(10) 0.0252(9) -0.0011(8) 0.0112(8) 0.0051(8)
C50 0.0598(15) 0.0183(11) 0.0236(10) -0.0002(9) 0.0112(10) -0.0055(11)
C51 0.0818(18) 0.0285(14) 0.0349(12) -0.0056(11) 0.0271(12)
-0.0003(13)
O34 0.0453(10) 0.0342(10) 0.0508(10) -0.0098(8) 0.0172(8) -0.0117(8)
O35 0.0288(7) 0.0297(9) 0.0288(7) 0.0027(7) 0.0090(6) 0.0110(7)
N32 0.0191(8) 0.0256(10) 0.0231(8) 0.0035(7) 0.0051(7) 0.0052(7)
N33 0.0249(8) 0.0285(10) 0.0223(8) 0.0014(8) 0.0064(7) 0.0019(8)
C52 0.0445(13) 0.0247(12) 0.0288(12) 0.0008(10) 0.0024(10) 0.0138(11)
S2 0.1029(5) 0.0329(4) 0.0350(3) 0.0024(3) 0.0339(3) 0.0095(4)
N34 0.0371(12) 0.0489(13) 0.0521(13) -0.0262(11) -0.0011(10)
0.0047(11)
C61 0.087(2) 0.0467(17) 0.0436(16) 0.0029(14) 0.0074(16) 0.0211(17)
C62 0.0573(15) 0.0407(16) 0.0417(14) -0.0094(12) 0.0193(12)
-0.0062(13)
O61 0.0879(17) 0.0528(14) 0.0835(17) 0.0012(13) 0.0140(14)
-0.0047(14)
O62 0.0440(9) 0.0380(10) 0.0389(9) 0.0016(8) 0.0102(8) 0.0083(8)
C63 0.0323(12) 0.0584(18) 0.0425(14) 0.0028(13) 0.0096(11) 0.0045(13)
C64 0.0437(14) 0.065(2) 0.0401(14) 0.0107(14) 0.0090(12) 0.0074(14)
O71 0.0243(7) 0.0348(9) 0.0320(8) -0.0089(7) 0.0044(6) 0.0037(7)
O72 0.175(2) 0.106(2) 0.174(3) 0.0533(19) 0.1234(19) 0.0877(19)
O73 0.189(4) 0.123(3) 0.337(6) 0.063(4) 0.154(4) 0.017(3)

_geom_special_details
;
All esds (except the esd in the dihedral angle between two l.s. planes) are
estimated using the full covariance matrix. The cell esds are taken into
account individually in the estimation of esds in distances, angles and

torsion angles; correlations between esds in cell parameters are only used
when they are defined by crystal symmetry. An approximate (isotropic)
treatment of cell esds is used for estimating esds involving l.s. planes.
;

loop_
 _geom_bond_atom_site_label_1
 _geom_bond_atom_site_label_2
 _geom_bond_distance
 _geom_bond_site_symmetry_2
 _geom_bond_publ_flag
C1 C2 1.390(3) . ?
C1 C6 1.394(3) . ?
C1 C7 1.515(3) . ?
C2 C3 1.386(3) . ?
C2 H2 0.9500 . ?
C3 O1 1.378(3) . ?
C3 C4 1.391(3) . ?
C4 O2 1.376(2) . ?
C4 C5 1.404(3) . ?
C5 O3 1.379(3) . ?
C5 C6 1.397(3) . ?
C6 C11 1.506(3) . ?
C7 C8 1.541(3) . ?
C7 H7A 0.9900 . ?
C7 H7B 0.9900 . ?
C8 C9 1.524(3) . ?
C8 H8A 0.9900 . ?
C8 H8B 0.9900 . ?
C9 N1 1.452(3) . ?
C9 C10 1.540(3) . ?
C9 H9 1.0000 . ?
C10 C16 1.368(3) . ?
C10 C11 1.429(3) . ?
C11 C12 1.371(3) . ?
C12 C13 1.414(3) . ?
C12 H12 0.9500 . ?
C13 C14 1.379(3) . ?
C13 H13 0.9500 . ?
C14 N2 1.371(3) . ?
C14 C15 1.462(3) . ?

C15 O5 1.264(2) . ?
C15 C16 1.433(3) . ?
C16 H16 0.9500 . ?
O1 C17 1.427(3) . ?
C17 H17A 0.9800 . ?
C17 H17B 0.9800 . ?
C17 H17C 0.9800 . ?
O2 C18 1.429(3) . ?
C18 H18A 0.9800 . ?
C18 H18B 0.9800 . ?
C18 H18C 0.9800 . ?
O3 C19 1.441(3) . ?
C19 H19A 0.9800 . ?
C19 H19B 0.9800 . ?
C19 H19C 0.9800 . ?
N1 C20 1.341(3) . ?
N1 H1 0.8800 . ?
C20 O4 1.230(3) . ?
C20 C21 1.505(3) . ?
C21 H21A 0.9800 . ?
C21 H21B 0.9800 . ?
C21 H21C 0.9800 . ?
N2 N3 1.394(2) . ?
N2 H2A 0.8800 . ?
N3 C22 1.339(3) . ?
N3 H3 0.8800 . ?
C22 N4 1.323(3) . ?
C22 S1 1.704(2) . ?
N4 H1NA 0.913(16) . ?
N4 H1NB 0.906(13) . ?
C31 C36 1.391(3) . ?
C31 C32 1.400(3) . ?
C31 C37 1.495(3) . ?
C32 C33 1.384(3) . ?
C32 H32 0.9500 . ?
C33 O31 1.376(3) . ?
C33 C34 1.390(4) . ?
C34 O32 1.380(3) . ?
C34 C35 1.397(3) . ?
C35 O33 1.406(4) . ?
C35 C36 1.411(3) . ?

C36 C41 1.497(3) . ?
C37 C38 1.537(3) . ?
C37 H37A 0.9900 . ?
C37 H37B 0.9900 . ?
C38 C39 1.539(3) . ?
C38 H38A 0.9900 . ?
C38 H38B 0.9900 . ?
C39 N31 1.450(3) . ?
C39 C40 1.535(3) . ?
C39 H39 1.0000 . ?
C40 C46 1.377(3) . ?
C40 C41 1.425(3) . ?
C41 C42 1.381(3) . ?
C42 C43 1.396(3) . ?
C42 H42 0.9500 . ?
C43 C44 1.372(3) . ?
C43 H43 0.9500 . ?
C44 N32 1.366(3) . ?
C44 C45 1.469(3) . ?
C45 O35 1.258(3) . ?
C45 C46 1.419(3) . ?
C46 H46 0.9500 . ?
O31 C47 1.432(3) . ?
C47 H47A 0.9800 . ?
C47 H47B 0.9800 . ?
C47 H47C 0.9800 . ?
O32 C48 1.434(3) . ?
C48 H48A 0.9800 . ?
C48 H48B 0.9800 . ?
C48 H48C 0.9800 . ?
O33 C49 1.271(5) . ?
C49 H49A 0.9800 . ?
C49 H49B 0.9800 . ?
C49 H49C 0.9800 . ?
N31 C50 1.349(3) . ?
N31 H31 0.8800 . ?
C50 O34 1.230(3) . ?
C50 C51 1.510(4) . ?
C51 H51A 0.9800 . ?
C51 H51B 0.9800 . ?
C51 H51C 0.9800 . ?

N32 N33 1.386(3) . ?
N32 H32A 0.8800 . ?
N33 C52 1.325(3) . ?
N33 H33 0.8800 . ?
C52 N34 1.324(4) . ?
C52 S2 1.694(3) . ?
N34 H2NA 0.898(16) . ?
N34 H2NB 0.893(16) . ?
C61 C62 1.493(4) . ?
C61 H61A 0.9800 . ?
C61 H61B 0.9800 . ?
C61 H61C 0.9800 . ?
C62 O61 1.179(4) . ?
C62 O62 1.297(4) . ?
O62 C63 1.467(3) . ?
C63 C64 1.478(4) . ?
C63 H63A 0.9900 . ?
C63 H63B 0.9900 . ?
C64 H64A 0.9800 . ?
C64 H64B 0.9800 . ?
C64 H64C 0.9800 . ?
O71 H1OA 0.88(3) . ?
O71 H1OB 0.85(3) . ?
O72 H2OA 0.9315 . ?
O72 H2OB 0.8794 . ?
O73 H3OA 0.9316 . ?
O73 H3OB 0.8798 . ?

loop_
  _geom_angle_atom_site_label_1
  _geom_angle_atom_site_label_2
  _geom_angle_atom_site_label_3
  _geom_angle
  _geom_angle_site_symmetry_1
  _geom_angle_site_symmetry_3
  _geom_angle_publ_flag
C2 C1 C6 120.29(18) . . ?
C2 C1 C7 120.40(19) . . ?
C6 C1 C7 119.31(19) . . ?
C3 C2 C1 120.0(2) . . ?
C3 C2 H2 120.0 . . ?

C1 C2 H2 120.0 . . ?
O1 C3 C2 123.1(2) . . ?
O1 C3 C4 116.18(18) . . ?
C2 C3 C4 120.7(2) . . ?
O2 C4 C3 122.7(2) . . ?
O2 C4 C5 118.4(2) . . ?
C3 C4 C5 118.73(18) . . ?
O3 C5 C6 121.67(19) . . ?
O3 C5 C4 117.58(17) . . ?
C6 C5 C4 120.71(19) . . ?
C1 C6 C5 119.11(19) . . ?
C1 C6 C11 119.57(17) . . ?
C5 C6 C11 121.19(18) . . ?
C1 C7 C8 111.82(17) . . ?
C1 C7 H7A 109.3 . . ?
C8 C7 H7A 109.3 . . ?
C1 C7 H7B 109.3 . . ?
C8 C7 H7B 109.3 . . ?
H7A C7 H7B 107.9 . . ?
C9 C8 C7 112.38(16) . . ?
C9 C8 H8A 109.1 . . ?
C7 C8 H8A 109.1 . . ?
C9 C8 H8B 109.1 . . ?
C7 C8 H8B 109.1 . . ?
H8A C8 H8B 107.9 . . ?
N1 C9 C8 109.04(15) . . ?
N1 C9 C10 114.09(17) . . ?
C8 C9 C10 111.24(17) . . ?
N1 C9 H9 107.4 . . ?
C8 C9 H9 107.4 . . ?
C10 C9 H9 107.4 . . ?
C16 C10 C11 127.72(19) . . ?
C16 C10 C9 117.64(17) . . ?
C11 C10 C9 114.64(17) . . ?
C12 C11 C10 125.98(19) . . ?
C12 C11 C6 115.46(17) . . ?
C10 C11 C6 118.46(18) . . ?
C11 C12 C13 131.39(19) . . ?
C11 C12 H12 114.3 . . ?
C13 C12 H12 114.3 . . ?
C14 C13 C12 129.9(2) . . ?

C14 C13 H13 115.1 . . ?
C12 C13 H13 115.1 . . ?
N2 C14 C13 121.02(18) . . ?
N2 C14 C15 111.47(17) . . ?
C13 C14 C15 127.44(19) . . ?
O5 C15 C16 119.41(18) . . ?
O5 C15 C14 116.68(19) . . ?
C16 C15 C14 123.87(18) . . ?
C10 C16 C15 133.55(18) . . ?
C10 C16 H16 113.2 . . ?
C15 C16 H16 113.2 . . ?
C3 O1 C17 116.83(17) . . ?
O1 C17 H17A 109.5 . . ?
O1 C17 H17B 109.5 . . ?
H17A C17 H17B 109.5 . . ?
O1 C17 H17C 109.5 . . ?
H17A C17 H17C 109.5 . . ?
H17B C17 H17C 109.5 . . ?
C4 O2 C18 114.73(18) . . ?
O2 C18 H18A 109.5 . . ?
O2 C18 H18B 109.5 . . ?
H18A C18 H18B 109.5 . . ?
O2 C18 H18C 109.5 . . ?
H18A C18 H18C 109.5 . . ?
H18B C18 H18C 109.5 . . ?
C5 O3 C19 114.20(16) . . ?
O3 C19 H19A 109.5 . . ?
O3 C19 H19B 109.5 . . ?
H19A C19 H19B 109.5 . . ?
O3 C19 H19C 109.5 . . ?
H19A C19 H19C 109.5 . . ?
H19B C19 H19C 109.5 . . ?
C20 N1 C9 121.40(16) . . ?
C20 N1 H1 119.3 . . ?
C9 N1 H1 119.3 . . ?
O4 C20 N1 121.6(2) . . ?
O4 C20 C21 122.6(2) . . ?
N1 C20 C21 115.78(18) . . ?
C20 C21 H21A 109.5 . . ?
C20 C21 H21B 109.5 . . ?
H21A C21 H21B 109.5 . . ?

C20 C21 H21C 109.5 . . ?
H21A C21 H21C 109.5 . . ?
H21B C21 H21C 109.5 . . ?
C14 N2 N3 120.05(17) . . ?
C14 N2 H2A 120.0 . . ?
N3 N2 H2A 120.0 . . ?
C22 N3 N2 121.89(18) . . ?
C22 N3 H3 119.1 . . ?
N2 N3 H3 119.1 . . ?
N4 C22 N3 118.78(19) . . ?
N4 C22 S1 122.00(18) . . ?
N3 C22 S1 119.21(16) . . ?
C22 N4 H1NA 120.9(13) . . ?
C22 N4 H1NB 125.8(17) . . ?
H1NA N4 H1NB 113(2) . . ?
C36 C31 C32 120.3(2) . . ?
C36 C31 C37 120.06(19) . . ?
C32 C31 C37 119.5(2) . . ?
C33 C32 C31 120.0(2) . . ?
C33 C32 H32 120.0 . . ?
C31 C32 H32 120.0 . . ?
O31 C33 C32 123.9(2) . . ?
O31 C33 C34 115.4(2) . . ?
C32 C33 C34 120.7(2) . . ?
O32 C34 C33 120.5(2) . . ?
O32 C34 C35 120.0(2) . . ?
C33 C34 C35 119.4(2) . . ?
C34 C35 O33 120.3(2) . . ?
C34 C35 C36 120.4(2) . . ?
O33 C35 C36 119.0(2) . . ?
C31 C36 C35 119.0(2) . . ?
C31 C36 C41 119.5(2) . . ?
C35 C36 C41 121.5(2) . . ?
C31 C37 C38 110.88(18) . . ?
C31 C37 H37A 109.5 . . ?
C38 C37 H37A 109.5 . . ?
C31 C37 H37B 109.5 . . ?
C38 C37 H37B 109.5 . . ?
H37A C37 H37B 108.1 . . ?
C37 C38 C39 112.5(2) . . ?
C37 C38 H38A 109.1 . . ?

C39 C38 H38A 109.1 . . ?
C37 C38 H38B 109.1 . . ?
C39 C38 H38B 109.1 . . ?
H38A C38 H38B 107.8 . . ?
N31 C39 C40 114.87(18) . . ?
N31 C39 C38 108.74(19) . . ?
C40 C39 C38 110.21(17) . . ?
N31 C39 H39 107.6 . . ?
C40 C39 H39 107.6 . . ?
C38 C39 H39 107.6 . . ?
C46 C40 C41 128.2(2) . . ?
C46 C40 C39 116.9(2) . . ?
C41 C40 C39 114.71(18) . . ?
C42 C41 C40 124.29(19) . . ?
C42 C41 C36 117.4(2) . . ?
C40 C41 C36 118.2(2) . . ?
C41 C42 C43 131.8(2) . . ?
C41 C42 H42 114.1 . . ?
C43 C42 H42 114.1 . . ?
C44 C43 C42 130.7(2) . . ?
C44 C43 H43 114.7 . . ?
C42 C43 H43 114.7 . . ?
N32 C44 C43 121.2(2) . . ?
N32 C44 C45 111.31(18) . . ?
C43 C44 C45 127.44(19) . . ?
O35 C45 C46 120.0(2) . . ?
O35 C45 C44 117.37(19) . . ?
C46 C45 C44 122.59(19) . . ?
C40 C46 C45 134.3(2) . . ?
C40 C46 H46 112.8 . . ?
C45 C46 H46 112.8 . . ?
C33 O31 C47 116.47(18) . . ?
O31 C47 H47A 109.5 . . ?
O31 C47 H47B 109.5 . . ?
H47A C47 H47B 109.5 . . ?
O31 C47 H47C 109.5 . . ?
H47A C47 H47C 109.5 . . ?
H47B C47 H47C 109.5 . . ?
C34 O32 C48 113.91(19) . . ?
O32 C48 H48A 109.5 . . ?
O32 C48 H48B 109.5 . . ?

H48A C48 H48B 109.5 . . ?
O32 C48 H48C 109.5 . . ?
H48A C48 H48C 109.5 . . ?
H48B C48 H48C 109.5 . . ?
C49 O33 C35 124.9(3) . . ?
O33 C49 H49A 109.5 . . ?
O33 C49 H49B 109.5 . . ?
H49A C49 H49B 109.5 . . ?
O33 C49 H49C 109.5 . . ?
H49A C49 H49C 109.5 . . ?
H49B C49 H49C 109.5 . . ?
C50 N31 C39 122.5(2) . . ?
C50 N31 H31 118.7 . . ?
C39 N31 H31 118.7 . . ?
O34 C50 N31 122.5(2) . . ?
O34 C50 C51 122.7(2) . . ?
N31 C50 C51 114.8(2) . . ?
C50 C51 H51A 109.5 . . ?
C50 C51 H51B 109.5 . . ?
H51A C51 H51B 109.5 . . ?
C50 C51 H51C 109.5 . . ?
H51A C51 H51C 109.5 . . ?
H51B C51 H51C 109.5 . . ?
C44 N32 N33 120.58(17) . . ?
C44 N32 H32A 119.7 . . ?
N33 N32 H32A 119.7 . . ?
C52 N33 N32 121.8(2) . . ?
C52 N33 H33 119.1 . . ?
N32 N33 H33 119.1 . . ?
N34 C52 N33 116.5(2) . . ?
N34 C52 S2 123.49(19) . . ?
N33 C52 S2 120.0(2) . . ?
C52 N34 H2NA 118.8(17) . . ?
C52 N34 H2NB 123(2) . . ?
H2NA N34 H2NB 115(2) . . ?
C62 C61 H61A 109.5 . . ?
C62 C61 H61B 109.5 . . ?
H61A C61 H61B 109.5 . . ?
C62 C61 H61C 109.5 . . ?
H61A C61 H61C 109.5 . . ?
H61B C61 H61C 109.5 . . ?

O61 C62 O62 123.7(3) . . ?
O61 C62 C61 123.9(3) . . ?
O62 C62 C61 112.2(3) . . ?
C62 O62 C63 116.7(2) . . ?
O62 C63 C64 107.6(2) . . ?
O62 C63 H63A 110.2 . . ?
C64 C63 H63A 110.2 . . ?
O62 C63 H63B 110.2 . . ?
C64 C63 H63B 110.2 . . ?
H63A C63 H63B 108.5 . . ?
C63 C64 H64A 109.5 . . ?
C63 C64 H64B 109.5 . . ?
H64A C64 H64B 109.5 . . ?
C63 C64 H64C 109.5 . . ?
H64A C64 H64C 109.5 . . ?
H64B C64 H64C 109.5 . . ?
H1OA O71 H1OB 103(3) . . ?
H2OA O72 H2OB 103.1 . . ?
H3OA O73 H3OB 103.1 . . ?

loop_
 _geom_torsion_atom_site_label_1
 _geom_torsion_atom_site_label_2
 _geom_torsion_atom_site_label_3
 _geom_torsion_atom_site_label_4
 _geom_torsion
 _geom_torsion_site_symmetry_1
 _geom_torsion_site_symmetry_2
 _geom_torsion_site_symmetry_3
 _geom_torsion_site_symmetry_4
 _geom_torsion_publ_flag
C6 C1 C2 C3 0.7(3) . . . . ?
C7 C1 C2 C3 -179.1(2) . . . . ?
C1 C2 C3 O1 -175.3(2) . . . . ?
C1 C2 C3 C4 4.9(4) . . . . ?
O1 C3 C4 O2 0.6(3) . . . . ?
C2 C3 C4 O2 -179.6(2) . . . . ?
O1 C3 C4 C5 174.9(4) . . . . ?
C2 C3 C4 C5 -5.3(4) . . . . ?
O2 C4 C5 O3 -3.1(3) . . . . ?
C3 C4 C5 O3 -177.7(2) . . . . ?

O2 C4 C5 C6 174.7(2) . . . . ?
C3 C4 C5 C6 0.2(3) . . . . ?
C2 C1 C6 C5 -5.8(3) . . . . ?
C7 C1 C6 C5 174.10(19) . . . . ?
C2 C1 C6 C11 170.10(19) . . . . ?
C7 C1 C6 C11 -10.0(3) . . . . ?
O3 C5 C6 C1 -176.91(19) . . . . ?
C4 C5 C6 C1 5.3(3) . . . . ?
O3 C5 C6 C11 7.3(3) . . . . ?
C4 C5 C6 C11 -170.5(2) . . . . ?
C2 C1 C7 C8 112.0(2) . . . . ?
C6 C1 C7 C8 -67.9(3) . . . . ?
C1 C7 C8 C9 44.9(2) . . . . ?
C7 C8 C9 N1 171.74(17) . . . . ?
C7 C8 C9 C10 45.1(2) . . . . ?
N1 C9 C10 C16 -24.0(2) . . . . ?
C8 C9 C10 C16 99.8(2) . . . . ?
N1 C9 C10 C11 156.31(17) . . . . ?
C8 C9 C10 C11 -79.8(2) . . . . ?
C16 C10 C11 C12 1.9(3) . . . . ?
C9 C10 C11 C12 -178.51(19) . . . . ?
C16 C10 C11 C6 -174.25(19) . . . . ?
C9 C10 C11 C6 5.4(3) . . . . ?
C1 C6 C11 C12 -120.8(2) . . . . ?
C5 C6 C11 C12 55.0(3) . . . . ?
C1 C6 C11 C10 55.8(3) . . . . ?
C5 C6 C11 C10 -128.5(2) . . . . ?
C10 C11 C12 C13 0.2(4) . . . . ?
C6 C11 C12 C13 176.4(2) . . . . ?
C11 C12 C13 C14 -1.8(4) . . . . ?
C12 C13 C14 N2 -177.7(2) . . . . ?
C12 C13 C14 C15 -1.0(4) . . . . ?
N2 C14 C15 O5 -0.8(3) . . . . ?
C13 C14 C15 O5 -177.8(2) . . . . ?
N2 C14 C15 C16 -178.45(19) . . . . ?
C13 C14 C15 C16 4.5(3) . . . . ?
C11 C10 C16 C15 0.4(4) . . . . ?
C9 C10 C16 C15 -179.2(2) . . . . ?
O5 C15 C16 C10 178.0(2) . . . . ?
C14 C15 C16 C10 -4.4(4) . . . . ?
C2 C3 O1 C17 7.7(3) . . . . ?

C4 C3 O1 C17 -172.5(2) . . . . ?
C3 C4 O2 C18 -68.2(3) . . . . ?
C5 C4 O2 C18 117.5(2) . . . . ?
C6 C5 O3 C19 64.9(3) . . . . ?
C4 C5 O3 C19 -117.3(2) . . . . ?
C8 C9 N1 C20 160.17(19) . . . . ?
C10 C9 N1 C20 -74.8(2) . . . . ?
C9 N1 C20 O4 0.0(3) . . . . ?
C9 N1 C20 C21 -179.8(2) . . . . ?
C13 C14 N2 N3 -13.2(3) . . . . ?
C15 C14 N2 N3 169.57(18) . . . . ?
C14 N2 N3 C22 114.6(2) . . . . ?
N2 N3 C22 N4 -7.8(3) . . . . ?
N2 N3 C22 S1 173.17(16) . . . . ?
C36 C31 C32 C33 1.0(3) . . . . ?
C37 C31 C32 C33 -175.0(2) . . . . ?
C31 C32 C33 O31 -179.8(2) . . . . ?
C31 C32 C33 C34 1.1(3) . . . . ?
O31 C33 C34 O32 -0.4(3) . . . . ?
C32 C33 C34 O32 178.8(2) . . . . ?
O31 C33 C34 C35 179.4(2) . . . . ?
C32 C33 C34 C35 -1.4(3) . . . . ?
O32 C34 C35 O33 -7.2(4) . . . . ?
C33 C34 C35 O33 173.0(2) . . . . ?
O32 C34 C35 C36 179.5(2) . . . . ?
C33 C34 C35 C36 -0.3(4) . . . . ?
C32 C31 C36 C35 -2.6(3) . . . . ?
C37 C31 C36 C35 173.3(2) . . . . ?
C32 C31 C36 C41 176.2(2) . . . . ?
C37 C31 C36 C41 -7.9(3) . . . . ?
C34 C35 C36 C31 2.3(4) . . . . ?
O33 C35 C36 C31 -171.0(2) . . . . ?
C34 C35 C36 C41 -176.5(2) . . . . ?
O33 C35 C36 C41 10.2(4) . . . . ?
C36 C31 C37 C38 -69.4(3) . . . . ?
C32 C31 C37 C38 106.5(2) . . . . ?
C31 C37 C38 C39 44.3(2) . . . . ?
C37 C38 C39 N31 172.39(17) . . . . ?
C37 C38 C39 C40 45.7(2) . . . . ?
N31 C39 C40 C46 -27.6(3) . . . . ?
C38 C39 C40 C46 95.6(2) . . . . ?

N31 C39 C40 C41 156.4(2) . . . . ?
C38 C39 C40 C41 -80.4(2) . . . . ?
C46 C40 C41 C42 7.8(4) . . . . ?
C39 C40 C41 C42 -176.8(2) . . . . ?
C46 C40 C41 C36 -169.3(2) . . . . ?
C39 C40 C41 C36 6.1(3) . . . . ?
C31 C36 C41 C42 -122.6(2) . . . . ?
C35 C36 C41 C42 56.2(3) . . . . ?
C31 C36 C41 C40 54.7(3) . . . . ?
C35 C36 C41 C40 -126.5(2) . . . . ?
C40 C41 C42 C43 -3.2(4) . . . . ?
C36 C41 C42 C43 174.0(2) . . . . ?
C41 C42 C43 C44 -3.7(4) . . . . ?
C42 C43 C44 N32 -176.7(2) . . . . ?
C42 C43 C44 C45 1.7(4) . . . . ?
N32 C44 C45 O35 1.2(3) . . . . ?
C43 C44 C45 O35 -177.2(2) . . . . ?
N32 C44 C45 C46 -176.2(2) . . . . ?
C43 C44 C45 C46 5.4(3) . . . . ?
C41 C40 C46 C45 -2.2(4) . . . . ?
C39 C40 C46 C45 -177.5(2) . . . . ?
O35 C45 C46 C40 176.5(2) . . . . ?
C44 C45 C46 C40 -6.1(4) . . . . ?
C32 C33 O31 C47 -0.3(3) . . . . ?
C34 C33 O31 C47 178.9(2) . . . . ?
C33 C34 O32 C48 -75.6(3) . . . . ?
C35 C34 O32 C48 104.6(3) . . . . ?
C34 C35 O33 C49 57.3(4) . . . . ?
C36 C35 O33 C49 -129.4(3) . . . . ?
C40 C39 N31 C50 -91.4(2) . . . . ?
C38 C39 N31 C50 144.6(2) . . . . ?
C39 N31 C50 O34 4.2(3) . . . . ?
C39 N31 C50 C51 -175.4(2) . . . . ?
C43 C44 N32 N33 -16.9(3) . . . . ?
C45 C44 N32 N33 164.52(18) . . . . ?
C44 N32 N33 C52 116.2(2) . . . . ?
N32 N33 C52 N34 -6.6(3) . . . . ?
N32 N33 C52 S2 175.74(16) . . . . ?
O61 C62 O62 C63 3.2(4) . . . . ?
C61 C62 O62 C63 179.2(2) . . . . ?
C62 O62 C63 C64 167.0(2) . . . . ?

_diffrn_measured_fraction_theta_max   0.994
_diffrn_reflns_theta_full   26.00
_diffrn_measured_fraction_theta_full   0.997
_refine_diff_density_max   0.747
_refine_diff_density_min   -0.496
_refine_diff_density_rms   0.061

3.4. Deposition of the X-ray crystallographic structure determination of **PT166**

Crystallographic data have been deposited with The Cambridge Crystallographic Data Centre (CCDC), 12 Union Road, Cambridge, CB2 1EZ, United Kingdom, as supplementary publication № **CCDC 1839505** (ID: **RIVGOW**). These data can be obtained free of charge from CCDC *via* https://www.ccdc.cam.ac.uk/structures/.

4. Experimental Instructions

4.1. Cytotoxicity and HIV-1$_{LAI}$ replication reverse transcriptase assays with **PT162**

The cytotoxicity and human immunodeficiency virus type 1 (HIV-1) strain LAI replication assays were performed in freshly explanted primary human peripheral blood mononuclear cells (PBM cells) according to published procedures [5]. The assays were conducted at least in triplicate and treated statistically (if possible). HIV-1$_{LAI}$ (= HIV-1$_{BRU}$ = LAV-1) was assayed in primary human peripheral blood lymphocyte (PBL) cells in the presence of a drug being evaluated. The parameter for antiviral activity was reduction of reverse transcriptase (RT) activity in the cell supernatant after Triton X–100-mediated lysis of released virions, as measured by [5α-^{3}H]dTTP (5α-tritiated thymidine 5′-triphosphate) incorporation into poly(rA)•poly(dT) directed by the primed RNA template poly(rA)•oligo(dT). It should be noted that the assay did not detect RT inhibition by potential RT inhibitors *per se*, but indirectly quantified the amount of released HIV-1 in the supernatant. The detailed assay methodology was reported by *Schinazi et al.* [6], as based on an older assay system of *Spira et al.* [7]. The experiments were conducted in triplicate and treated statistically by regression curve analysis (r^2 coefficient of determination). The RT inhibitor AZT (zidovudine, 3'-azido-3'-deoxythymidine; RETROVIR™) served as a positive control. Cytotoxicity on PBL and the other cells (CCRF–CEM, Vero) exerted by the test compounds was determined as described by *Stuyver et al.* [8], by application of the CellTiter 96® AQ$_{ueous}$ One Solution Cell Proliferation Assay (Promega Corp., Madison, WI, USA). Briefly, the phenazine ethosulfate (PES)-coupled reduction of the tetrazolium salt 3-(4,5-dimethylthiazol-2-yl)-5-(3-carboxymethoxyphenyl)-2-(4-sulfophenyl)-2*H*-tetrazolium (MTS) to a purple, water-soluble formazan by living, undamaged cells was measured.

4.2. Cytochrome *c* assay (mitochondrial and cytosolic)

Cell numbers of 2×10^6 PC-3 and DU-145 cells were seeded into a 100-well plate. At the next day cells were treated with either dimethyl sulfoxide (DMSO) or 6 concentrations of compound **1** (**PT162**), compound **2** (**PT166**), and compound **3** (**PT167**) (500 nM, 1 µM, 5 µM, 25 µM, 50 µM, 75 µM) dissolved in DMSO for a time of 48 h. The concentrations of 25 µM, 50 µM and 75 µM of compound **1** (**PT162**), compound **2** (**PT166**) and compound **3** (**PT167**) were found to be highly toxic for both cell lines 48 h post-treatment. The enzyme-linked immunosorbent assay (ELISA) for cytochrome *c* was performed according to the manufacturer's instructions [Cytochrome *c* (human), ELISA kit (Enzo Life Sciences, Inc., Farmingdale, NY, USA)] with two fractions (mitochondrial and cytosolic) of each cell line at the concentrations of compound **1** (**PT162**), compound **2** (**PT166**), and compound **3** (**PT167**) of 500 nM, 1 µM, 5 µM, and 25 µM. The protein content for each fraction was calculated to determine the mass content of cytochrome c in each fraction (pg cytochrome c/mg total protein). The mass content of cytochrome c (pg cytochrome c/mg total protein) was normalized towards the corresponding blank DMSO control and is given in percent (%) of blank DMSO control.

4.3. National Cancer Institute (NCI) Developmental Therapeutics Program (DTP) 60-cancer cell 5-dose testing

Compounds which exhibit significant growth inhibition in the one-dose screen are evaluated against the 60-cell panel at five concentration levels. The human tumor cell lines of the cancer screening panel are grown in RPMI 1640 medium containing 5% fetal bovine serum and 2 mM L-glutamine. For a typical screening experiment, cells are inoculated into 96-well microtiter plates in 100 µl at plating densities ranging from 5,000 to 40,000 cells/well depending on the doubling time of individual cell lines. After cell inoculation, the microtiter plates are incubated at 37 °C, 5 % CO_2, 95% air and 100% relative humidity for 24 h prior to addition of experimental drugs. After 24 h, two plates of each cell line are fixed *in situ* with trichloroacetic acid (TCA), to represent a measurement of the cell population for each cell line at the time of drug addition (T_z). Experimental drugs are solubilized in dimethyl sulfoxide at 400-fold the desired final maximum test concentration and stored frozen prior to use. At the time of drug addition, an aliquot of frozen concentrate is thawed and diluted to twice the desired final maximum test concentration with complete medium containing 50 µg/ml gentamicin. Additional four, 10-fold or ½ log serial dilutions are made to provide a total of five drug concentrations plus control. Aliquots of 100 µl of these different drug dilutions are added to the appropriate microtiter wells already containing 100 μl of medium, resulting in the required final drug concentrations.

Following drug addition, the plates are incubated for an additional 48 h at 37 °C, 5% CO_2, 95% air, and 100% relative humidity. For adherent cells, the assay is terminated by the addition of cold TCA. Cells are fixed *in situ* by the gentle addition of 50 μl of cold 50% (*m/v*) TCA (final concentration, 10% TCA) and incubated for 60 minutes at 4 °C. The supernatant is discarded, and the plates are washed five times with tap water and air dried. Sulforhodamine B (SRB) [C.I. (Colour Index) 45100, Kiton Red 620, C.I. Acid Red 52, $C_{27}H_{30}N_2O_7S_2$,   2-{3-(diethylamino)-6-[(diethylazanium) ylidene]xanthen-9-yl}-5-sulfobenzenesulfonate] solution (100 μl) at 0.4% (*m/v*) in 1% acetic acid is added to each well, and plates are incubated for 10 minutes at room temperature [9]. After staining, unbound dye is removed by washing five times with 1% acetic acid and the plates are air dried. Bound stain is subsequently solubilized with 10 mM trizma®-base [tris base, 2-amino-2-(hydroxymethyl)-1,3-propandiol],   and   the absorbance is read on an automated plate reader at a wavelength of λ = 515 nm. For suspension cells, the methodology [9] is the same except that the assay is terminated by fixing settled cells at the bottom of the wells by gently adding 50 μl of 80% (*m/v*) TCA [final concentration, 16% TCA]. Using the seven absorbance measurements [time zero, (T_z), control growth, (C), and test growth in the presence of drug at the five concentration levels, (T_i)], the percentage growth is calculated at each of the drug concentrations levels. Percentage growth inhibition is calculated as:

$[(T_i - T_z)/(C - T_z)] \times 100$; for concentrations for which $T_i \geq T_z$

$[(T_i - T_z)/T_z] \times 100$; for concentrations for which $T_i < T_z$.

Three dose response parameters are calculated for each experimental agent. Growth inhibition of 50% (**GI50**) is calculated from $[(T_i - T_z)/(C - T_z)] \times 100 = 50$, which is the drug concentration resulting in a 50% reduction in the net protein increase (as measured by SRB staining) in control cells during the drug incubation. The drug concentration resulting in total growth inhibition (**TGI**) is calculated from $T_i = T_z$. The **LC50** (concentration of drug resulting in a 50% reduction in the measured protein at the end of the drug treatment as compared to that at the beginning) indicating a net loss of cells following treatment is calculated from $[(T_i - T_z)/T_z] \times 100 = -50$. Values are calculated for each of these three parameters if the level of activity is reached; however, if the effect is not reached or is exceeded, the value for that parameter is expressed as greater or less than the maximum or minimum concentration tested.

5. Supplementary Data

5.1. Table of contents

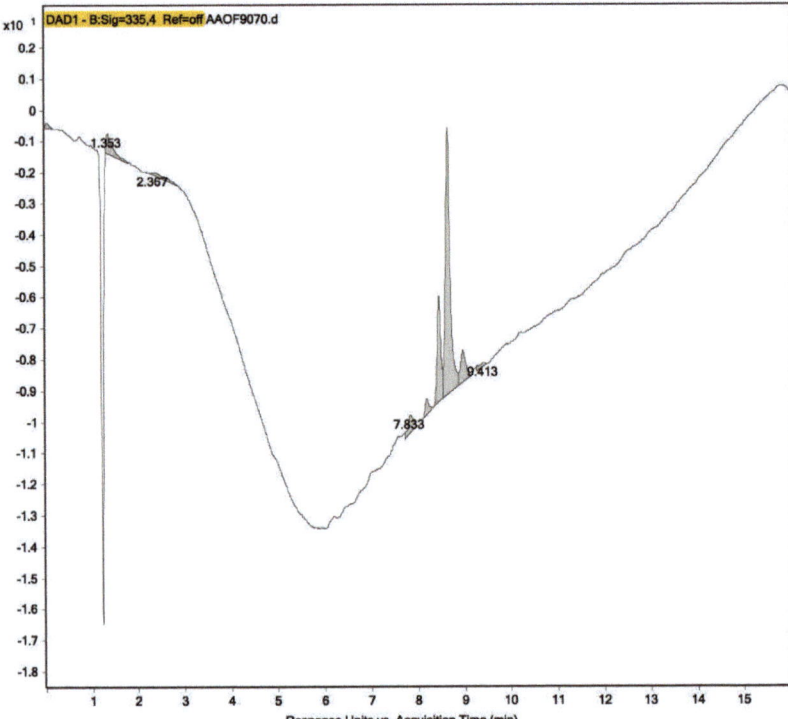

Fig. S1. The liquid chromatographic (HPLC) investigation of **PT167** (**NSC 799315**) with UV detection at λ = 335 nm, after storing the substance over six years at +0–4 °C in the refrigerator. The high-performance liquid chromatography (HPLC) of **PT167** (**NSC 799315**) was performed on a reversed phase C_8 (RP8) column with gradient elution [eluent A = water/0.1% (v/v) formic acid (HCOOH), eluent B = acetonitrile/0.1% (v/v) formic acid (HCOOH)]. The flowrate was 0.5 ml/min and the linear eluent gradient was t_{0min} = 95% eluent A/5% eluent B to t_{13min} = 5% eluent A/95% eluent B, t_{16min} = stop.

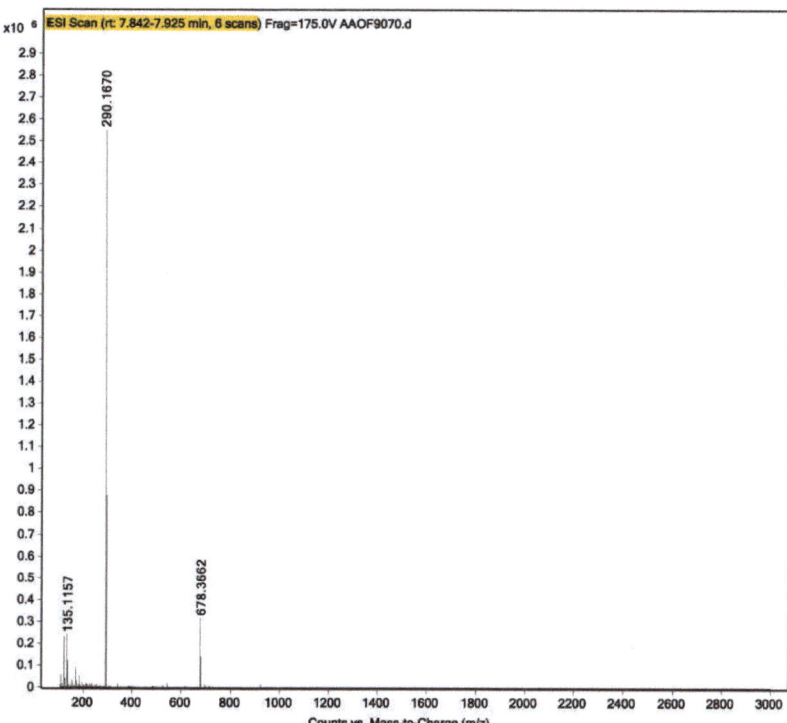

Fig. S2. The ESI mass spectrum of the separated HPLC peak region
7.842–7.925 min (see Fig. 29) with the ammonium trication ionization
species of **PT167** (**NSC 799315**). The ESI–MS fragment peaks (relative
intensity of the 100% base peak) were m/z 290.1670 (100%), 678.3662
(12.5%), and 135.1157 (9.6%).

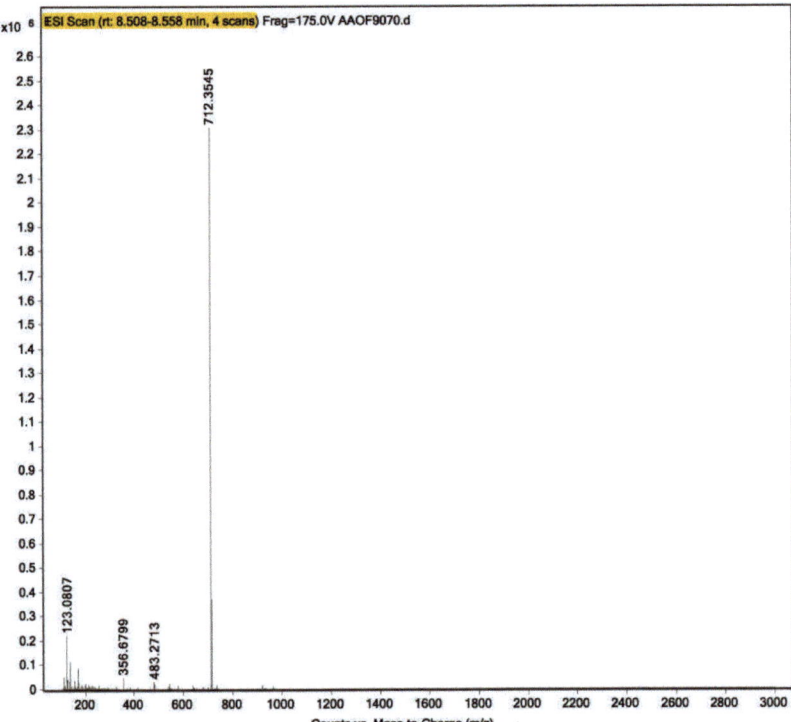

Fig. S3. The ESI mass spectrum of the separated HPLC peak region 8.508–8.558 min (see Fig. 29) with the ammonium dication ionization species of **PT167** (**NSC 799315**). The ESI−MS fragment peaks (relative intensity of the 100% base peak) were m/z 712.3545 (100%), 123.0807 (16.5%), 356.6799 (2.1%), and 483.2713 (1.3%).

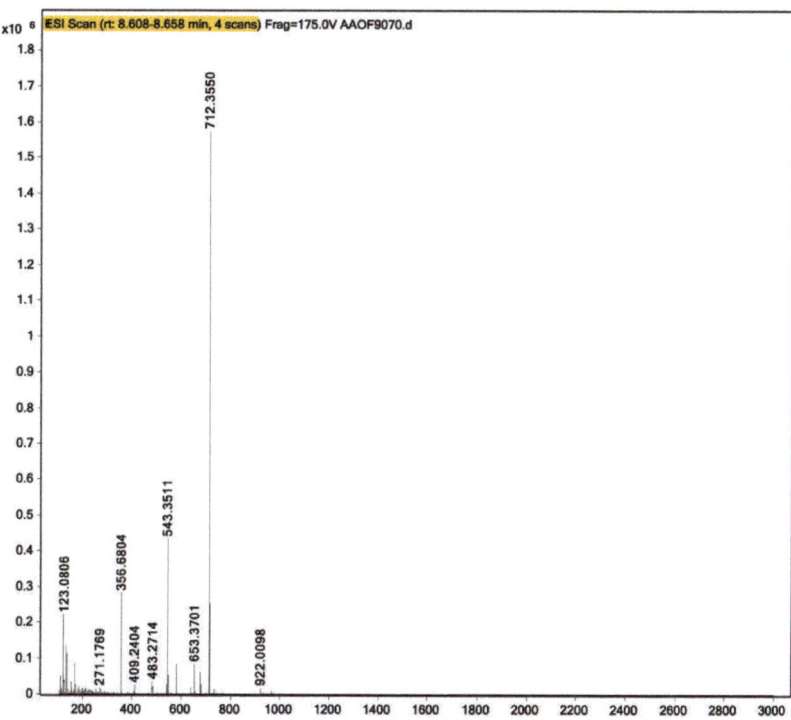

Fig. S4. The ESI mass spectrum of the separated HPLC peak region
8.608−8.658 min (see Fig. 29) with the ammonium monocation ionization
species of **PT167** (**NSC 799315**). The ESI−MS fragment peaks (relative
intensity of the 100% base peak) were m/z 712.3550 (100%), 543.3511
(27.9%), 356.6804 (18.1%), 123.0806 (14.2%), 653.3701 (5.4%),
483.2714 (2.5%), and 409.2404 (1.7%). The m/z 922.0098 is an internal
control substance (reference cation) added to the analysis for auto-
calibration of the mass spectrometer.

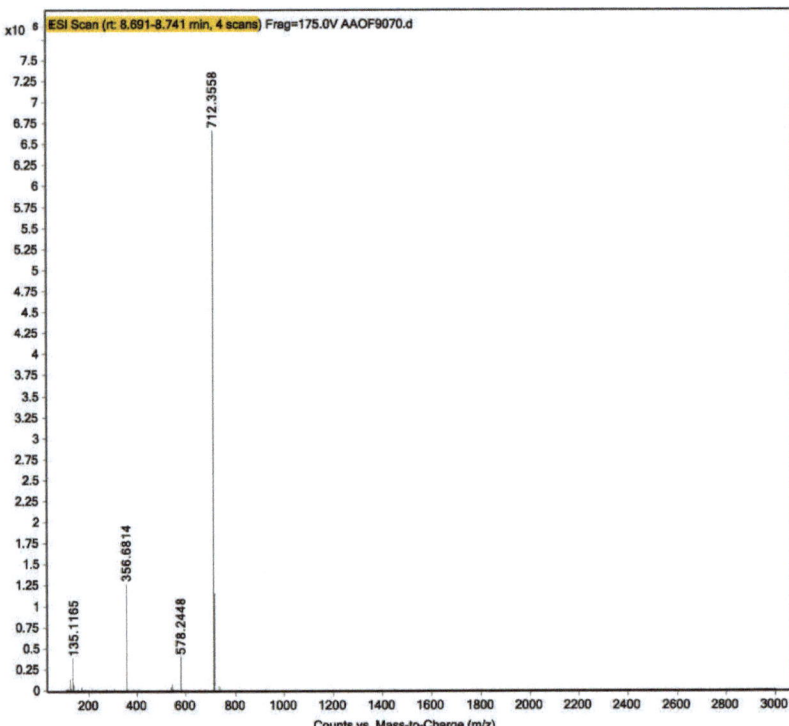

Fig. S5. The ESI mass spectrum of the separated HPLC peak region 8.691−8.741 min (see Fig. 29) with the ammonium monocation ionization species of **PT167** (**NSC 799315**). The ESI−MS fragment peaks (relative intensity of the 100% base peak) were *m/z* 712.3558 (100%), 356.6814 (19.1%), 578.2448 (6.3%), and 135.1165 (5.8%).

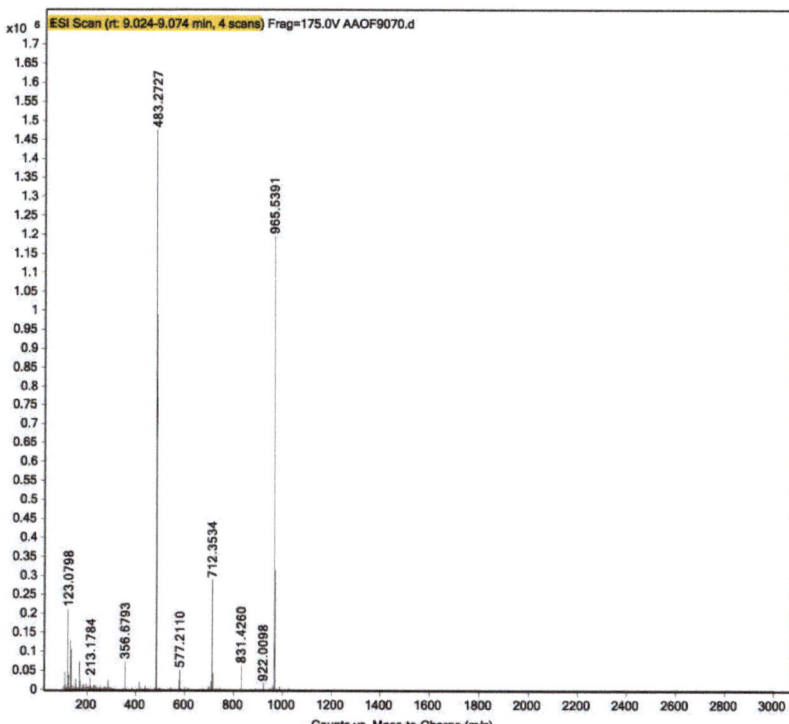

Fig. S6. The ESI mass spectrum of the separated HPLC peak region
9.024−9.074 min (see Fig. 29) with the ylide dication ionization species of
PT167 (**NSC 799315**). The ESI−MS fragment peaks (relative intensity of
the 100% base peak) were m/z 483.2727 (100%), 965.5391 (80.9%),
712.3534 (19.5%), 123.0798 (14.1%), 356.6793 (5.0%), 831.4260 (4.3%),
577.2110 (3.4%), and 213.1784 (2.3%). The m/z 922.0098 is an internal
control substance (reference cation) added to the analysis for auto-
calibration of the mass spectrometer.

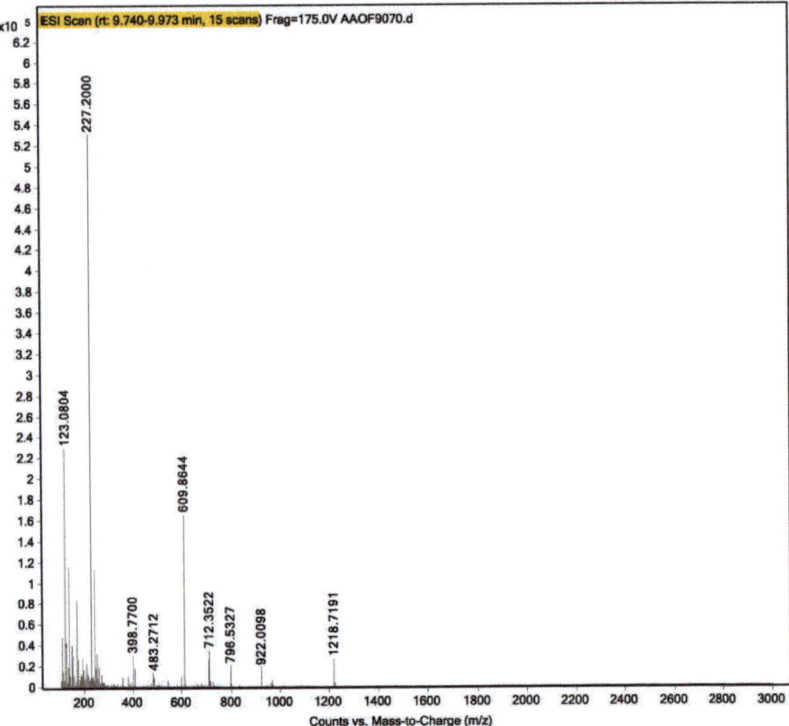

Fig. S7. The ESI mass spectrum of the separated HPLC peak region 9.740−9.973 min (see Fig. 29) with the ylide monocation ionization species of **PT167** (**NSC 799315**). The ESI−MS fragment peaks (relative intensity of the 100% base peak) were *m/z* 227.2000 (100%), 123.0804 (47.2%), 609.8644 (31.0%), 712.3522 (6.6%), 398.7700 (5.8%), 1218.7191 (5.0%), 796.5327 (4.0%), and 483.2712 (2.5%). The *m/z* 922.0098 is an internal control substance (reference cation) added to the analysis for auto-calibration of the mass spectrometer.

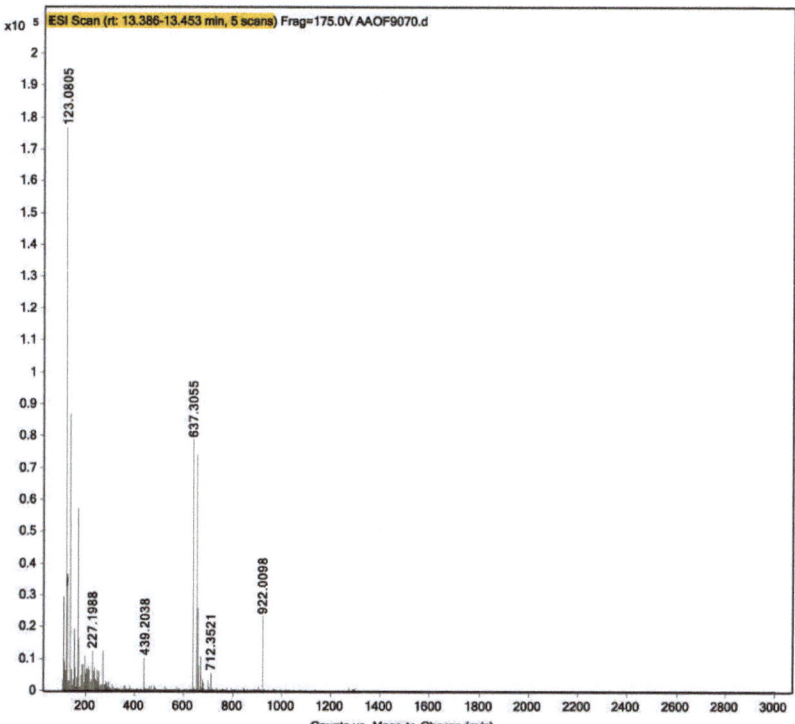

Fig. S8. The ESI mass spectrum of the separated HPLC peak region
13.386–13.453 min (see Fig. 29) with the neutral ylide ionization species
of **PT167** (**NSC 799315**). The ESI–MS fragment peaks (relative intensity
of the 100% base peak) were m/z 123.0805 (100%), 637.3055 (45.6%),
227.1988 (7.1%), 439.2038 (5.8%), and 712.3521 (3.2%). The m/z
922.0098 is an internal control substance (reference cation) added to the
analysis for auto-calibration of the mass spectrometer.

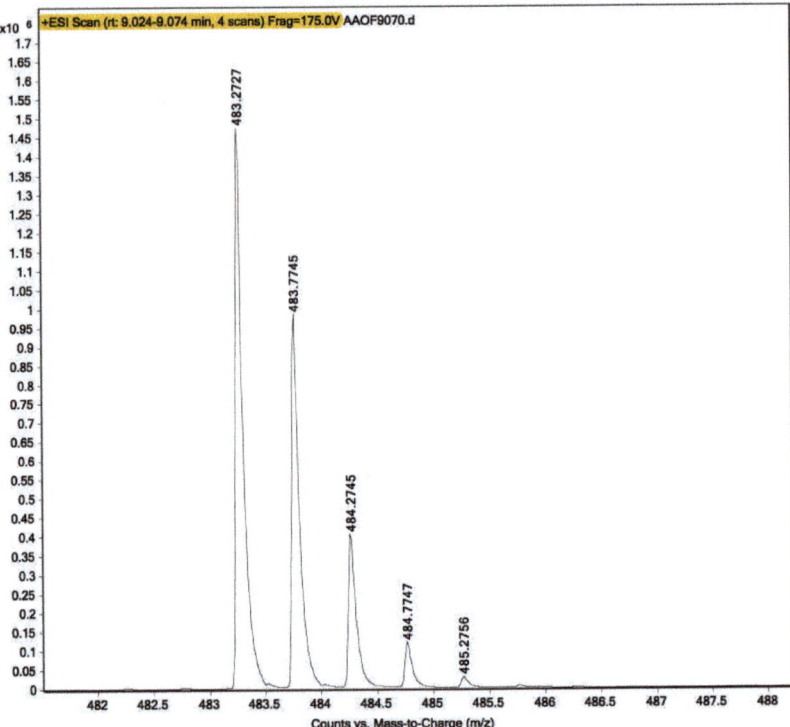

Fig. S9. The enlargement of the ESI mass spectrum of the separated HPLC peak region 9.024−9.074 min (see Fig. 29) with the ylide dication ionization species of **PT167** (**NSC 799315**), showing the 0.5 Da isotope peak spacing of the dication $(C_{58}H_{74}N_6O_5S)^{2+}$ m/z 483.2727 Da.

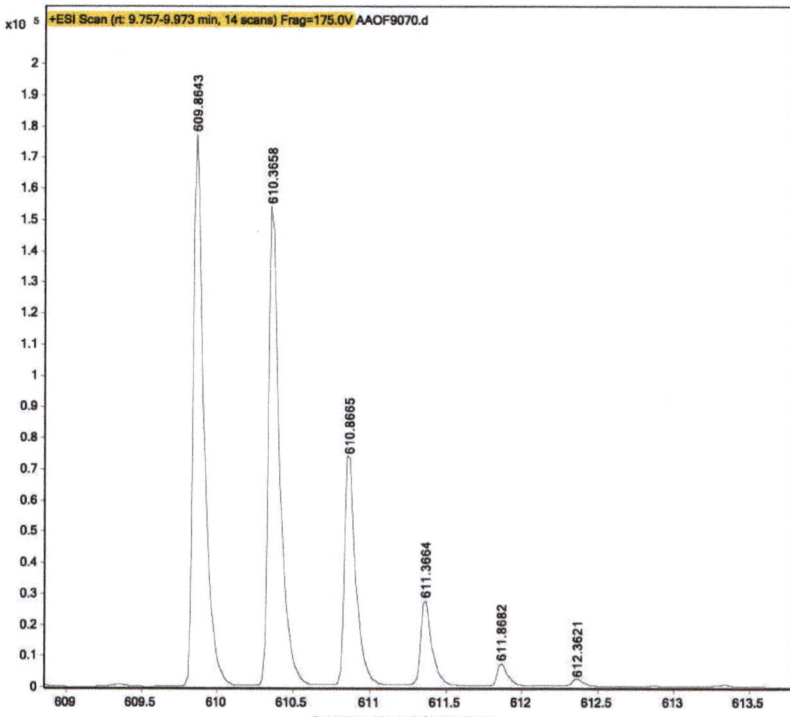

Fig. S10. The enlargement of the ESI mass spectrum of the separated HPLC peak region 9.757−9.973 min (see Fig. 29) with the ylide monocation ionization species of **PT167** (**NSC 799315**), showing the 0.5 Da isotope peak spacing of the dication $(C_{74}H_{89}N_7O_7S)^{2+}$ m/z 609.8643 Da.

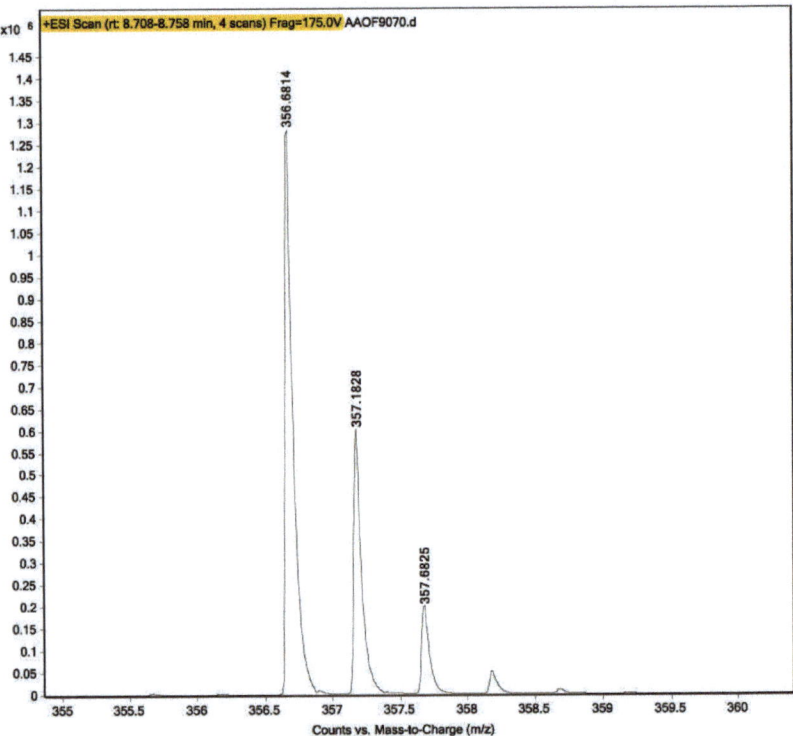

Fig. S11. The enlargement of the ESI mass spectrum of the separated HPLC peak region 8.706–8.758 min (see Fig. 29) with the ammonium monocation ionization species of **PT167** (**NSC 799315**), showing the 0.5 Da isotope peak spacing of the dication $(C_{40}H_{49}N_4O_6S)^{2+}$ m/z 356.6814 Da.

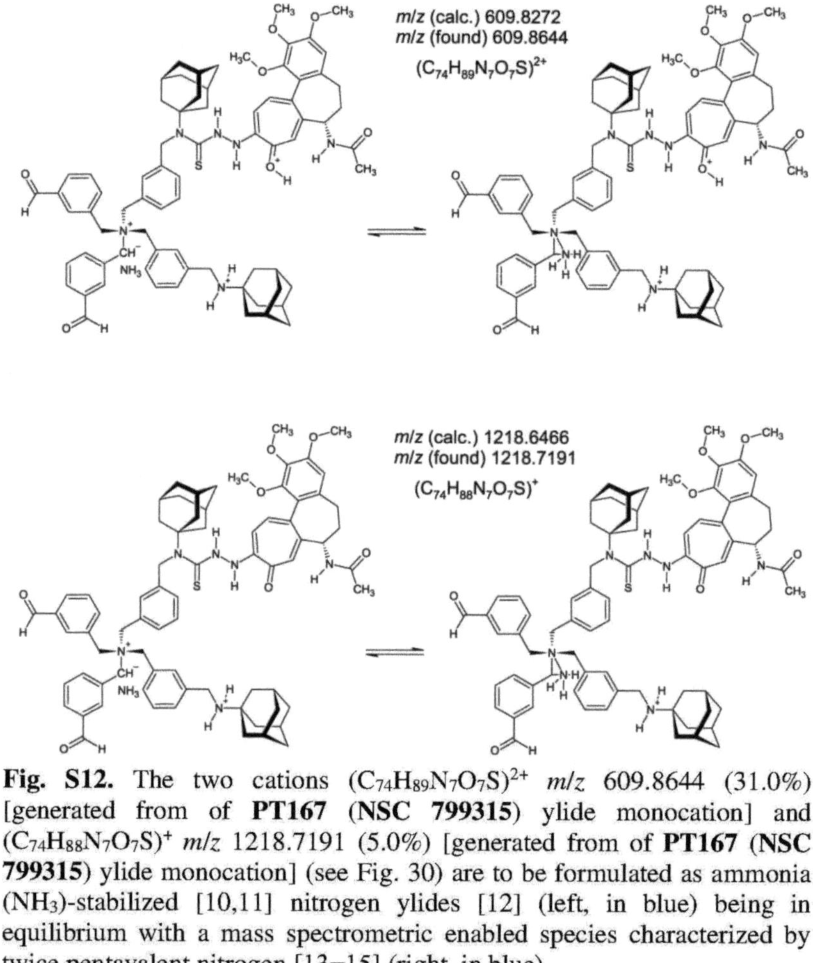

Fig. S12. The two cations $(C_{74}H_{89}N_7O_7S)^{2+}$ m/z 609.8644 (31.0%) [generated from of **PT167** (**NSC 799315**) ylide monocation] and $(C_{74}H_{88}N_7O_7S)^+$ m/z 1218.7191 (5.0%) [generated from of **PT167** (**NSC 799315**) ylide monocation] (see Fig. 30) are to be formulated as ammonia (NH_3)-stabilized [10,11] nitrogen ylides [12] (left, in blue) being in equilibrium with a mass spectrometric enabled species characterized by twice pentavalent nitrogen [13–15] (right, in blue).

Table S1. Cytotoxicity and antiviral activity of tetrakis{3-[(tricyclo [3.3.1.1^{3,7}]decan-1-ammonio)methyl]benzyl}ammonium   pentachloride (**PT162, NSC 796018**) versus human immunodeficiency virus type 1 strain LAI (HIV-1$_{LAI}$) in mammalian cells.

Drug	Cytotoxicity CC$_{50}$ (μM) and CCRF–CEM growth inhibition at fixed 1 μM concentration (%, in parentheses)			Anti-HIV-1$_{LAI}$ activity EC$_{50}$ (μM)/EC$_{90}$ (μM) in PBM cells			
	PBM cells	CCRF–CEM	Vero	EC$_{50}$	EC$_{90}$	SI$_{50}$	r^2
PT 162	2.2	< 1 (60.0)	1.8	0.56	4.3	3.9	0.93
AZT*	> 100	14.3	56.0	0.0044 ± 0.0018	0.031 ± 0.015	> 22,727	0.99

CC$_{50}$, cytotoxic concentration 50%. EC$_{50}$, effective inhibitory concentration 50%. EC$_{90}$, effective inhibitory concentration 90%. SI$_{50}$, selectivity index CC$_{50}$/EC$_{50}$. r^2, coefficient of determination (r^2 measure of goodness–of–fit) on EC$_{50}$ and EC$_{90}$. AZT, zidovudine (3′-azido-3′-deoxythymidine).

* The given effective inhibitory concentrations (μM ± s.d.) for the positive control AZT were averaged and treated statistically from four ($n = 4$) independent determinations.

5.2. Supplementary References

[1]   R. Burger, P. Bigler, DEPTQ: Distorsionless enhancement by polarization transfer including the detection of quaternary nuclei, *J. Magn. Res.* **135** (1998) 529–534.

[2]   S. Berger, S. Braun, 200 and more NMR experiments. A practical course, 1st ed., Wiley-VCH Verlag GmbH & Co. KGaA, Weinheim, 2004, 854 pp., ISBN 978-3527310678.

[3]   G.M. Sheldrick, A short history of *SHELX*, *Acta Crystallogr. A* **64** (2008) 112–122.

[4]   H.D. Flack, On enantiomorph-polarity estimation, *Acta Crystallogr. A* **39** (1983) 876–881.

[5]   A.J. Kesel, et al., Retinazone inhibits certain blood-borne human viruses including Ebola virus Zaire, *Antivir. Chem. Chemother.* **23** (2014) 197–215.

[6]   R.F. Schinazi, et al., Activities of 3′-azido-3′-deoxythymidine nucleotide dimers in primary lymphocytes infected with human immunodeficiency virus type 1, *Antimicrob. Agents Chemother.* **34** (1990) 1061–1067.

[7]   T.J. Spira, L.H. Bozeman, R.C. Holman, D.T. Warfield, S.K. Phillips, P.M. Feorino, Micromethod for assaying reverse transcriptase of human T-cell lymphotropic virus type III/lymphadenopathy-associated virus, *J. Clin. Microbiol.* **25** (1987) 97–99.

[8]   L.J. Stuyver, et al., Antiviral activities and cellular toxicities of modified 2′,3′-dideoxy-2′,3′-didehydrocytidine analogues, *Antimicrob. Agents Chemother.* **46** (2002) 3854–3860.

[9]   V. Vichai, K. Kirtikara, Sulforhodamine B colorimetric assay for cytotoxicity screening, *Nat. Protoc.* **1** (2006) 1112–1116.

[10] A.W. Johnson, Organic chemistry, Vol. 7, Ylid chemistry, 1st ed., Academic Press, New York, London, 1966, pp. 251–283, ISBN 978-0123864505.

[11] W.K. Musker, R.R. Stevens, Nitrogen ylides. V. Coordination chemistry of trimethylammonium methylide, *Inorg. Chem.* **8** (1969) 255–264.

[12] G. Wittig, M.-H. Wetterling, Darstellung und Eigenschaften des Trimethyl-ammonium-methylids, *Justus Liebigs Ann. Chem.* **557** (1947) 193–201.

[13] B.V. Nekrasov, Pentavalent nitrogen, *Bull. Acad. Sci. U. S. S. R., Div. Chem. Sci. (Russ. Chem. Bull.)* **28** (1979) 1789–1790, https://doi.org/10.1007/BF00952448.

[14] D. Kurzydłowski, P. Zaleski-Ejgierd, Hexacoordinated nitrogen(V) stabilized by high pressure, *Sci. Rep.* **6** (2016), 36049, https://doi.org/10.1038/srep36049.

[15] C. Yan, et al., Synthesis and properties of hypervalent electron-rich pentacoordinate nitrogen compounds, *Chem. Sci.* **11** (2020) 5082–5088, https://doi.org/10.1039/D0SC00002G.